T0202000

Oxford Handbook of Rehabilitation Medicine

THIRD EDITION

Manoj Sivan

Associate Clinical Professor in Rehabilitation Medicine,
University of Leeds; Honorary Consultant Leeds Teaching
Hospitals and Community NHS Trusts; Honorary Senior
Lecturer, University of Manchester, UK

Margaret Phillips

Consultant in Rehabilitation Medicine, University Hospitals
of Derby and Burton Foundation NHS Trust, Derby, UK

Ian Baguley

Clinical Associate Professor, Macquarie University;
Clinical Senior Lecturer in Rehabilitation Medicine,
Westmead Clinical School, The University of Sydney,
Sydney, Australia

Melissa Nott

Senior Lecturer in Occupational Therapy, Charles Stuart
University, Albury-Wodonga, Australia

OXFORD
UNIVERSITY PRESS

OXFORD
UNIVERSITY PRESS

Great Clarendon Street, Oxford, OX2 6DP,
United Kingdom

Oxford University Press is a department of the University of Oxford.
It furthers the University's objective of excellence in research, scholarship,
and education by publishing worldwide. Oxford is a registered trade mark of
Oxford University Press in the UK and in certain other countries

Published in the United States of America by Oxford University Press
198 Madison Avenue, New York, NY 10016, United States of America

British Library Cataloguing in Publication Data
Data available

Library of Congress Control Number: 2019944686

ISBN 978–0–19–878547–7

Printed and bound in China by
C&C Offset Printing Co., Ltd.

Foreword

Many clinicians in practice today will remember their first Oxford Handbook. The familiar cover and easily accessible layout was ground-breaking in its day, providing valuable clinical information in emergencies before the electronic resources that we take for granted today existed. Many of us learnt our medicine from carrying it about in a white-coat pocket where it could be accessed soon after seeing a patient. My abiding memory of my own first handbook is the exhortation in the early chapters 'not to blame the sick for being sick'. This is a very powerful concept that resonated with me deeply and confirmed my choice of career in rehabilitation medicine where we can do so much with medical interventions to alleviate the impact of disabling conditions and where the cause of the disability cannot be cured. Over the years, the Oxford Handbook stable has increased, encompassing many clinical areas, and I was delighted when the first edition of the rehabilitation medicine handbook was published.

Rehabilitation is an educational and problem-solving clinical intervention that aims to reduce the impact of disabling conditions on people's functioning. This is achieved through three main strategies—restoration of the function of impaired structures, reorganization of impaired pathways to deliver improved abilities, and reducing the discrepancy between the limited ability of disabled people and the demands of their environment.

Manoj, Margaret, Ian, and Melissa in editing this handbook have brought together a distinguished group of contributors who comprehensively cover the widest possible syllabus of topics in rehabilitation medicine—the medical management of disabling conditions. The topics included in the handbook encompass a broader spectrum of conditions than most of the rehabilitation medicine curricula across Europe and North America, providing an invaluable insight into the rehabilitation of these conditions.

Rehabilitation starts with a thorough understanding of the impact of the condition on people and their families. The early chapters of the handbook in Section 1 take us through the inclusive evaluation of the needs of the person with a disability. Each topic-specific chapter includes further information on assessment in that clinical area. The chapters in Section 2 provide valuable overviews of the management strategies of specific impairments that cut across a range of disabling conditions. The condition-specific chapters provide a succinct, yet comprehensive, overview of the impact of each diagnosis on the person and how to limit its impact.

This edition has reviewed the state-of-the-art in rehabilitation medicine once more and provides an update to all clinicians interested in the field of rehabilitation from medical students through to senior consultants—we all have something to learn from the knowledge in this useful volume.

Professor Rory J. O'Connor
Charterhouse Professor and
Head of the Academic Department of Rehabilitation Medicine,
University of Leeds, and Lead Clinician in Rehabilitation,
the National Demonstration Centre in Rehabilitation,
Leeds Teaching Hospitals NHS Trust, Leeds, UK

Preface

The *Oxford Handbook of Rehabilitation Medicine* is designed to provide concise information on rehabilitation aspects of care for adults with long-term medical conditions. The second edition was published in 2009, and since then, there have been advances in the management of medical conditions and new rehabilitation approaches and technologies have emerged. New guidelines and treatment protocols have been agreed based on emerging evidence and consensus. An updated edition of the handbook was therefore much needed to cover all these aspects.

Rehabilitation medicine is an expanding medical specialty, and worldwide, there is a wide scope of practice in the specialty, particularly in the fields of pain, musculoskeletal medicine, trauma, cancer, cardiopulmonary rehabilitation, and rehabilitation technology. We have made a sincere effort to include all the relevant areas by adding 14 new chapters in this new edition. Colour pictures, diagrams, and management flowcharts/algorithms have been introduced to make the information easily accessible. The handbook luckily manages to retain its pocket size in spite of our enthusiasm to cover everything new and novel in rehabilitation.

The book has two sections: Section 1 on common clinical approaches and Section 2 on condition-specific approaches. The clinical approach section outlines the management of common symptoms encountered in rehabilitation settings. The subsequent section on specific conditions provides information that will enable the reader to put the symptoms in context with the condition and provide direct management in a comprehensive and holistic manner. Every chapter has list of further reading resources that includes journal articles, textbooks, and online material.

This handbook, although aimed at medical doctors, will prove useful to other members of the multidisciplinary rehabilitation team such as physiotherapists, occupational therapists, nurses, psychologists, speech and language therapists, dieticians, support workers, and other allied healthcare professionals. The handbook will also appeal to doctors in the related specialties such as neurology, orthopaedics and trauma, palliative medicine, geriatrics, and pain medicine.

The new editorial team have enjoyed bringing together British and Australian perspectives on various aspects of rehabilitation and it is hard to believe we never had any disagreement during the years of preparing this new edition. The four of us have worked extremely hard in ensuring that every chapter is reviewed meticulously by each of us and meets the standards we had set for this handbook. We hope our readers find the new edition up to date and useful in their everyday practice of improving the lives of individuals with long-term conditions.

Acknowledgements

We would like to dedicate this work to our patients and their families who keep us motivated and inspired by their resilience and determination to improve their abilities even when the odds are all stacked against them. The material presented in this handbook has been written by experts in their areas and we would like to express our gratitude to all the contributing authors for their time and efforts. We are grateful to our reviewers who provided valuable insights and suggestions to improve the quality and scope of the chapters. This work would not have been possible without the support and encouragement from our families and friends who did not mind us working over the years in the small hours after busy clinical commitments. We would like to particularly thank the Oxford University Press team for their help, guidance, and patience throughout the process as this edition has been an ambitious revamp of the previous edition and needed energies and efforts of essentially writing a new book.

Contents

Symbols and abbreviations

⊃	cross reference		CSF	cerebrospinal fluid
♨	website		CT	computed tomography
ABI	acquired brain injury		DAI	diffuse axonal injury
ACE	angiotensin-converting enzyme		DALY	disability-adjusted life year
ACS	acute coronary syndrome		DFLE	disability-free life expectancy
ADLS	activities of daily living		DM1	myotonic dystrophy type 1
ADRT	advance decision to refuse treatment		DM2	myotonic dystrophy type 2
AED	antiepileptic drug		DMARD	disease-modifying antirheumatic drug
AFO	ankle–foot orthosis		DMT	disease-modifying treatment
ARDS	acute respiratory distress syndrome		DOLS	Deprivation of Liberty Safeguards
ASIA	American Spinal Injury Association		DVT	deep venous thrombosis
AT	assistive technology		DXA	dual energy X-ray absorptiometry
ATA	Assistive Technology Assessment		ECG	electrocardiogram
BMI	body mass index		EEG	electroencephalography
BONT	botulinum toxin		EMG	electromyography/ electromyogram
CABG	coronary artery bypass surgery		ES	electrical stimulation
CBR	community-based rehabilitation		ESD	early supported discharge
CBT	cognitive behaviour therapy		ESR	erythrocyte sedimentation rate
CFS	chronic fatigue syndrome		FSH	facioscapulohumeral muscular dystrophy
CGA	Comprehensive Geriatric Assessment		GABA	gamma-aminobutyric acid
CGRP	calcitonin gene-related peptide		GBS	Guillain–Barré syndrome
CHD	coronary heart disease		GCS	Glasgow Coma Scale
CHF	chronic heart failure		GI	gastrointestinal
CK	creatine kinase		GMFCS	Gross Motor Function Classification System
CNS	central nervous system		GP	general practitioner
COPD	chronic obstructive pulmonary disease		GS	grip strength
CP	cerebral palsy		HD	Huntington's disease
CRP	C-reactive protein		HKAFO	hip–knee–ankle–foot orthosis
CRPS	complex regional pain syndrome		HLA	human leucocyte antigen
			IADLS	instrumental activities of daily living

ICF	International Classification of Functioning, Disability and Health
ICU	intensive care unit
INR	international normalized ratio
ITB	intrathecal baclofen
IV	intravenous
KAFO	knee–ankle–foot orthosis
KO	knee orthosis
LIS	locked-in syndrome
LL	lower limb
LMN	lower motor neuron
LOS	length of stay
LRTI	lower respiratory tract infection
MCP	metacarpophalangeal
MCS	minimally conscious state
MDT	multidisciplinary team
MFS	Miller Fisher syndrome
MI	myocardial infarction
MMSE	Mini-Mental State Examination
MND	motor neuron disease
MODS	multiple organ dysfunction syndrome
MRC	Medical Research Council
MS	multiple sclerosis
MSK	musculoskeletal
NDGC	neurodegenerative condition
NG	nasogastric
NHS	National Health Service
NICE	National Institute for Health and Care Excellence
NIV	non-invasive ventilation
NSAID	non-steroidal anti-inflammatory drug
OA	osteoarthritis
PA	physical activity
PCI	percutaneous coronary intervention
PCS	post-concussive syndrome
PD	Parkinson's disease
PDOC	prolonged disorder of consciousness
PE	pulmonary embolus
PEG	percutaneous gastrostomy
PSH	paroxysmal sympathetic hyperactivity
PTA	post-traumatic amnesia
PTSD	post-traumatic stress disorder
QALY	quality-adjusted life year
QOL	quality of life
RA	rheumatoid arthritis
REM	rapid eye movement
ROM	range of motion
SCI	spinal cord injury
SCPE	Surveillance of Cerebral Palsy in Europe
SMART	Sensory Modality and Assessment Rehabilitation Technique
SSRI	selective serotonin reuptake inhibitor
TBI	traumatic brain injury
TENS	transcutaneous electrical nerve stimulation
TIA	transient ischaemic attack
TN	trigeminal neuralgia
TUG	Timed Up and Go
UL	upper limb
UMN	upper motor neuron
UTI	urinary tract infection
VO2 MAX	maximal oxygen uptake
VR	vocational rehabilitation
VS	vegetative state
WHO	World Health Organization
WS	walking speed

Contributors

Dr Stephen Ashford
NIHR Clinical Lecturer and
Consultant Physiotherapist
and Regional Hyper-acute
Rehabilitation Unit, Northwick
Park Hospital, Harrow, UK
10: Spasticity and contractures

Dr Hannah Barden
Adjunct Researcher, Charles
Stuart University, Albury-
Wodonga; Occupational
Therapist, Westmead Hospital,
Westmead, New South Wales,
Australia
*10: Spasticity and contractures;
40: Burns rehabilitation*

Dr Angela Clough
Clinical Lead, Musculoskeletal
Physiotherapist, Hull & East
Yorkshire NHS Trust, and Co-
Chair, Yorkshire & Humber
Regional Network of Chartered
Society of Physiotherapists, UK
*35: Musculoskeletal problems of
upper limb; 36: Musculoskeletal
problems of lower limb*

Dr Catherine D'Souza
Palliative Care Lead, South
Canterbury District Health
Board, New Zealand
31: Neurodegenerative conditions

Dr Hanain Dalal
Honorary Clinical Associate
Professor, University of Exeter
Medical School, Truro Campus,
and Knowledge Spa, Royal
Cornwall Hospital, Truro, UK
16: Cardiac Rehabilitation

Dr Laura Edwards
Clinical Associate Professor
in Rehabilitation Medicine,
University of Nottingham and
Honorary Consultant, University
Hospitals of Derby and
Burton Foundation NHS Trust,
Derby, UK
31: Neurodegenerative conditions

Dr Helen Evans
Highly Specialist Physiotherapist,
Gait and FES Service, University
Hospitals of Derby and
Burton Foundation NHS Trust,
Derby, UK
18: Mobility and Gait

Mr Jonathan Flynn
Programme leader for
Physiotherapy, University of
Huddersfield, Huddersfield, UK
*35: Musculoskeletal problems of
upper limb; 36: Musculoskeletal
problems of lower limb*

Dr Lorraine Graham
Lead Consultant in Amputee
Rehabilitation Medicine,
Musgrave Park Hospital, Belfast,
Northern Ireland, UK
41: Amputee rehabilitation

Ms Alison Howle
Speech and Language Therapist,
Westmead Hospital, Westmead,
New South Wales, Australia
*8: Speech and language;
9: Swallowing*

Ms Trina Phuah
Lecturer in Occupational
Therapy, School of Community
Health, Charles Sturt University,
Albury, New South Wales,
Australia
*23: Technical aids and assistive
technology*

Dr Ng Yee Sien
Senior Consultant in
Rehabilitation Medicine,
Singapore General Hospital,
Singapore
39: Geriatric rehabilitation

Mrs Alison Smith
Rehabilitation Nurse
Specialist, University Hospitals
of Derby and Burton
Foundation NHS Trust,
Derby, UK
29: Multiple sclerosis

Dr Matthew Smith
Consultant in Rehabilitation
Medicine, Leeds General
Infirmary, Leeds, UK
28: Stroke

Mr Matthew Sproats
Head of Department,
Occupational Therapy,
Westmead & Auburn Hospitals,
Western Sydney Local Health
District, New South Wales,
Australia
21: Orthotics and prosthesis

Professor Rod Taylor
Chair of Health Services
Research and Academic Lead,
Exeter Clinical Trials Support
Network; and NIHR Senior
Investigator, University of Exeter
Medical School, Exeter, UK
16: Cardiac rehabilitation

Section 1

Common clinical approaches

Concepts of rehabilitation

Introduction

There is a lot of variation in what people understand by 'rehabilitation'. This is probably due to the perspective they are coming from and the system or setting in which rehabilitation might occur. The origins of the word are thought to be from the Latin noun '*habilitas*', meaning ability, skill, or aptitude, adjective '*habilis*' meaning skilful, capable, and verb '*habilitare*', meaning to enable. This chapter focuses on the concepts behind rehabilitation and rehabilitation medicine, and how these concepts are operationalized.

In healthcare, rehabilitation has been defined as 'a general health strategy with the aim of enabling persons with health conditions experiencing, or likely to experience, disability to achieve and maintain optimal functioning'[1]. This means that an understanding of the concepts of disability and of optimal functioning are central to understanding the concept of rehabilitation, and are described later in this chapter. In addition, several models of disability exist and will also be described. 'Optimal functioning' is a less well-defined phrase—for the purposes of this handbook, it is taken to mean not just a utilitarian concept of functioning but an engagement of the individual in life in an autonomous way. Importantly, this differentiates a person's ability to perform activities useful to self or society from their ability to meaningfully engage in life in their chosen way. This difference can become crucially important in those who have lost physical and cognitive abilities. The World Health Organization (WHO) International Classification of Functioning, Disability and Health (ICF), described later in this chapter, a concept that serves as a theoretical underpinning for rehabilitation, makes this apparent through the description of 'participation'.

Rehabilitation, specialist rehabilitation, and rehabilitation medicine are different, but related, concepts that are relevant to the content of this handbook. Rehabilitation, as an overall term, covers aspects of healthcare that any healthcare practitioner can and should engage in, as it leads to intervention being made with a purpose in mind that includes optimal functioning in its widest sense, and not just the management of a specific impairment. For example, it is the difference between optimum control of a person's asthma enabling them to work and participate in sport, rather than merely maximizing peak flow readings. Specialist rehabilitation often describes a more complex situation, where multiple factors impact rehabilitation across simultaneous and diverse rehabilitation goals. Of necessity, this 'complex' rehabilitation requires different healthcare professionals working as a team to achieve optimum outcomes. Rehabilitation medicine describes the medical specialty driven by this more sophisticated rehabilitation philosophy, rather than using an organ-based, medical model. Rehabilitation medicine works across the whole spectrum, from specialist rehabilitation through to having a basic rehabilitation role and possibly an educational role in enabling any type of rehabilitation to occur. Rehabilitation medicine has similarities to specialities which cover a specific phase of life or disease trajectory, such as palliative care, but differs in that rehabilitation can be part of condition management at any time.

Models of disability

Traditional biomedical model

The biomedical model of disability is focused on pathology and impairment. It assumes several unhelpful notions about the nature of disability (Box 1.1).[2]

The philosophy of Western medicine has traditionally been to treat and to cure, but in rehabilitation these outcomes are unlikely and the aim has often been to 'normalize'. This philosophy was reinforced by the initial WHO classification that produced a distinction between impairment, disability, and handicap. The biomedical model of disability usually implies that the physician takes a leading role in the entire rehabilitation process—being team leader, organizing programmes of care, and generally directing the delivery of services for the person with disabilities. The doctor/patient relationship was the senior relationship in the medical model. Rehabilitation was born around the time of the First World War when there was a strong philosophy of the doctor telling injured servicemen how to behave, how to get better, and how to get back as quickly as possible to active duty. Such a model may have been appropriate in that cultural context but not in wider society today.

Social model of disability

The social model of disability understands disability as secondary to the social, legislative, and attitudinal environment in which the person lives and not any underlying medical condition. Although a person's abilities may be different, the disability is because society either actively discriminates against the person with a disability or it fails to account for their different needs. The key features of the social model are listed in Box 1.2.[2]

Biopsychosocial model of disability

The biopsychosocial model of disability is an attempt to account for both the social and biomedical models of disability. The WHO ICF[3] uses the biopsychosocial model. There is controversy over this approach, and some who use the social model of disability disagree with approaches that include

---

Box 1.1 Unhelpful assumptions of the medical model of disability

- Disability is regarded as a disease state that is located within an individual: the problem and solution are found solely within that person.
- Disability is a deviation from the norm that inherently necessitates some form of treatment or cure.
- Being disabled, a person is regarded as biologically or psychologically inferior to those who are able-bodied and 'normal'.
- Disability is viewed as a personal tragedy. It assumes the presence of a victim. The objective normality state that is assumed by professionals gives them a dominant decision-making role often noted in a typical doctor/patient relationship.

Box 1.2 Assumptions of the social model of disability
- A person's impairment is not the cause of restriction of activity.
- The cause of restriction is the organization of society.
- Society discriminates against people with disabilities.
- Attitudinal, sensory, architectural, and economic barriers are of equal, if not greater, importance than health barriers.
- Less emphasis is placed on the involvement of health professionals in the life of the person with disabilities.

aspects of health within a model of disability, as they would define disability as being solely due to a lack of response in changing the environment to accommodate the needs of the person. There are weaknesses in the ICF model, principally around personal context and well-being, and philosophies around the biopsychosocial model are still developing.[4,5]

The definitions used in the ICF are shown in Box 1.3[3] and described in the following paragraphs.

Impairment is a medically descriptive term that says nothing about consequence. For example, a right hemiparesis, a left-sided sensory loss, and a homonymous hemianopia are all impairments but the consequences of each of these will depend on many other factors, such as the person's environment, their job, family role, lifestyle, and expectations.

Activity describes the everyday tasks that any person, wherever they live, would be expected to do as a basic part of life, for instance, walking or eating. There is an overlap with participation and there is a judgement involved in relation to societal norms as to what these everyday tasks are.

Participation is defined as involvement in a life situation. It will vary considerably between people, for instance, having a mild right hemiparesis may have profound implications for a young person wanting to join the armed forces, as such occupations may be closed to him/her or an existing job may be lost. However, for a retired person with comorbidities, a similar

Box 1.3 International Classification of Functioning, Disability and Health
- Impairment: loss or abnormality of a body structure or of a physiological or psychological function.
- Activity: the execution of a task or action by an individual. Thus, activity limitations are difficulties an individual may have in executing activities.
- Participation: involvement in a life situation and thus participation restrictions are problems an individual may experience in such involvement.
- Contextual factors: includes the features, aspects, and attributes of, or objects, structures, human-made organizations, service provision, and agencies in, the physical, social, and attitudinal environment in which the people live and conduct their lives. Contextual factors include both environmental and personal factors.

impairment may have no perceptible impact on lifestyle. Participation is often optimized by changing environmental factors, for example, a receptionist with a hemiparesis remains capable of undertaking the job and being a valuable member of the workforce if appropriate modifications are made to IT equipment. Another example is a person who needs to use a wheelchair but cannot move around the office because it is not wheelchair accessible. In both cases, the employer's attitude may cause the person to be moved elsewhere or even lose their job. The change necessary here is attitudinal, legislative, or both. Therefore, rehabilitation includes addressing aspects such as societal attitudes and the physical environment, which are traditionally outside the realm of medicine. A rehabilitation medicine doctor would not undertake that change themselves, as that is not where their skills lie. However, part of their duty is to identify the issue, give appropriate information, and send appropriate referrals to advocate on the patient's behalf.

The full ICF is a detailed and lengthy document. The ICF recognizes the importance not only of describing the functioning of an individual but also placing such functioning into its social context. Fig. 1.1 is reproduced from the WHO website and provides a useful summary.

Rehabilitation medicine focuses not on the impairments and pathologies, but rather on activity and participation, attempting to optimize these according to what is felt to be important by the individual involved. This is operationalized by identifying the aims or goals the person may have (⊃ see 'Goals and habits'). This may include addressing aspects of pathology and impairment, but the overall aim or goal is at the level of activity

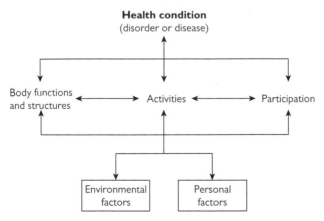

Fig. 1.1 Interactions between the components of the ICF.

or participation. Changing aspects of the environment or the ways in which a person performs an activity are often the key changes that lead to that person achieving their goal. Rehabilitation medicine does not minimize the importance of diagnosis and impairment but sees addressing these as part of a whole spectrum of ways to achieve a person's goals. As the primary skills of a doctor are often in the area of pathology and impairment whereas those of allied health professionals are more in activity and participation, it often falls to the doctors within the multidisciplinary team to be the professionals who are most involved with pathology and impairment, and this can cause a tendency to revert to the medical model. The skill of a rehabilitation doctor is dependent on being able to take an informed overview of the whole ICF spectrum.

At times, a sense of antagonism has existed between health professionals involved in disability and activists in the disability movement. These two extreme positions have softened over time: people with disabilities realize that health professionals have a clear and important role in helping to optimise abilities, while health professionals realize the rights of the person with disabilities to make decisions about their rehabilitation. Nevertheless, it can be difficult to maintain these ideals in practice. Multidisciplinary rehabilitation is often based within a healthcare system predominantly using the biomedical model; coupled with resource constraints, this can lead to focusing on very narrow aspects of a person's health.

Terminology

In the disability literature and in clinical practice it is vital to use the correct terminology. This is not mere political correctness. Incorrect terminology can not only be demeaning but can indicate an unhelpful philosophy or attitude from the individual concerned or from the multidisciplinary team.

It is important to avoid terminology that implies dependency or terminology which just categorizes all people with disabilities. The word 'patient', for example, may be entirely appropriate for someone who is acutely ill and is dependent upon medical and health professionals or where interventions affecting pathology are made. However, in rehabilitation, using the philosophy underlying the social model of disability, people with disabilities are not ill and thus the term 'patient' is inappropriate. When the rehabilitation process is striving to give that person independence and develop new skills, terminology that implies the opposite should be avoided. There are a number of other group classifications to be avoided including:

- epileptics
- stroke sufferers
- multiple sclerosis (MS) sufferers
- spastics
- young chronic sick
- the handicapped
- the disabled.

Although there is no universally accepted terminology, it does seem reasonable to use the term 'person with a disability'. Correct terminology simply means that the person is being treated as an individual and not just labelled as an example of a particular group.

As with many sections of society, it does seem acceptable for the group members themselves to use self labelling terms, for instance, people with spinal cord injuries will often refer to themselves as 'paras' or 'tetras' or even 'crips'.

Disability terminology is a minefield waiting to trap the unwary. The strength of feeling on these issues should not be underestimated. A useful approach in clinical practice may be to ask the clients you are working with if they have a preferred term to use when collectively referring to people with that specific condition.

Approaches to rehabilitation

At its core, rehabilitation involves assisting the person with a disability in making plans and setting goals that are important and relevant to their own circumstances. Rehabilitation is not a process that is done *to* the person but it is a process that is done *by* the person with a disability, in collaboration *with* a wide range of professionals as well as family and friends who offer guidance, support, and assistance. Of necessity, rehabilitation goes beyond the narrow confines of physical disease and deals with the psychological consequences of disability, as well as the social milieu in which the person has to function. A key factor that differentiates rehabilitation from many other areas of medicine is that it cannot be carried out by medical and nursing practitioners alone, but requires the active partnership of a whole range of health and social service professionals.

The characteristics of rehabilitation are listed in Box 1.4. Rehabilitation is primarily an educational process so that the person can manage their life with as little support as possible.

Rehabilitation can also be defined as an active and dynamic process by which a person with disabilities is helped to acquire knowledge and skills in order to maximize physical, psychological, and social function. The process maximizes functional ability and minimizes disability—thus promoting activity and participation. There are three basic approaches in rehabilitation:
- Restoration of previous abilities.
- Acquiring new skills and strategies.
- Altering the physical and social environment to optimize participation.

Box 1.4 Characteristics of rehabilitation
- It is an educational process.
- There is crucial involvement of the person with disabilities in programme planning.
- There is key involvement of family, friends, and colleagues.
- It is a process that requires clear goals to be set and measured.
- It is a multidisciplinary process.
- It is a process based on the concepts of activity and participation.

Box 1.5 shows an example of these three approaches in action.

Box 1.5 Case study

A middle-aged man has MS. He has been working in the post room of a large factory. He is married with two children and has an active social life. However, in recent months he has developed increasing problems with walking secondary to developing paraparesis complicated by spasticity. In addition, he has recently developed difficulties with urinary frequency and urgency. Rehabilitation, using our three basic approaches, could be structured as follows:

- Attempts could be made to restore some of his previous abilities and health by appropriate treatment of his spasticity and use of medication to control his bladder symptoms.
- He could learn new skills, for example, to walk with external support such as a stick or to use a wheelchair for longer distances such as from the office car park to his place of work. He could learn intermittent self-catheterization to assist his urinary problems.
- His work environment could be altered, for example, he could be advised on the use of a perching stool so he can support himself while sorting the post. He may need to approach his employer to change or reduce his hours if prolonged periods of standing are leading to increasing fatigue. At home, there may be a need to provide grab rails in the toilet or other adaptations to the bathroom or kitchen. His wife and family will need to be involved in order to understand his condition and possibly adjust the family lifestyle.

Thus, there are many simple pointers that could help him to minimize the impact of his condition on his work, on his family, and on his leisure time. The rehabilitation team needs to keep in mind these three basic approaches when planning the rehabilitation programme.

Goals and habits

Rehabilitation aims to optimize functioning and participation in life. Goal planning, or at least establishing goals, is the chief method by which a person can operationalize their rehabilitation. Apart from achieving specific aims of rehabilitation, the therapeutic process of goal planning itself is known to enhance self-efficacy and engagement in rehabilitation. Establishing effective 'habits' allows a person to maintain function once they have achieved a goal.

The first goal to be established is often the final strategic aim. This can vary significantly. For some, a long-term goal would be returning to a completely normal lifestyle. For others, it may simply be to return to and remain at home with the help of carers. In other situations, it may be to take up part-time employment or resume a leisure interest. Sometimes much discussion, and disagreement, is necessary in order that all parties can agree a realistic, long-term, strategic goal. Occasionally, parties have to 'agree to disagree' while choosing to work on shorter-term goals. After a long-term goal has been established, steps need to be identified in order to achieve that goal. For example, a long-term goal of independent mobility without the use of aids can be broken down into a number of shorter-term goals. This may, for example, start with sitting without support, then standing with support, then walking with assistance of therapists, then walking with aids, and finally independent walking over increasing distances and different surfaces. Goals should be precise. It is inappropriate, for example, to set a goal to walk with an improved gait. This could be the start of defining a goal, but it is not specific or measurable and is obviously open to considerable subjective interpretation. A more specific goal would be to walk 20 metres with the aid of a stick within a period of 30 seconds. Thus, goals need to be specific and measurable. They also need to be achievable within the context of the underlying natural history or pathophysiology of the condition—and this is often where there is disagreement. In order for progress to be seen, it is also useful for goals to be time limited. In a post-acute rehabilitation setting, it is useful to plan for goals that can be achieved in a period of 1 or 2 weeks, whereas when working with people in the community such goals could be set over a much longer timescale. Finally, each goal must be relevant for that individual. It may be relevant for some people to learn how to make a cup of tea but for others it may be more relevant to learn how to open a can of lager! It is useful to remember the mnemonic 'SMART' when goals are being established. All goals should be:
- Specific
- Measurable
- Achievable
- Relevant
- Time limited.

Usually a person is working on several goals concurrently—hence the usefulness of a coordinated interdisciplinary approach to rehabilitation.

The process by which goals are planned and negotiated with the person is vital. Engagement of the person and their family with goal planning improves the outcome, and it is disagreement concerning goals that is often the source of dissatisfaction and complaints. However, the practicality of fully engaging the person in the goal-planning process is challenging, especially when resources are scarce, and when impaired cognition affects the ability of the person to participate. Deliberately building goal planning into the culture and process of the rehabilitation service helps, for instance, discussing goals with patients as a routine part of any clinical encounter; incorporating goals in letter templates, leaflets about the service, and team meeting paperwork; and staff training concerning goals. Goals can be measured using Goal Attainment Scaling[6].

Habits are also important in rehabilitation. Once a person has reached a certain level, especially if they have a degenerative condition, further goals are often not helpful and the process of continuing to improve to reach a specific goal can be demoralizing. Developing lifelong habits that maintain a goal or health is important—for instance, habits surrounding daily or weekly exercise or relaxation, maintaining continence, or a healthy diet. Habits can used to maintain performance within the cycle of rehabilitation and reassessment, and can assist in self-management.

Outcome measurement

Outcome measures can serve several purposes, can be used in different environments, and can measure different aspects of rehabilitation. Although this is a simple statement, it is vital to remember that an outcome measure can only be useful where there is a clear idea of the question to be answered, matched with a valid and reliable outcome measure. There are three broad purposes, which may overlap, for which outcome measures are used:

• Research, where the outcome measure may be more detailed and take a longer time to complete.
• Clinical practice, where the outcome measure will have to be completed in a shorter period of time and by a greater variety of users.
• Development and auditing of services, where the outcome measure needs to be time efficient, and reflect specific aspects related to service delivery, adherence to standards, and health economics.

Ideally, an outcome measure should include just one ICF domain of pathology, impairment, activity or participation, or quality of life (which may overlap with participation). In order to gain a full picture of a person's rehabilitation, several outcome measures encompassing different ICF domains may be required. The different domains, although related, have no necessary causality between them, making measurement of all domains necessary. As the boundary between activity and participation is blurred, some measures will combine activity and participation domains, for example, the Functional Independence Measure/Functional Assessment Measure (FIM/FAM). Other measures can be individualized according to the aspect being measured—so it is the method of individualizing the measure that is the common aspect of the scale—for instance, Goal Attainment Scaling or the Canadian Occupational Performance Measure. Table 1.1 gives examples of different outcome measures.

The person themselves might complete an outcome measure, or a relative or carer, researcher, or clinician may do so on their behalf. It is important that the person using the scale has been instructed in its use. Outcome measures may measure the details of individuals participating in rehabilitation, the effects of rehabilitation, or the process of rehabilitation. While outcome measures are a vital part of assessing rehabilitation, it is important to remember that some aspects of rehabilitation are difficult to measure, so it is important that rehabilitation is not just led by what is measurable. Measures should be used alongside subjective perceptions of rehabilitation.

Outcome measures relating to specific conditions or aspects of rehabilitation are discussed in the relevant chapters of this handbook.

Table 1.1 Examples of measures relevant to different ICF domains and different processes

Domain	Measure
Impairment	Medical Research Council scale of muscle strength
	Vital capacity
	Goniometry
	Modified Ashworth Scale
	Pain Visual Analogue Scale
Activity	Timed walk
	Timed up and go
	Barthel Index
Participation	Stroke Impact Scale (some items)
	Community Integration Questionnaire
	EQ-5D
	Assessment of Life Habits scale
	Fatigue Severity Scale (some items are activity related)
Process	Rehabilitation Complexity Scale
	Northwick Park Therapy Dependency Scale

Benefits of rehabilitation

The specific benefits of rehabilitation will become self-evident in the later sections of this handbook. However, in general terms the benefits of rehabilitation can be summarized as follows:

Functional benefit

There is now significant evidence that a coordinated interdisciplinary rehabilitation approach produces better functional outcomes than traditional unidisciplinary service delivery. In terms of stroke, for example, a rehabilitation unit will produce greater functional gain, more quickly, with a better chance of the person returning home and with decreased morbidity and mortality. This is similar in the context of traumatic brain injury. There is also evidence of a functional benefit of multidisciplinary rehabilitation in degenerative conditions, such as MS. These specific conditions are discussed in later chapters. There is also evidence that short-term gains in a rehabilitation unit can generalize into longer-term functional improvements, but if longer contact with the rehabilitation team is not established, then any short-term functional gains and new skills may fade with time. This emphasizes the importance of not only post-acute rehabilitation units but also longer-term community support, as well as rehabilitation for those with degenerative conditions. What is not known is which elements of the rehabilitation process produce such functional benefits: is it the basic rehabilitation process or is it the interdisciplinary team—or both combined?; what is the relative effectiveness of individual elements and how do they interact? There is room for much more research on this subject but it is very likely that it is the whole rehabilitation process outlined in preceding sections that is the key to such functional benefit.

Reduction of unnecessary complications

It is possible to predict what problems may occur for a person with a disability and seek to avoid them. Coordinated rehabilitation services can minimize the risk that such problems remain unrecognized or untreated. An example is that untreated spasticity can lead to muscle contracture which further worsens function, increases dependence, and places the person at a risk of even more complications, such as pressure sores. The different chapters in this handbook outline many such examples.

General health benefits of rehabilitation

The general lifestyle recommendations on diet and physical activity that aim to reduce cardiovascular and metabolic disease are just as applicable to those with disabilities, or possibly more so. Rehabilitation assists in combining beneficial habits of diet and exercise with a person's lifestyle, and advising where modifications may have to be made.

Quality of life

Many trials of rehabilitation interventions have shown that improving participation and reducing dependence are likely to result in an improved quality of life. Some recent examples are from areas as diverse as group exercise in MS, adding in rehabilitation on a Saturday in addition to weekdays for inpatients, and early home-based rehabilitation following stroke.

Better coordination and use of resources

The person with complex and severe disabilities needs a variety of health, social, and other services. There is the clear potential for unnecessary overlap of assessment, treatment, and follow-up. The rehabilitation team should act as a single point of contact and information for the person and their family. The team should be in the best position to coordinate the various services. A case manager whose key role is to coordinate the different health and social inputs can be extremely beneficial in this regard.

Better use of resources

There is good evidence of the cost-effectiveness of inpatient rehabilitation[7] in reducing dependency and lifetime care costs, especially for those who have the greatest disability. There is also some evidence for different aspects of community rehabilitation in different conditions. Cost-effectiveness is higher when rehabilitation occurs as a continuous process rather than a broken chain of events[8]. Factors such as length of stay are also improved. Cost gains from rehabilitation are spread across several different sectors, for instance, if a person can be assisted into work, even on a part-time basis, then it is a major cost saving for the national economy; and if a person requires fewer care costs, this can reduce costs in the social care sector, and may allow relatives to continue working. This is a strength but it can also be a disadvantage to rehabilitation services when their funding comes from a single sector of the economy, such as the health sector.

Education, training, and research

There is a need for further studies in the whole realm of rehabilitation. Much more education, training, and research are needed. A rehabilitation team can act in such an education and research capacity and can help to enhance knowledge, reduce ignorance, and go some way to reducing disability discrimination.

Summary

This introductory chapter has outlined the concepts, principles, and pro-cesses of rehabilitation and illustrated some of the benefits. Rehabilitation is a process of education and enablement that centres on the person with disabilities and their family. It is a process that must be conducted through a series of specific goals leading to a long-term strategic aim. We now know that rehabilitation can produce real benefits in terms of functional improve-ment, fewer unnecessary complications, better coordination of services, and cost-effectiveness as well as providing a key role in general education, training, and research for both professionals and disabled people.

In summary, the basic tasks of rehabilitation are to:
- work in partnership with the person with disabilities and their family
- give accurate information and advice about the nature of the disability, natural history and prognosis
- listen to the needs and perceptions of the person and their family
- assist in the establishment of realistic rehabilitation goals appropriate to that person's disability, family, social, and employment needs
- establish appropriate measures so that the person with a disability and the rehabilitation team know when such goals have been obtained
- work with all colleagues in an interdisciplinary fashion
- liaise with carers and advocates of the person with disabilities
- foster appropriate education and training of health and social service professionals as well as helping to meet the educational requirements of the person with disabilities
- foster research into the many aspects of the rehabilitation service—from scientific principles to basic service delivery.

Rehabilitation has in the past been viewed as a rather vague and woolly process—sometimes with justification. However, modern rehabilita-tion should be a combination of the science and art of enabling optimal functioning.

References

1. Meyer T, Gutenbrunner C, Kiekens C, et al. (2014). ISPRM discussion paper: Proposing a conceptual description of health-related rehabilitation services. *Journal of Rehabilitation Medicine* 46, 1–6.
2. Laing R (1998). A critique of the disability movement. *Asia Pacific Disability and Rehabilitation Journal* 9, 4–8.
3. World Health Organization (WHO). (2018). *International Classification of Functioning, Disability and Health (ICF)*. WHO, Geneva. ℬ http://www.who.int/classifications/icf.
4. Wade DT (2015). Rehabilitation—a new approach. Part one: the problem. *Clinical Rehabilitation* 29, 1011–1050.
5. Wade DT (2015). Rehabilitation—a new approach. Part two: the underlying theories. *Clinical Rehabilitation* 29, 1145–1154.
6. Cicely Saunders Institute of Palliative Care, Policy & Rehabilitation. *GAS - Goal Attainment Scaling in Rehabilitation*. ℬ http://www.kcl.ac.uk/lsm/research/divisions/cicelysaunders/resources/tools/gas.aspx [information about Goal Attainment Scaling].
7. Turner-Stokes L, Williams H, Bill A, et al. (2016). Cost-efficiency of specialist inpatient rehabilitation for working-aged adults with complex neurological disabilities: a multicentre cohort analysis of a national clinical data set. *BMJ Open* 6, e010238.
8. Andelic N, Ye J, Tornas S, et al. (2014). Cost-effectiveness analysis of an early-initiated, continuous chain of rehabilitation after severe traumatic brain injury. *Journal of Neurotrauma* 31, 1313–1320.

Further reading

Dobkin BH (ed) (2003). *The Clinical Science of Neurologic Rehabilitation*, 2nd edn. Oxford University Press, Oxford.
Greenwood RJ, Barnes MP, MacMillan M, et al. (eds) (2003). *Handbook of Neurological Rehabilitation*. Psychology Press, Hove.
Shakespeare T (2006). *Disability Rights and Wrongs*. Routledge, Oxford.
Wade DT (ed) (1996). *Measurement in Neurological Rehabilitation*. Oxford University Press, Oxford.

Websites

ℬ http://www.direct.gov.uk/en/DisabledPeople—a useful generic website produced by the UK government.
ℬ http://www.disabilityresources.org—a very useful website that provides access to many hundreds of resources on the web regarding disability issues.

Epidemiology

Introduction

Epidemiology is the study of the frequency and distribution of disease, and of the causes, associations, and effects of those diseases. It allows us to think of how these aspects of a condition apply to whole populations. In rehabilitation this helps with the following:

- Planning of rehabilitation services at international, national, regional, and local levels.
- Identifying deficits in service provision to assist in advocacy and to highlight where change may be needed.
- Comparing services in different areas in order to explore different models of practice.
- Identifying future trends.

Definitions

Incidence
The number of new cases appearing in a certain period of time.

Prevalence
The number of affected people in a population at any one time. On a worldwide basis, disability affects between 15% and 20% of the world's population (World Health Survey and Global Burden of Disease).

Disability
A negative interaction between a person's health and the physical, social, and legislative environment in which they live. For a more detailed discussion on disability, ➲ see Chapter 1.

Disability-free life expectancy (DFLE)
The number of years a person spends without disability from a specific point in their lifetime.

Years living with a disability (YLD)
The number of years spent living with a disability.

Quality-adjusted life years (QALYs)
This adjusts the number of years of life following an event to take account of the health-related quality of life during those years. It does this by assigning a year lived in perfect quality of health as 1.0, and poorer quality of health being assigned numbers less than 1.0 according to values termed as 'health utilities'. There are various ways to calculate health utilities, such as using a rating scale, commonly the EQ-5D, or direct measurement or utility valuation. A QALY is the product of life expectancy in years multiplied by health utility.

Disability-adjusted life years (DALYs)
The number of years of life lost due to premature mortality due to the condition plus the number of years living with a disability. This gives an impression of the total burden of mortality and disability associated with a condition. There are a wide variety of physical and mental health conditions that cause significant disability which is reflected in the ten highest leading causes of DALYs worldwide. In 2012 these were (in order from highest to lowest) ischaemic heart disease, lower respiratory tract infections, stroke, preterm birth complications, diarrhoeal diseases, chronic obstructive pulmonary disease, HIV/AIDS, road injury, unipolar depressive disorders, and birth trauma/asphyxia.[1] Differences between regions reflect some important inequalities in health: the African region has the world's highest DALYs per 1000 of population, being three times the level in some countries, but it also experienced the most marked decline in DALYs between 2000 and 2012. Fig. 2.1 shows the DALYs standardized for age in different countries.

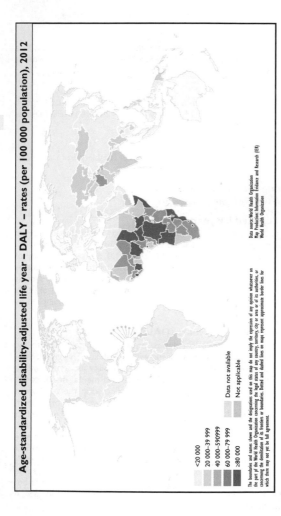

Age-standardized disability-adjusted life year – DALY – rates (per 100 000 population), 2012

<20 000
20 000–39 999
40 000–590999
60 000–79 999
≥80 000

Data not available

Not applicable

The boundaries and names shown and the designations used on this map do not imply the expression of any opinion whatsoever on the part of the World Health Organization concerning the legal status of any country, territory, city or area or of its authorities, or concerning the delimitation of its frontiers or boundaries. Dotted and dashed lines on maps represent approximate border lines for which there may not yet be full agreement.

Data source: World Health Organization
Map Production: Information Evidence and Research (IER)
World Health Organization

Fig. 2.1 Global rates of disability-adjusted life years standardized for age.

Reproduced with permission from World Health Organization (WHO). *Map Production Health Statistics and Information Systems*. Geneva, Switzerland: World Health Organization. Copyright © 2014 WHO. http://gamapserver.who.int/gho/interactive_charts/mbd/as_daly_rates/atlas.html [accessed 05/11/2018].

How epidemiological data are collected

The WHO collects data on high-level aspects of disability using the World Health Survey and the Global Burden of Disease and publishes these on its website and in the *World Report on Disability* (2011). Individual countries collect and publish their own data, for instance, in the UK, the Office for National Statistics collects data relevant to disability and rehabilitation that is published by theme, such as the example in Fig. 2.2 on years free from disability. Many countries have government-sponsored equivalents, such as Health Canada and the Australian Institute of Health and Welfare. Non-governmental organizations such as the Joseph Rowntree Foundation in the UK collect data on aspects of disability and rehabilitation in society.

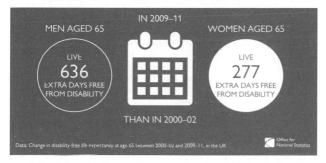

Fig. 2.2 Years free from disability for a 65-year-old in 2009–2011 compared to 2000–2002.

Source: data from Office for National Statistics (ONS). *6 facts about healthy and disability-free life expectancy, at birth and at age 65, in the UK*. Newport, UK: Office for National Statistics. © Crown copyright 2015. http://www.ons.gov.uk/ons/rel/disability-and-health-measurement/health-expectancies-at-birth-and-age-65-in-the-united-kingdom/2009-11/sty-facts-about-healthy-and-disability-free-life-expectancy.html. Contains public sector information licensed under the Open Government Licence v3.0.

Epidemiology of different conditions causing disability

Although disability is associated with a wide range of conditions (as shown in Table 2.1), those that are more relevant to rehabilitation medicine are those which are more complex or cause a greater degree of acute and/or chronic disability. Disability is a multidimensional construct. It does not result from medical condition/s, but from the interaction between different diseases, environmental factors, and personal factors. This means that knowing the epidemiology of one specific condition does not allow a detailed understanding of the need for rehabilitation. Furthermore, information can be patchy, as recording methods and definitions vary widely, and most figures are from studies in specific countries rather than any national or international methods of recording data. Examples of the prevalence and incidence of some conditions seen by rehabilitation medicine specialists are given in Table 2.2. It can be seen from these data that more detail than just whole population data is often important—for instance, knowing the spread of incidence and prevalence across the age range or in important groups that have specific risk factors for the condition.

The environment has a major impact on disability and may be the main focus of rehabilitation. It is known that difficulties in access to basic household and health facilities and poverty are associated with the development of disability and are affected by the presence of disability. In the UK there is a 15-year difference in DFLE between the least and most deprived areas of the country. The prevalence of disability also increases with age, and this is an important future trend in the many countries where the age of the population is increasing.

Table 2.1 Prevalence of moderate and severe disability (in millions) by leading health condition associated with disability, and by age and income status of countries

Health condition[a, b]	High-income countries[c] (with a total population of 977 million)		Low-income and middle-income countries (with a total population of 5460 million)		World (population 6437 million)
	0–59 years	60 years and over	0–59 years	60 years and over	All ages
1. Hearing loss[d]	7.4	18.5	54.3	43.9	124.2
2. Refractive errors[e]	7.7	6.4	68.1	39.8	121.9
3. Depression	15.8	0.5	77.6	4.8	98.7
4. Cataracts	0.5	1.1	20.8	31.4	53.8
5. Unintentional injuries	2.8	1.1	35.4	5.7	45.0
6. Osteoarthritis	1.9	8.1	14.1	19.4	43.4

Table 2.1 *(Contd.)*

Health condition[a, b]	High-income countries[c] (with a total population of 977 million)		Low-income and middle-income countries (with a total population of 5460 million)		World (population 6437 million)
7. Alcohol dependence and problem use	7.3	0.4	31.0	1.8	40.5
8. Infertility due to unsafe abortion and maternal sepsis	0.8	0.0	32.5	0.0	33.4
9. Macular degeneration[f]	1.8	6.0	9.0	15.1	31.9
10. Chronic obstructive pulmonary disease	3.2	4.5	10.9	8.0	26.6
11. Ischaemic heart disease	1.0	2.2	8.1	11.9	23.2
12. Bipolar disorder	3.3	0.4	17.6	0.8	22.2
13. Asthma	2.9	0.5	15.1	0.9	19.4
14. Schizophrenia	2.2	0.4	13.1	1.0	16.7
15. Glaucoma	0.4	1.5	5.7	7.9	15.5
16. Alzheimer and other dementias	0.4	6.2	1.3	7.0	14.9
17. Panic disorder	1.9	0.1	11.4	0.3	13.8
18. Cerebrovascular disease	1.4	2.2	4.0	4.9	12.6
19. Rheumatoid arthritis	1.3	1.7	5.9	3.0	11.9
20. Drug dependence and problem use	3.7	0.1	8.0	0.1	11.8

[a] Global Burden of Disease disability classes III and above.

[b] Disease and injury associated with disability. Conditions are listed in descending order by global all-age prevalence.

[c] High-income countries are those with 2004 gross national income per capita of US$10,066 or more in 2004, as estimated by the World Bank.

[d] Includes adult-onset hearing loss, excluding that due to infectious causes; adjusted for availability of hearing aids.

[e] Includes presenting refractive errors; adjusted for availability of glasses and other devices for correction.

[f] Includes other age-related causes of vision loss apart from glaucoma, cataracts, and refractive errors.

Reproduced with permission from World Health Organization (WHO). *World report on disability.* Geneva, Switzerland: World Health Organization. Copyright © 2011 WHO. http://www.who.int/disabilities/world_report/2011/en/ [accessed 06/11/2018].

Table 2.2 Approximate prevalence and incidence of conditions seen frequently by specialists in rehabilitation medicine

Condition	Prevalence/1000	Incidence/1000/year
Musculoskeletal conditions	300	–
Ischaemic heart disease	40	–
Cancer	3.8 (diagnosed in the previous 5 years)	1.7
Stroke	15	2
Lower limb amputation	5.3	–
Diabetic population	–	2.0
Non-diabetic population	–	0.2
Traumatic brain injury	3.2	2.3
Parkinson's disease	3	0.08–0.18
All ages	10	
Over 60 years		
Multiple sclerosis	0.8–2	0.02–2
Amyotrophic lateral sclerosis	0.04–0.07	0.004–0.02

Activities and participation in people with disabilities

Understanding how activity and participation are affected across the whole population of people with disabilities helps in focusing rehabilitation input and services. One way of doing this is by noting which tasks people with disabilities find difficult, and the results of that from the Labour Force Survey in Scotland are shown in Fig. 2.3.

Work is an important barometer of how successful rehabilitation is in helping people with disabilities stay or get into work. Fig. 2.4 shows there are higher numbers of disabled than non-disabled people who want to find work or are in low-paid jobs, with this disparity being worse for those with no higher qualification.

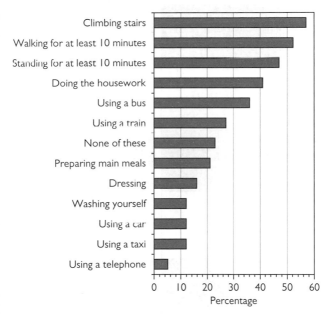

Fig. 2.3 Tasks normally found difficult. Equality in Scotland—disabled people (1999) Labour Force Survey.

Source: data from Scottish Government. Edinburgh, UK: Scottish Government. © Crown copyright 2015. http://www.gov.scot/Topics/People/Equality/Equalities/DataGrid/Disability. Contains public sector information licensed under the Open Government Licence v3.0.

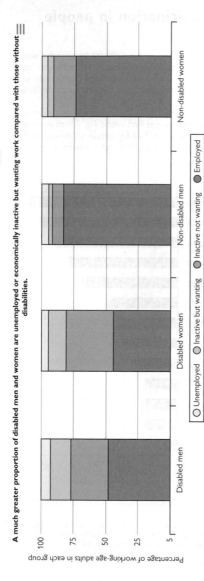

Fig. 2.4 Proportions of disabled and non-disabled people wanting work in relation to qualification level (a level 3 qualification is a higher qualification).

Source: Labour Force Survey; the data is the four quarter average to Q2 2015; the data is for the UK.

Cost of living for those with disabilities

The cost of living increases for many people who become acutely disabled for many different reasons, such as healthcare, equipment, transport, schooling, diet, domestic tasks, heating, and personal care.

Taking the example of personal care, the majority of costs associated with disability are paid for by the person with the disability and their family. Data from the 2011 UK census showed that 5.8 million people, about 10% of the population, were providing unpaid care, including 1.4 million providing 50 hours or more per week. In addition, family income often falls due to difficulties in finding and maintaining the previous level of employment, both for the person with a disability and family members who are carers.

Rehabilitation needs and services

Services for rehabilitation vary from country to country. For instance, in Europe the number of rehabilitation medicine/physical medicine and rehabilitation doctors varies from 11.7 per 100,000 population in Estonia to 0.25 per 100,000 in Malta, with the UK being 0.27 per 100,000. The number of therapists also varies, as can be seen in Fig. 2.5 which shows the number of occupational therapists per 10,000 of population.

Needs and unmet needs can indicate where rehabilitation can best be focused. They can also be used to explore differences in provision in different geographical areas and between different conditions.

Needs will be linked to the prevalence of different conditions in a particular country and to the environmental issues within that country. For example, the optimum prosthetic limb for a person living in a developed country may differ from that in a less developed country where the physical environment may place more stress on the limb, the physical activities of the user may be different, and maintenance is less easy to access. An example is the Jaipur limb, which was specifically designed for use in a developing country (Fig. 2.6).

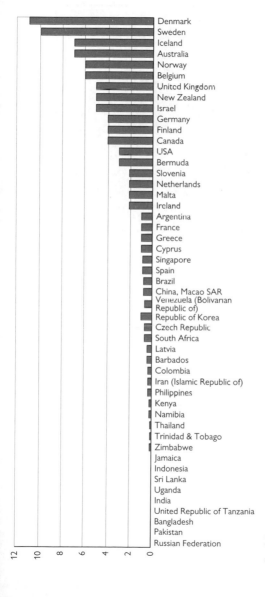

Fig. 2.5 Occupational therapists per 10,000 population.

Reproduced with permission from World Health Organization (WHO). *World report on disability*. Geneva, Switzerland: World Health Organization. Copyright © 2011 WHO. http://www.who.int/disabilities/world_report/2011/en/ [accessed 06/11/2018].

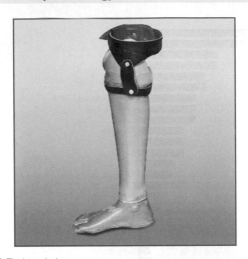

Fig. 2.6 The Jaipur limb.

Reference

1. World Health Organization. Disease burden and mortality estimates. ✑ http://www.who.int/healthinfo/global_burden_disease/estimates/en/index2.html.

Further reading

Epidemiology concerning specific conditions

Bray F, Ren JS, Masuyer E, et al. (2012). Global estimates of cancer prevalence for 27 sites in the adult population in 2008. *International Journal of Cancer* 5, 1133–1145.

Krishnamurthi RV, Moran AE, Feigin VL, et al. (2015). Stroke prevalence, mortality and disability-adjusted life years in adults aged 20–64 years in 1990–2013: data from the global burden of disease 2013 study. *Neuroepidemiology* 45, 190–202.

Woolf AD, Pflegr W (2003). Burden of major musculoskeletal conditions. *Bulletin of the World Health Organization* 81, 646–656.

World Health Organization topic pages and reports

Health topics—disabilities: ✑ http://www.who.int/topics/disabilities/en/

World Health Survey: ✑ http://www.who.int/healthinfo/survey/en/

Global Burden of Disease: ✑ http://www.who.int/topics/global_burden_of_disease/en/.

World Report on Disability (2011): ✑ http://www.who.int/disabilities/world_report/2011/report/en/.

Examples of government-sponsored statistics websites

UK Office for National Statistics: ✑ http://www.ons.gov.uk.

Health Canada: ✑ http://www.statcan.gc.ca/eng/health/index.

The Australian Institute of Health and Welfare: ✑ http://aihw.gov.au/.

Example of health services research regarding rehabilitation needs and services

Foster M (2015). Unmet health and rehabilitation needs of people with long term neurological conditions in Queensland, Australia. *Health and Social Care in the Community* 23, 292–303.

Example of a non-governmental organization involved in health epidemiology research

Joseph Rowntree Foundation: ✑ http://www.jrf.org.uk/.

Other relevant source

European Board of Physical and Rehabilitation Medicine (2006). *White Book on Physical and Rehabilitation Medicine in Europe*. ✑ https://www.euro-prm.org/docs/white_book_v_5_2.pdf.

Rehabilitation team

Rehabilitation teams

A disabling event impacts the way a person manages across many domains of life (e.g. physical, psychological, and so on) but also on how they and others see their place in society. The enormous breadth of impact means that no one clinician can provide all the expertise necessary to maximize positive change. This predetermines the need for clinicians from a wide range of disciplines to facilitate rehabilitation goals, that is, to enable the person to return to as much of their previous life function as possible. For these reasons, the concept of teamwork has been at the core of rehabilitation since its inception following the Second World War.

Why have teams?

In most circumstances, coordinated rehabilitation will be provided by a team. The essence of the rehabilitation team is that it is not simply a collection of different professionals, but a group of professionals working together for the common good of the individual receiving rehabilitation. There is evidence that effective teamwork can produce functional benefit over and above a collection of individuals working together as a group. The benefits of effective team work are likely to include:

- establishment of and working towards common goals
- exposure to different points of view
- integration of knowledge among people of different disciplines
- brainstorming novel solutions to complex problems
- detecting flaws in proposed solutions
- improved communication
- consistency in approach and better continuity of care
- promotion of a 'whole-person' perspective
- creation of an 'esprit de corps' that leads to a mutually supporting atmosphere.

These characteristics emphasize the importance of the rehabilitation team for the individual receiving rehabilitation. In addition, the team has both practical and psychological advantages for its constituent members. Rehabilitation is a broad subject and no individual can carry all the necessary knowledge and information required to provide a comprehensive and thorough rehabilitation programme. Single practitioners working by themselves, often in the community, can become isolated. Part of a team's function is mutual support, recognition of problems, and development of a team culture where individuals feel empowered to further enhance their own skills by working with others.

Definition of a team

In the context of rehabilitation, the main characteristics of a rehabilitation team include the following:

- A dedicated group of people from different disciplines who meet regularly, contributing their individual knowledge and skills towards improving the patients function.
- Agreement to work together cohesively on mutually agreed objectives or goals.
- Agreed delineation of responsibilities for those skills and roles that are specific and unique to individual members, as well as recognition of those roles that may be shared.
- Sufficient allocation of time by each member towards achieving the team's objectives.
- Adequate administrative and clinical coordination to support the work of the team.
- A defined geographical base.

Team members

Members of a rehabilitation team have to be carefully selected with regard to the team's purpose, in that the full range of knowledge and skills required must be present and the team composition well balanced. One conceptual way of looking at this is to divide the team into two parts—the core team and the support team. The core team are the individuals that have a direct, 'hands-on' relationship with the client, while the support team often facilitate the core team capacity to accomplish their task, such as secretarial and administrative staff. Effective teamwork of both parts of the rehabilitation team is necessary in order to provide comprehensive management.

A non-exhaustive list of rehabilitation team members includes:
- client and family
- rehabilitation nurse/doctor/pharmacist
- physical/occupational/speech language therapist
- social worker/discharge planner/case manager/care coordinator
- clinical psychologist/psychiatrist/neuropsychologist
- dietician/audiologist/orthoptist/orthotist/prosthetist/rehabilitation engineer
- recreation/music/art therapist
- vocational counsellor/case coordinator
- chaplain
- client advocate.

Team membership often evolves over time, for example, where access to other subspecialties such as urology or orthopaedic surgery becomes necessary. Team membership will also vary by the phase of rehabilitation being undertaken. In the post-acute rehabilitation setting, the rehabilitation team is often health orientated, the person is a patient in hospital, the intensity of therapy is high, and the goals will include the discharge of the person to an appropriate setting. In the community, there often needs to be a broader network of core individuals as a focus on health requirements moves towards social or vocational goals, for example, through the addition of vocational rehabilitation or other voluntary providers, lawyers, social security staff, disability support groups, etc. These changing goals require effective management of teamwork to maintain flexibility and continuity of service.

Team structures

In the same way that different team members are needed at different stages of rehabilitation, the team should also be structured in a way that maximizes the person's recovery at that point in time. One way of examining this issue is to look at the patterns within interprofessional collaborations. These interprofessional collaborations tend to fit into two inter-related dominant themes: communication structures (both formal and informal) and the culture within the team. These will be examined in turn.

Communication structures

The traditional medical model is not well suited to rehabilitation practice. In this model, there is a strong emphasis on medical diagnosis and medical interventions from the treating physician, while also providing instruction to the therapists without involving teamwork in the usual sense of the term. The medical model is potentially more relevant to solo practitioners, with each clinician following their own agenda.

Within rehabilitation circles, the basic team structure became the multi-disciplinary team—multiple members working independently with the client/family, and who may or may not have team conferences and meetings. In this older style, the team leader (often the treating physician) would direct the other members' behaviour, each of whom would largely work in parallel to each other. This model was improved upon with the development of the interdisciplinary team. The main point of difference compared to the multidisciplinary team is that the interdisciplinary team pursues client (and family)-centric goals as a coherent whole, requiring interventions that may blur professional roles while still preserving the separate identity and expertise of individual professions. Interdisciplinary team meetings involve communication and planning between team members to produce an integrated assessment and a unified treatment plan that is jointly carried out by all team members. This plan is then reviewed and modified over the course of the person's rehabilitation. This structure also directly recognizes the need for family members to understand the goals and the methods by which they are being achieved. Such understanding can only occur if the family is an integral part of the rehabilitation team. Interdisciplinary teams require a higher degree of group interaction and focused teamwork compared to the simpler multidisciplinary team.

The logical extension of the interdisciplinary team requires the reconsideration of artificially contrived 'professional boundaries'. This concept is thought of as the transdisciplinary team, a structure which encourages team members to blur the lines between craft specialities. It is potentially a more efficient way of working but requires greater team commitment to communication and flexibility. In a transdisciplinary team, it is not possible, or indeed desirable, to define the optimal disciplines to be included in the rehabilitation team. Indeed, a list of such disciplines will inappropriately emphasize professional boundaries.

Commonly, this model will utilize a keyworker or case manager who acts as a central point of contact with other team members. In theory, the keyworker can be any team member as long as he/she has an appropriate range of interpersonal skills and broad background knowledge of the needs and requirements of the client. Team members may come from a recognized craft group, but in other situations, most of the day-to-day rehabilitation can be carried out by generic healthcare workers who work under the guidance of the qualified therapist. This model can be less resource intensive and has been utilized in countries such as Hungary and South Africa.

In some cases, the role of the keyworker can be extended to that of a case manager. The concept of case management has been developed as a way of assisting the individual with disability with the coordination of the necessary professional staff. Case management can include:

- simple coordination within a single agency
- coordination across agency boundaries
- service brokerage in which the case manager negotiates with the key agencies on the client's behalf
- budget-holding responsibility where services can be purchased on behalf of the client from statutory bodies or other voluntary and private agencies.

Although there have been few controlled studies of the efficacy of case management, it is now a widely practised role and almost certainly provides a better and more coherent service and assists people, particularly those with cognitive impairment, to find their way through the maze of services.

Team culture

The second domain of team culture can be divided into leadership, care philosophy, relationships, and the context of practice. It involves the concept of team management, that is, the ability of an individual or an organization to administer and coordinate the group of individuals who perform a task. With respect to rehabilitation, the formal management of the team most usually involves the use of the team meeting.

The rehabilitation team meeting

Most rehabilitation teams have meetings to discuss various aspects of a client's care. The frequency of meetings will vary (e.g. weekly, biweekly, or monthly) depending on the setting. Topics covered at team meetings often include:

- client and family education needs (e.g. prognosis and length of stay)
- setting short- and long-term SMART goals (specific, measurable, appropriate, realistic, and timely)
- treatment planning and how to achieve the goals
- problem-solving around issues limiting progression of rehabilitation
- discharge planning
- team debriefing in difficult interpersonal or clinical situations.

Team leadership

The single most important determinant of team culture is the how well the team is led. In this context, a team leader is the person who takes responsibility to provide guidance, instruction, direction, and leadership to other members of the team. In many situations, historical, cultural, or political factors dictate that the leader of the rehabilitation team is the physician. There are potential advantages to rehabilitation physicians acting as the team leader: medical training gives a broad overview of any particular disorder rather than the potentially narrower perspective of other professional disciplines. The doctor is often at a stage of their career where they can offer wide-ranging experience across disability of the 'whole person', along with some grasp of the role of other professionals, and an understanding of the complementary role of team members. However, these factors are not as important as leadership style, which is in turn based on personality variables and self-awareness that may be completely unrelated to medical competence. There are many situations where non-medical team leaders will be more effective, particularly in community settings. Overall, there is no doubt that the right leader is more important than their professional background.

A number of different leadership styles are recognized in the literature, most of which are not suitable to the rehabilitation setting. These styles include the following:

- Command and control—based on military constructs, team management is centralized under the team leader who makes decisions without consultation. This is an autocratic leadership style involving one-way communication. This approach can work well in crisis situations, but is otherwise inefficient, ignores team members' expertise, and leads to poor team morale.
- Participative—the leader shares decision-making with group members by encouraging team members to provide input and voice their opinions. This two-way communication approach values the contribution of team members and tends to enhance group identity and productivity, but can slow down the decision-making process.
- Laissez-faire—here the team leader provides little to no management, and decision-making is passively delegated to the team members who carry out their duties independently and at their own pace. This style of leadership is said to stimulate creativity; however, it relies on team members having a strong work ethic and effective communication/negotiation skills with each other.
- Transformational—these leaders hold positive expectations of their team members and work to encourage the team to exceed normal levels of performance. Transformational leaders inspire, empower, and motivate the team, enhancing motivation and morale.

A leader has usefully been described as someone tolerant enough to listen to others but strong enough to reject their advice. Qualities that should be present in a good team leader include the following:
- At a client/individual level:
  - Communicates team decisions well to the client/family.
  - Ability to establish rapport with people of diverse education and cultural backgrounds.
- At the team level.
  - Technical knowhow and skill.
  - Good interpersonal and social skills
  - Excellent speaking and listening skills.
  - Relationship building—engendering trust, mutual respect, and team cohesiveness.
  - Creativity and critical thinking.
  - Flexibility—the ability to listen to others and adjust the direction of the team according to the thoughts and views of other team members.
  - Good time management—being able to devote enough time to the team activities rather than just clinical tasks.
  - Toughness—to be able to make difficult decisions when necessary.
- At the organizational level:
  - Financial and budgetary understanding.
  - Political skills—to influence colleagues and managers and direct maximum resources to the team.
  - A long-term vision for the team.

When teams go wrong ...

While effective rehabilitation teams tend to embody the previously mentioned principles, there are times when rehabilitation teams do not work well. Such breakdowns of team dynamics may be due to the particulars of the person being treated but could just as likely come from the team members themselves. Examples of these sorts of issues include:

- interpersonal conflict with clients/family or between team members
- absence of trust
- fear of conflict
- lack of commitment
- avoidance of accountability
- poor leadership (e.g. poor choice of leadership style, or not accommodating personal factors of the client)
- insistence of functioning within professional boundaries
- staff shortages and difficulty recruiting appropriate staff
- problems in team management.

The common thread through these issues is negotiating with people with a difficult personality, irrespective of whether they are a staff member or a client. People with personality disorders or other non-typical personality limitations (e.g. personal insecurity, defensiveness, etc.) add complexity to their interactions. Where related to the personality of the client, it is important to remember to 'play the ball and not the man' (to borrow from football). It is important to remember that aggressive, bullying, dictatorial, or defensive clients behave like this due to their own anxiety or personality limitations, and that the team members do not take on ownership of the other person's issues.

However, such behavioural traits are not limited to clients, and on occasion team conflict will occur. Low-level conflict is a standard part of life, and should be thought of as important to decision-making and personal growth. Where this happens openly with trust, mutual respect, communication, knowledge, shared responsibility, and collaboration, low levels of stress can lead to increased work satisfaction. However, high levels of conflict adversely affect team care, damage team cohesiveness, and disempower individuals within the team, for example, ineffective or insecure team leaders will stifle team efficacy. In these circumstances, formal skills training in conflict resolution should be sought, with such courses being offered in many institutions.

Further reading

Abreu BC, Zhang L, Seale G, et al. (2002). Interdisciplinary meetings: investigating the collaboration between persons with brain injury and treatment teams. *Brain Injury* 16, 691–704.

Sinclair LB, Lingard LA, Mohabeer RN (2009). What's so great about rehabilitation teams? An ethnographic study of interprofessional collaboration in a rehabilitation unit. *Archives of Physical Medicine and Rehabilitation* 90, 1196–1201.

Wood RL (2003). The rehabilitation team. In: Greenwood RJ, Barnes MP, McMillan TM, et al. (eds), *Handbook of Neurological Rehabilitation*, 2nd edn, pp. 41–50. Psychology Press, Hove.

Chapter 4

47

Organization of services

Principles of service delivery

This chapter examines ways in which a comprehensive rehabilitation service can be organized and delivered. There is no single way to develop a rehabilitation service and the physical base, team, structure, and scope and range of the services provided will clearly vary. This chapter will outline some of the possibilities for the organization of services and discuss the merits and drawbacks of different systems. Guiding principles for rehabilitation teams are discussed in ➔ Chapter 3.

No matter how the team is structured, it should first establish the basic principles under which it chooses to work. A useful set of principles was produced by the Prince of Wales' Advisory Group on Disability in 1985.[1]

These are as follows:

- People with disabilities and their family should be consulted as services are planned.
- Information should be clearly presented and readily available to all.
- The life of people with disabilities in the local and national community should be promoted with respect to both responsibilities and benefits.
- Disabled people should have a choice as to where to live and how to maintain independence, including help in learning how to choose.
- There should be recognition that long-term disability is not synonymous with illness and that the medical model of care is inappropriate in the majority of cases.
- The service should provide autonomy for the freedom to make decisions regarding a way of life best suited to an individual's circumstances.

Although not part of the Advisory Group's principles, a seventh principle could be added:

- A fully comprehensive range of rehabilitation services should be provided as close to an individual's home as possible.

Most comprehensive rehabilitation systems are based on a two-tier service. The majority of rehabilitation can and should be carried out either at home or in the individual's own neighbourhood. Thus, each community should have an accessible and local rehabilitation team. However, an estimated 10% of disabled people will require the expertise and facilities of a more specialist service. While some elements of a specialist service can be delivered locally, subspecialty and complex rehabilitation needs will be best served by a regional specialist rehabilitation centre to complement and supplement local services.

The range and type of services required at regional and local levels will depend on the availability of appropriately trained staff, resources, and facilities and will vary from area to area. Close links between the regional and local services are vital. The person with disabilities should be able to move seamlessly from one service to the other with continuity of care. However, resources are scarce and an ideal, fully interlinked, two-tier rehabilitation system is difficult to achieve and maintain.

Regional or subregional rehabilitation services

The regional, sometimes subregional, specialist rehabilitation centre should work on the same underlying principles of rehabilitation as any local team, namely interdisciplinary team working, goal setting, an emphasis on participation, and well-documented outcome measures (see ➔ Chapter 3). The regional team will consist of more specialist allied health professionals, physicians, and nurses and will contain a more specialist range of equipment and assessment facilities. The population served by each centre will vary considerably according to the range and scope of the local teams, geography, demography, and resources. However, the following list of services is likely to be better provided at a regional or subregional level as the frequency with which the skills or equipment are required means that provision over a larger population can be more effective and of better quality:

- A inpatient specialist rehabilitation unit for people with the most complex multiple disabilities, often associated with acquired brain injury, particularly those with a combination of physical, psychological and behavioural problems, and medical instability.
  An inpatient service for assessment, and perhaps long-term care, of people with prolonged disorders of consciousness (PDOC).
- A spinal injury service—for example, in the UK there is a network of separate spinal injury regional centres.
- A specialist service for complex wheelchair and special seating needs.
- A regional bioengineering service.
- A communication aids centre to provide specialist equipment for those with the most complicated communication problems.
- A centre for advice and assessment on specialist assistive technology.
- An information, advice, and assessment service for car driving for disabled people.
- A service for persons with limb loss, including provision of prosthetic limbs.
- A range of specialist outpatient services that are not provided more locally. The range of outpatient support will vary considerably but potential services are likely to include the following:
  - A specialist orthotic service.
  - Specialist neuropsychological clinics for those with cognitive impairment and to promote psychological well-being.
  - A specialist neurobehavioural service (both inpatient and outpatient) for people with behavioural problems, for instance following traumatic brain injury.
  - Specialist services for the rehabilitation needs of those with rarer conditions.
  - Specialist services according to local need and resources for other conditions where multidisciplinary rehabilitation is required, for example, musculoskeletal or neuromuscular rehabilitation, or complex pain management services.

The regional centre should be a focus for education and training for health professionals, both within the centre and for the local teams, and indeed other health and social services professionals around the region. Thus, lecture facilities and appropriate libraries and other Internet resources should be provided. Finally, the regional centre could also act as a focus for rehabilitation research and provide a link with local academic centres.

The design of the regional centre is also important. It should include realistic assessment areas such as kitchens, bathrooms, toilets, and bedrooms. It requires a wide range of specialist equipment, such as specialist wheelchairs and assistive technology for assessment and demonstration purposes. Outdoor areas need to be provided for outdoor walking training, with different surfaces, and potentially access to a car driving track to allow the range of driving adaptation equipment to be properly demonstrated. Suitable overnight facilities or facilities for relatives to stay for a period of time would also be desirable for families who are travelling a considerable distance.

Local rehabilitation services

The local rehabilitation team should be able to deliver all standard post-acute inpatient rehabilitation and provide an outpatient service for individuals in the locality. There would be a general trend towards the local services meeting needs that are less specialist and more frequent, but the detail of this will vary, chiefly dependent on geography and the previous development of services. There should be links in both directions with the subregional or regional centre.

There are various models of such services, as described later in this chapter, some of which are more community based and some secondary care based.

With regard to the types of service, a local rehabilitation team should be able to provide, or work closely with services that provide, all or most of the following:

- An inpatient post-acute rehabilitation service for patients with more complex rehabilitation requirements where an inpatient stay in a specialist unit would be more beneficial than rehabilitation in the community.
- A spasticity service (discussed in detail in ➔ Chapter 10).
- Access to a continence service (see ➔ Chapter 12).
- Orthotic and prosthetic services..
- A prescription and maintenance service for wheelchairs and specialist seating.
- Access to a tissue viability service.
- A counselling service that helps individuals with adjustment and coping problems in the context of physical disability—including sexual counselling.
- An appropriate range of outpatient services for rehabilitation, which could be further subdivided according to needs, impairments, or conditions, or a combination of these.
- A rehabilitation liaison service with the acute medical, surgical, and psychiatric wards for those with cognitive and physical disabilities who require hospital admission.
- An aids and equipment service, including for electronic assistive technology. There is international variation in the extent of such services and the sector responsible for providing them.
- An information and advice service.
- A range of settings outside of secondary care in which the service can work, for instance, in a person's own home, care homes, health centres, gyms, etc.

The local team will need to maintain a broad network of contacts with other relevant professionals and departments, including social services, the housing department, and the local employment service. Disability groups should also be associated with the team and can provide invaluable peer support and information.

Local rehabilitation unit

There are many advantages to the creation of a dedicated rehabilitation unit working from a physical base. A physical unit is required for a post-acute inpatient facility; however, all teams need a physical base to provide consultation and therapy rooms for seeing clients, displaying equipment, and organizing seminars as well as providing necessary administrative support. Thus, every locality should have a clearly identified physical base. Ideally, the rehabilitation unit needs to have the following facilities:

- An appropriate number of inpatient beds—the figure will vary according to country, regional population, local needs, and resources. For example, around 20 beds would probably meet the post-acute neurological disability rehabilitation needs for a population of approximately 250,000 people.
- Communal living spaces.
- Practice kitchen, bedroom, and living areas.
- A self-contained flat to allow further practice at daily living skills for individuals about to return to the community.
- Space for appropriate outpatient clinics—although many services ought to be provided either in the home or even more local facilities, such as the general practitioner (GP) surgery or other community centre.
- Space for information displays.
- Seminar and teaching space as well as meeting areas for the local team and perhaps local voluntary and disability groups.
- Plenty of appropriate car parking and links to accessible transport.
- An outdoor green area, accessible to inpatients.
- A physiotherapy gym, with specialist equipment such as a partial body-weight support treadmill and exercise equipment.
- Space for splinting, casting, and orthotic fabrication.
- A hydrotherapy pool.
- Access to assistive technology.

The unit itself should obviously be fully accessible for people with a whole range of disabilities.

The presence of a physical unit enhances the development of an identifiable rehabilitation service, which should promote staff morale and stimulate education, training, and research. There are advantages if the unit is based separately from acute hospital wards. Moving to a separate rehabilitation unit can be a step towards return to the community and might allow for more appropriate 'non-hospital' design.

Early supported discharge services

Early supported discharge (ESD) provides a method of bridging the gap between inpatient and community rehabilitation while simultaneously reducing inpatient length of stay. The initial research has been with regard to people with stroke, but the principles are likely to be similar for other patients. Research has shown such models to be effective, providing there is adequate staffing, frequency of intervention, and expertise. Important features of ESD programmes include the following:

- An interdisciplinary team that includes occupational therapists, nurses, a social worker, physiotherapists, speech and language therapists, and a physician.
- A keyworker for each patient and a coordinator for the team.
- Team meetings each week.
- Specific criteria supplemented by team discussion regarding which patients would benefit from entry to an ESD programme. Current evidence suggests that people with mild to moderate disability benefit most. The evidence around the impact of cognitive impairment is less certain, with many studies not including those with greater degrees of cognitive impairment.
- Involvement of the ESD team in both discharge from hospital and provision of rehabilitation in the community.
- A home environment which is suitable for rehabilitation and close enough to the ESD team base to be practical.
- The provision of adequate care.
- Patients who are medically stable.
- There is variation in the level of disability that patients entering an ESD programme might have, but a consensus statement[2] suggested a Barthel score of between 10 and 17 out of 20.
- The duration of provision and frequency of visits vary between services, depending on local factors such as the existence of other services. Duration in studies has varied between 4 weeks and 4 months.

The outpatient clinic

Equality in delivery of healthcare to people with disabilities is relevant to a substantial proportion of the population. About 14% of the adult population have a disability and at least 2–3% of the population have a severe disability, so it is clear that a local rehabilitation service will need to see a large number of people—often on an ongoing basis. There are many different models of service delivery and no single model is preferable to another. The service design must meet the local needs and take into account other local and regional resources, staffing, and facilities. Even in one area it is likely that several of the service models described in the following sections could apply.

The traditional model for short- and long-term support of people with disabilities is through a hospital-based outpatient clinic.

The *advantages* of the outpatient service include the following:
• Economies of scale—it is logistically easier to see people in one physical setting from the point of view of maximum use of staff time.
• It may be possible for the same inpatient team who looked after an individual in the post-acute setting to continue to see that individual on an outpatient basis—thus ensuring continuity of care.
• It may be possible to arrange outpatients so that individuals with the same sort of problem can attend for a specific clinic—for example, to provide an MS clinic or a Parkinson's disease clinic, or alternatively symptom-based clinics, for instance, to address continence or spasticity-related needs. This service would enable an expert multidisciplinary team to be on hand at each clinic and provide the necessary assessment and treatment as well as providing appropriate information and advice. Such a clinic could act as a focus for the relevant local self-help group.

However, there are *disadvantages* to an outpatient system:
• It may be difficult to involve relevant members of the multidisciplinary team who do not work in the hospital.
• Some patients find it distressing to see individuals with the same condition in a more disabled state.
• The length of time and difficulty the patient may have in travelling to and from the hospital.
• Provision of adequate parking.
• Some patients cannot get to a clinic.
• It may be more advantageous to assess rehabilitation needs and provide rehabilitation services/intervention in a person's own environment.
• The patient may feel less empowered in a hospital setting.

Primary care team

The practitioner with overall responsibility for a person's health is their GP and so clear communication and understanding of responsibilities between the rehabilitation team and the GP is important for effective healthcare and rehabilitation. There are some important principles that can help this interaction:

- Clear communication by letter with the GP. This can be assisted by rehabilitation departments agreeing a standard format for GP letters that will document the interaction with the patient, give results of assessments, and communicate rehabilitation goals, actions, investigations, and referrals.
- Timely correspondence between the GP and the rehabilitation team in both directions.
- An understanding with the patient on when they should contact the rehabilitation team rather than their GP. Sometimes, especially if there is frequent interaction with the rehabilitation team, there is a possibility that the person can become overdependent on that team for their general health needs rather than using their GP. However, there are also important situations where contacting the rehabilitation team rather than the GP is appropriate and can mean the person receives the appropriate rehabilitation more quickly—for instance, if they experience an increase in number of falls or in spasticity. In some more complex situations this may require a formal agreement about 'shared care' with the GP.
- Some patients may need an emergency care plan agreed with the GP, such as patients with neurogenic respiratory impairment or those with indwelling catheters who are prone to infection.
- Being mindful that 'diagnostic overshadowing' can occur in people with long-term conditions. In other words, symptoms that are not related to the person's long-term condition may be ascribed to it, especially by those less familiar with the condition. One role of the rehabilitation physician is often to clarify for the GP when a symptom is not associated with a person's long-term condition.
- Communication by phone with the GP when a conversation is required about the person's rehabilitation or care.
- An understanding by the rehabilitation team of what the primary care team do not know. Many disabling conditions are quite rare. The GP, for example, is likely to only see one new person with MS every 20 years. Sometimes rehabilitation teams forget that aspects of care that are obvious to them are not obvious to the primary care team.
- Outreach clinics at specific primary care centres can be a way of reaching patients more easily in rural areas.
- At a healthcare system level, the rehabilitation physician can advocate for equal access for people with disabilities to primary care and healthcare screening.
- Education for primary healthcare regarding when to refer to rehabilitation medicine services.

Community rehabilitation team

Full interdisciplinary rehabilitation teams can be provided in the local community. The team would clearly need close liaison and good working relations with the local primary care teams in that area as well as the local hospital and regional units. One example, in the UK, is a local community MS team. The team has a physical base in the rehabilitation centre but assessment and ongoing therapy is mainly conducted in the individual's home. A weekly social/support group is run at the centre. The team itself, consisting of a physiotherapist (team manager), occupational therapist, therapy assistant, and secretary, are all employed on a full-time basis as well as part-time input from a counsellor, social worker, MS nurse, clinical neuropsychologist, and rehabilitation physician. The team has access to wider specialist support and respite beds are provided in a local rehabilitation centre. The team accepts referrals from a variety of sources, particularly GPs and neurologists as well as the local MS society (which part funds the team). The team has good links with local social services department and the necessity for double assessment by the health team and then the social services team is avoided. The potential disadvantages of such a team are that:

- the team may only deal with a specific disability (such as MS) to the detriment of people with other conditions
- the provision of a comprehensive community rehabilitation team in every locality may be impractical—although comprehensive economic studies have yet to be conducted to compare such models of service.

Specialist allied health professionals and nurses

In recent years there has been a growth in the concept of the specialist practitioner. There are specialist nurses with expertise in such conditions as Parkinson's disease, epilepsy, and MS as well as symptom-based specialist nurses working in fields such as pain management, continence, and stoma care. There are physiotherapists working at specialist level, such as in spasticity, and occupational therapists in areas such as vocational rehabilitation. While some of these specialist allied health professionals and nurses are still hospital based, many work in a community setting. Some are attached to the primary care team while others perform outreach work from the rehabilitation centre. There are a number of *advantages* to this model:

- A broad range of disorders and symptoms can be covered.
- It is clearly less expensive to provide a single broadly trained practitioner in the community rather than the full community rehabilitation team.
- The practitioner can act as a single point of contact/keyworker/ caseworker for people within their expert area. Many problems can be addressed by the practitioner, but onward referral to the local or regional teams can still be made.
- Close links can be maintained with the primary care team.
- Individuals can be seen in their own home—thus saving unnecessary trips to hospital outpatient departments or unnecessary hospital admission.

However, there are obvious *disadvantages*:

- One individual cannot provide all the necessary expertise to an entire diagnostic group.
- Individuals are working in isolation and do not have the advantages of working as a member of an interdisciplinary rehabilitation team.
- Individuals would require lengthy training and considerable effort would need to be expended on continuing professional development. At the moment, at the least in the UK, such comprehensive training and support programmes are not yet widely available.
- The service may become over-reliant on individual practitioners, with consequent problems in providing cover and in succession planning.

Given relatively limited resources in health, however, the concept of the independent specialist practitioner working in the community who links to the local and regional centre is worth pursuing as long as such development goes hand in hand with a proper high-quality training programme.

Empowering people with disabilities

The person who has a disability and who needs to access rehabilitation services should have a role in the development and maintenance of such services and be in control of how they access such services. However, this can be a difficult ideal to meet, for several reasons:

- Balancing the differing needs of individuals.
- Allowing for personal differences in ability to access the services needed.
- Individuals having different levels of knowledge in how to best manage their condition.
- Entrenched working patterns in health and social services.
- Some health conditions may impose barriers to accessing services, even if services are designed to reduce those barriers—such as when a person has cognitive impairment.
- Finances may be such that only a very basic level of service can be provided.
- One reason that funding for services for people with disabilities can be low is paradoxically because of the wide-ranging benefits of intervention. When such benefits reduce costs across healthcare, social care, benefit provision, employment, education, and housing, the spread of economic advantage can mean that no one sector sees a large economic benefit or that the service provision in one sector leads to economic benefit in another sector. If budgets are devolved between these different sectors, this means that the activity and cost may be in one budget and the savings made in another, so that the overall impact is not understood by either service, and there is less incentive to invest in a service that will result in a saving for another sector. An example is health service input that enables return to work results in reduced benefit provision and an increase in taxes paid.

These issues can be minimized by:

- Sharing of community facilities across different patient groups (e.g. information services, exercise facilities, or disability living centres).
- Educating and facilitating people to move towards self-management of their condition, such the Expert Patients Programme in the UK.
- Minimizing environmental and procedural barriers to accessing services or centres.
- Integrating healthcare and local authority budgets.
- Developing a culture of integrating users into the running of services that involve them.

Community rehabilitation in developing countries

Most of the examples in the preceding sections are applicable to health systems in more developed countries, particularly in Europe, the US, Australia, and Canada. However, people living in many developing countries have limited or no ability to access rehabilitation resources and facilities. If they are able to get into a hospital rehabilitation unit then there is often no community support after discharge. Thus, other models have been developed to overcome these difficulties in the developing world. The WHO developed the concept of *community-based rehabilitation* (CBR) (Fig. 4.1). The model is open to different interpretations but the general approach is for the local community to be the main supporter of its own disabled population. Local village workers are given basic disability training—perhaps just lasting a few weeks. In many parts of the world, one or more individuals in the local village are already involved in some aspect of basic healthcare or childbirth. These people are given further training, generally supported by non-governmental organizations, and are provided with further background disability knowledge. At this basic level of training it has been shown that such people can deal with about 80% of the needs of a disabled population in their own village. The village workers may need support and ongoing training and supervision which is usually provided by a more trained individual who covers several local villages—perhaps visiting them on a regular basis to deal with more complex problems and make appropriate referrals to the local hospital or a regional centre.

The CBR model has been developed in many places to establish disabled groups in individual villages to provide economically viable employment for themselves. The groups, perhaps with some external support, are trained and provided with basic tools for such skills as woodworking, dressmaking, and bicycle repairing. These groups then contribute a small sum to a central pool so that a few members of the group needing medicine or external referral can be supported. Obviously, such basic training and support of disabled people is far from ideal but nevertheless such systems have been shown to be viable, cheap, and offer sustainable solutions for many disabled people in terms of healthcare and employment. The concept also goes some way to reducing the stigma of disability—disabled people in many cultures are marginalized from their own communities. There is a great need for much more to be done on a global basis and very significant investment is required in developing countries for the establishment of an appropriate disability infrastructure. However, CBR is a start and in many parts of the world is still the only means of long-term support for disabled people.

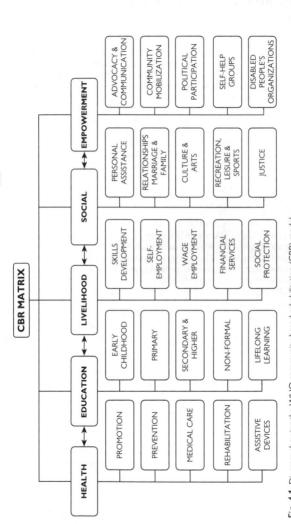

Fig. 4.1 Diagram showing the WHO community-based rehabilitation (CBR) model.
Reproduced with permission from World Health Organization (WHO). *The Community-based rehabilitation matrix.* Geneva, Switzerland: World Health Organization. Copyright © 2018 WHO. http://www.who.int/disabilities/cbr/matrix/en/ [accessed 06/11/2018].

References

1. Prince of Wales' Advisory Group on Disability (1985). *Living Options: Guidelines for Those Planning Services for People with Severe Physical Disabilities*. Prince of Wales' Advisory Group on Disability, London.
2. Fisher RJ, Gaynor C, Kerr M, et al. (2011). A consensus on stroke: early supported discharge. *Stroke* 42, 1392–1397.

Further reading

Department of Health (2005). *The National Service Framework for Long Term Conditions*. Department of Health, London. ℘ https://www.gov.uk/government/publications/quality-standards-for-supporting-people-with-long-term-conditions.

Meyer MJ, Teasell R, Thind A, et al. (2016). A synthesis of peer-reviewed literature on team-coordinated and delivered early supported discharge after stroke. *Canadian Journal of Neurological Sciences* 43, 353–359.

NHS England. Commissioning: Rehabilitation and Disability. ℘ https://www.england.nhs.uk/commissioning/spec-services/npc-crg/group-d/d01/.

History and examination

History taking in rehabilitation

This is an essential part of a comprehensive assessment of an individual by a rehabilitation physician. The approach taken in eliciting a history in rehabilitation settings is unique in that there is equal emphasis on understanding the impact of any illness on body function, activities, and participation in the context of that particular individual in the unique environment they live in. The format or template might differ depending on whether the individual is being assessed in an outpatient setting or inpatient ward and also on the underlying health condition. The history might be obtained by the physician on his/her own or by the multidisciplinary team (MDT) members.

Presenting complaints

The main complaints of individuals seeking rehabilitation interventions are generally pain, weakness, cognitive problems, or loss of function in activities/vocation. The symptoms can be ranked in the order of choice of the individual depending on the extent they affect the individual's function and quality of life. Every complaint is further explored in terms of time of onset, nature of onset, location, extent, duration, severity, aggravating or relieving factors, and associated symptoms.

Assessment of body function, activities, and participation

The physician (or team) has to gather information about cognition and communication problems the individual might have. Cognition is a term used to include mental functions such as orientation, memory, attention, concentration, calculation, and executive skills. Communication is an ability to convey information and interact with others. The presence of cognition and communication problems might actually make the history taking challenging and the physician might have to use a range of alternative communication methods such as sign language, gestures, writing, and electronic aids to communicate with the individual. The physician might need to obtain information form carers, family, and other members of the rehabilitation team.

Mobility is vital for an individual's independence and needs to be determined in the history. The individual might be using a mobility aid such as crutch, stick, frame, or walker. There might be a need for assistance from others to mobilize. A wheelchair (manual/powered) might be being used. The type of transfer from bed to chair (pivot/slide board/standing frame/hoist) and assistance required is a reflection of the extent of participation by the individual in transfers. Bed mobility should be explored in people with significant motor restrictions (e.g. tetraparesis). Stair mobility and driving ability can also be explored.

Activities of daily living (ADLs) is a term used for activities related to personal care such as feeding, toileting, bathing, transfers, mobility indoors, using stairs, dressing and grooming. Extended ADL (E-ADLs), also referred to as instrumental ADLs (I-ADL), are those tasks and activities required for independent living. These include walking further distances, preparing a meal, house cleaning, laundry, using information technology, managing finances, getting in and out of a car, driving, shopping, or using public transport. Understanding the individual's ability and limitations in ADLs and E-ADLs can help the rehabilitation team plan interventions to not only increase the individual's independence but also plan appropriate supportive care.

Past medical and functional history

The presence of co-morbidities can inform decisions on rehabilitation goal planning. For example, an individual with ischaemic heart disease and heart failure will need a cautious approach in terms of planning a physical rehabilitation programme that matches the individual's cardiac reserve. Assessment of previous functional history is another key determinant of rehabilitation potential of the individual. An elderly individual with previous declining mental function due to dementia might not have the same rehabilitation potential as a young, fit road traffic victim if both were being assessed for rehabilitation after traumatic brain injury.

Pre-existing neurological and musculoskeletal problems can have an impact on function and will require modifications in the approach to rehabilitation. For example, knowledge of previous contractures and arthritis in joints helps in ongoing management of pain and spasticity. All medications the individual has been on in the past and is currently using need to be documented, with reference to any drug or food allergies.

Review of symptoms

All major systems should be reviewed to ensure better understanding of the conditions that could influence the presenting health condition and vice versa (impact of the health condition on systems). This also enables assessment of preventable risks. Cardiovascular, respiratory, gastrointestinal, genitourinary, musculoskeletal, neurological, endocrine, psychological, dermatological, and immune systems are some of the key systems. For example, some symptoms such as urinary or bowel urgency might not be the main presenting symptom unless specifically asked about by the physician. Management of neurogenic bladder or bowel can have a significant impact on the individual's functioning and quality of life.

Personal and environmental history

The individual's educational background, vocation, leisure interests, alcohol history, and smoking history should be sought. The physician should ask about cultural background and family members in order to better understand the inter-relationships of the person with their family and friends. This will assist in determining the available support from family and friends, possible conflicting interests, and the individual's role within that network. The home design should be assessed for any potential barriers in anticipation of discharge from rehabilitation. Information about other environments that are important to the person's independence may be collected at this stage or may become more important later on in their rehabilitation.

The individual's perception of their condition

In order to use the information gathered in the history and examination to negotiate goals and a rehabilitation plan it is important to gain an understanding of how the person views the impact of their condition(s), their psychological and emotional reaction to the situation they are in, factors that motivate them, and their factual knowledge of their condition(s). Assessing this will be an iterative process throughout the person's rehabilitation, but a lot of information can be gained during the initial history taking and examination and this also helps to establish a therapeutic relationship with the patient.

Neurological examination

Most patients seen in rehabilitation settings already have a diagnosis. The examination is therefore more focused on understanding the impairment patterns and their impact on functioning. An upper motor neuron (UMN) syndrome pattern is seen in lesions in the central nervous system and is characterized by hypertonia, hyperreflexia, spasticity, or weakness. In lesions to the anterior horn cell and peripheral nerve, a lower motor neuron (LMN) syndrome with hypotonia, absent reflexes, muscle atrophy, or fasciculations is seen. The distinction is not always clear and there can be a combination of UMN and LMN findings in many conditions, for example, the amyotrophic lateral sclerosis form of motor neuron disease (MND).

General mental status can be assessed by the Mini-Mental State Examination (MMSE), a brief 30-item measure that assesses orientation to time and place, registration, language function, short-term memory, working memory, and construction skills (Fig. 5.1). A cut-score of 24 is used to indicate cognitive impairment. The scale does not capture frontal lobe functioning/executive skills well. The Montreal Cognitive Assessment (MoCA) is a similar brief measure that has been shown to be more sensitive than the MMSE to identify mild cognitive impairment. The Addenbrooke's Cognitive Examination (ACE-R) is used for more detailed cognitive assessment that includes executive skills. Assessment of mood should be conducted in conjunction with the cognitive assessment and can be done by simply asking 'Do you feel low or depressed?' or using validated scales such as the Hospital Anxiety and Depression Scale (HADS). Refer to ➲ Chapter 7 for detailed information on cognitive assessment.

Language and speech function can be assessed by an individual's ability to name objects, repeat words/sentences, read, and write. Further details on patterns of communication problems and assessment methods can be found in ➲ Chapter 8.

Cranial nerve examination includes testing of smell (olfactory nerve), visual acuity and field (optic nerve), eye movements (oculomotor, trochlear, and abducens nerves), pupillary light reflex (optic and oculomotor nerve), sensation to face (trigeminal nerve), muscles of facial expression (facial nerve), hearing (cochlear nerve), nystagmus with head manoeuvres (vestibular nerve), gag reflex (glossopharyngeal and vagus nerves), shrugging of shoulders (accessory nerve), and movements of the tongue (hypoglossal nerve).

Motor system examination involves testing muscle tone, muscle strength (Table 5.1 and 5.2), coordination, and reflexes (Table 5.2). Assessment of the sensory system includes testing dermatomes (Figs. 5.2 and 5.3) for superficial sensation and testing vibration and position sense for deep sensation. Apraxia is the loss of ability to carry out a sequence of planned movements in spite of no motor or sensory weakness. Involuntary movements such as tremor, chorea, athetosis, dystonia, and hemiballismus should be identified and diagnosed. Spasticity is common in UMN syndrome and is described in more detail in ➲ Chapter 10.

Domain tested	Score

Orientation

- Year, month, day, date, season —/5
- Country, county (district), town, hospital, ward (room) —/5

Registration (memory)

- Examiner names three objects (e.g. lemon, key, ball).
  Patient asked to repeat three names —/3

Attention

- Subtract 7 from 100, then repeat from result, etc.
  Stop after five trials: 100, 93, 86, 79, 72, 65 (do not correct if errors made)
  (alternative if unable to perform serial subtraction: spell 'world' backwards: DLROW).
  Score the best performance on either task —/5

Recall (memory)

- Ask for the names of the three objects learned earlier. /3

Language

- Name a pencil and a watch. —/2
- Repeat 'No ifs, ands, or buts'. —/1
- Give a three-stage command. Score one for each stage
  (e.g. 'Take this piece of paper in your right hand, fold it in half, and place it on hte chair next to you.'). —/3
- Ask patient to read and obey a written command on a piece of paper that states:
- 'Close your eyes.'
- Ask patient to write a sentence. Score if it sensible, and has a subject and a verb. —/1

Copying

- Ask patient to copy intersectiong pentagons (Figure 6.1). —/1

Total Score —/30

Fig. 5.1 The MMSE questionnaire.

Table 5.1 Medical Research Council (MRC) scale for muscle strength

0	No muscle contraction
1	Flicker or trace of muscle contraction
2	Active movement possible only with gravity eliminated
3	Active movement possible against gravity, but not against resistance
4	Active movement against resistance possible but power reduced
5	Normal power against resistance

Table 5.2 Superficial and deep tendon reflexes

	Reflex	Root level
Superficial	Corneal	Pons
	Abdominal	T8–12
	Cremasteric	L1, L2
	Plantar	L5, S1
Muscle/tendon	Biceps	C5, C6
	Supinator	C6, C7
	Triceps	C7, C8
	Patella (quadriceps)	L3, L4
	Achilles	S1, S2

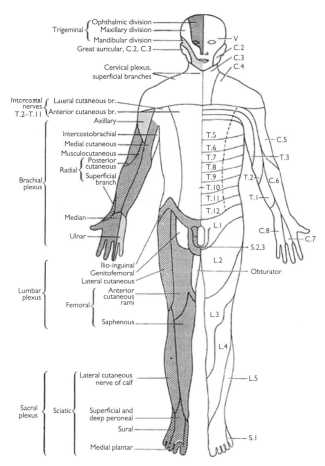

Fig. 5.2 Dermatomes anterior aspect.

Reproduced with permission from Wilkinson I.B. et al. 'Neurology' in *Oxford Handbook of Clinical Medicine* (10 ed.). Oxford, UK: Oxford University Press. © 2017 Oxford University Press. Reproduced with permission of Oxford University Press through PLSclear. http://oxfordmedicine.com/view/10.1093/med/9780199689903.001.0001/med-9780199689903-chapter-10.

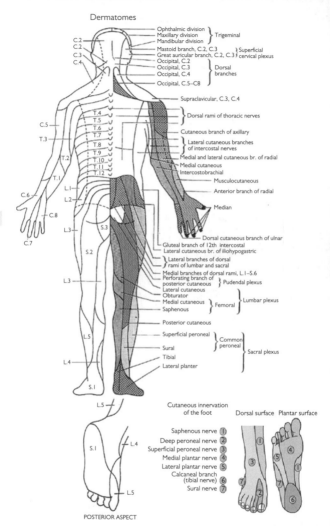

Dermatomes

Ophthalmic division
Maxillary division } Trigeminal
Mandibular division
C.2 — Mastoid branch, C.2, C.3 } Superficial
C.2 — Great auricular branch, C.2, C.3 } cervical plexus
C.3 — Occipital, C.2
C.4 — Occipital, C.3 } Dorsal
Occipital, C.4 } branches
Occipital, C.5–C8

Supraclavicular, C.3, C.4

C.5 — Dorsal rami of thoracic nerves
T.3 — Cutaneous branch of axillary
T.2 — Lateral cutaneous branches of intercostal nerves
Medial and lateral cutaneous br. of radial
T.1 — Medial cutaneous
Intercostobrachial
Musculocutaneous
C.6 — Anterior branch of radial
C.8 — Median
C.7 —

L.1 — Dorsal cutaneous branch of ulnar
L.2 — Gluteal branch of 12th intercostal
Lateral cutaneous br. of iliohypogastric
L.3 — Lateral branches of dorsal rami of lumbar and sacral
S.3 — Medial branches of dorsal rami, L.1–S.6
S.2 — Perforating branch of posterior cutaneous } Pudendal plexus
Lateral cutaneous
L.3 — Obturator
Medial cutaneous } Femoral } Lumbar plexus
Saphenous

Posterior cutaneous

Superficial peroneal } Common peroneal
L.5 — Sural } Sacral plexus
Tibial
L.4 — Lateral planter

S.1 —

L.5 —

Cutaneous innervation
of the foot

Dorsal surface   Plantar surface

Saphenous nerve ①
S.1 — Deep peroneal nerve ②
L.4 — Superficial peroneal nerve ③
Medial plantar nerve ④
Lateral plantar nerve ⑤
Calcaneal branch (tibial nerve) ⑥
Sural nerve ⑦
L.5 —

POSTERIOR ASPECT

Fig. 5.3 Dermatomes posterior aspect.

Musculoskeletal examination

A comprehensive musculoskeletal examination is an important component of examination in rehabilitation. The individual may present with a primary musculoskeletal problem or with a secondary musculoskeletal complication in a neurological condition. It involves inspection, palpation, active and passive range of movements, muscle strength testing, and joint- or condition-specific tests (otherwise called special tests).

Even though inspection should focus on the area relevant to the individual's complaints, it is better to inspect the entire musculoskeletal system as it functions in a kinetic chain with each joint linked in series to proximal and distal joints and pathology in one having an impact on others. The spine should be inspected for abnormal curvatures (kyphosis/lordosis or scoliosis). Limbs should be inspected for abnormal contour, joint swelling or deformity, muscle wasting, or atrophy. Trophic changes and scars also help in diagnosis. Gait pattern and use of walking aids should be assessed (see ➲ Chapter 18 for more details).

Next in the assessment is palpation of relevant structures to confirm the impressions made in inspection. The bones, joints, ligaments, muscles, and tendons must be palpated for any abnormal swelling, tenderness, warmth, movement, or trigger points. Tenderness over a tendon can suggest either tendinopathy or tenosynovitis (inflammation of tendon sheath). In the presence of swelling around a joint, displacement of fluid is attempted to see whether it has communication with the joint capsule. Fractures are tender to palpate with abnormal movement at the fracture site.

Leg length discrepancy must be noted and measured. A rough estimate would be to observe the pelvic obliquity in standing and further measured in the supine position. The distance from the anterior superior iliac spine to the medial joint line is used to measure the thigh segment and the distance from the medial joint line to the tip of the medial malleolus to measure the leg segment. Comparison between the two sides might help understand the discrepancy and the involved segment. Up to 1.5 cm of limb length difference is considered normal and does not need correction.

Joint range of movement needs to be assessed in both active and passive modes. Active range of movement is a reflection of muscle power, pain, and joint/soft tissue pathology. It is generally less than the passive range where the examiner takes the joint through the full range assessing the feel and judging blocks, if any, in the movement. A soft block could be due to capsular tightness, muscle tightness/spasm, or pain inhibition. A hard block is seen in arthritis or heterotopic ossification. Hypermobility implies additional range than expected and the examiner can use the Beighton score to diagnose joint hypermobility (Fig. 5.4). The range of movements can be measured using a goniometer and compared with the corresponding joint on the other side (Figs. 5.5 and 5.6).

A contracture or deformity is used to describe a lack of a full range of motion (ROM). The various reasons for this could be muscle hypertonia, soft tissue contracture, or bony contracture. The muscle tone can be reduced by a nerve block to assess the extent of soft tissue or bony abnormality. Soft tissue shortening yields to prolonged stretch whereas bony deformity does not. The Thomas test is a famous special test used to reveal

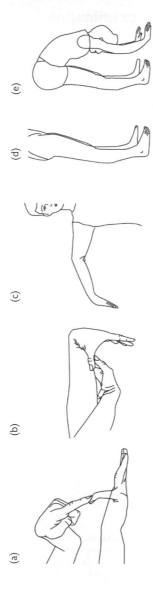

Fig. 5.4 Beighton tests (score of ≥4 suggests joint hypermobility and additional polyarthralgia suggests benign joint hypermobility syndrome).

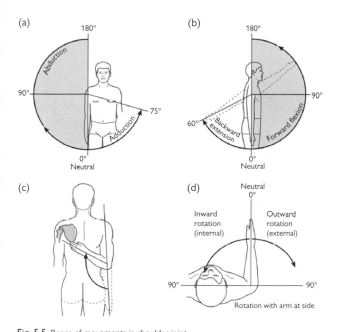

Fig. 5.5 Range of movements in shoulder joint.

Reproduced with permission from Baldwin A. et al. 'Orthopaedics' in *Oxford Handbook of Clinical Specialties* (10 ed.). Oxford, UK: Oxford University Press. © 2016 Oxford University Press. Reproduced with permission of Oxford University Press through PLSclear. http://oxfordmedicine.com/view/10.1093/med/9780198719021.001.0001/med-9780198719021-chapter-11.

the true flxed flexion deformity at the hip by obliterating the exaggerated lumbar lordosis by flexing the hip on the other side.

There are various other special tests for specific joints and conditions: Neer and Hawkins tests for shoulder impingement syndrome, Hoffman's test for cervical myelopathy, straight leg raise test for lumbar nerve root compression, and Phalen's test for carpal tunnel syndrome are a few examples. These tests have reasonable sensitivity and specificity for specific conditions that can help in diagnosis and requesting relevant investigations.

Dynamic tests/assessments are sometimes used to reproduce symptoms that might not be present at the time of examination. For example, an individual with knee impingement syndrome may be asked to walk up and down stairs or perform squats until symptomatic and then further evaluated. The dynamic assessment can also be repeated after diagnostic anaesthetic injection to the area that might help in diagnosis. Spastic dystonia on walking is another such example where a dynamic assessment is helpful in diagnosis and intervention.

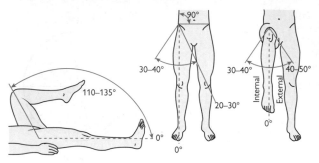

Fig. 5.6 Range of movements in hip joint.

Reproduced with permission from Baldwin A. et al. 'Orthopaedics' in *Oxford Handbook of Clinical Specialties* (10 ed.). Oxford, UK: Oxford University Press. © 2016 Oxford University Press. Reproduced with permission of Oxford University Press through PLSclear. http://oxfordmedicine.com/view/10.1093/med/9780198719021.001.0001/med-9780198719021-chapter-11.

Rehabilitation plan

After eliciting a history and performing a comprehensive examination, the rehabilitation physician (along with his/her team) should summarize the important findings and formulate a rehabilitation plan with the individual. A sample rehabilitation plan for an individual presenting for stroke rehabilitation is shown in Box 5.1. The rehabilitation plan can be operationalized by negotiating goals with the patient. The manner in which this first step in developing a rehabilitation plan with the patient is conducted is vital in commencing a therapeutic relationship with the patient.

Box 5.1 Example of rehabilitation plan

Summary

A 56-year-old electrician assessed 3 days post stroke after left middle cerebral artery infarction. Weakness on right side with sensory loss. Visual field defect on right. Global dysphasia. Bladder incontinence. Atrial fibrillation, on rate-controlling medications. Elevated serum cholesterol. Echocardiogram shows mild systolic dysfunction. History of hypertension, smoking, and moderate alcohol intake. Self-employed. Lives alone in flat. Family and friends live nearby and willing to help when he returns home. Currently, some function returning on right side, shoulder and neuropathic pain on right side, hoisted for transfers, needs help with toilet care, and independent in feeding and drinking.

Problems and rehabilitation plan

1. Secondary prevention—ensure on antiplatelets, statin, and antihypertensive medications. Plan for long-term anticoagulation given atrial fibrillation. Optimization of blood pressure control. Smoking cessation plan.
2. Pain—shoulder suprascapular nerve block to help relieve pain of impingement and commence neuropathic analgesic medications.
3. Urinary incontinence—check residual volume and formulate incontinence plan based on findings.
4. Right visual field defect—visual field tests and visual aids to improve field of vision.
5. Mood—screen for depression and offer psychological support.
6. Right side motor and sensory deficits—therapy to improve power and function, sensory training, improve posture, maintain range of motion.
7. Transfers and mobility—therapy to improve independence, and gait retraining and gait aids.
8. ADLs—therapy to retrain in ADLs and improve participation.
9. Swallow—therapy to assess swallow and recommend dietary modifications.
10. Family and friends—arrange MDT meeting with them to update on progress in rehabilitation and plan for future placement.
11. Home adaptations and community reintegration—involve social services to facilitate adaptations and care at home.
12. Driving—inform driving licensing agency and plan for retraining and retesting if required.
13. Vocation—counselling and plan for vocational training. Support for ill health benefits and insurance.

Further reading

Feinberg JH, Moley PJ (2010). Physical examination. In: *DeLisa's Physical Medicine and Rehabilitation*, 5th edn, pp. 45–59. Lippincott Williams and Wilkins, Philadelphia, PA.

O'Dell MW, Lin CD, Panagos A (2011). The physiatric history and physical examination. In: Bradom RL (ed), *Physical Medicine and Rehabilitation*, 4th edn, pp. 22–33. Elsevier, Philadelphia, PA.

Useful website

◎ http://asia-spinalinjury.org—International Standards for Neurological Classification of SCI (ISNCSCI) worksheet, autonomic standards assessment form, urodynamics basic data set form.

Rehabilitation assessment and evaluation

Assessment processes

The processes of rehabilitation and evaluation of outcomes can be difficult to quantify. Measurement is the quantification of an observation, usually based on measurement tools and techniques to provide numerical or descriptive data. Processes for measuring rehabilitation outcomes are being increasingly applied in clinical practice due to increased quality control and audit procedures. In addition, assessment and outcome measurement has become fundamental to the practice of evidence-based medicine. Assessment forms an integral part of the treatment planning and rehabilitation process. In this chapter, we will explore various assessment processes and purposes.

Initial assessment is a process engaged in by MDT members. Each team member uses a discipline-specific process for collecting initial information with a unique focus. For example, medical staff may focus on the patient's current medical condition, symptoms, and previous medical history, while a social worker may focus on availability of social supports and current living arrangements. Initial assessment serves many purposes including (1) defining the current problem, (2) identifying the need for further investigations or in-depth assessment, (3) facilitating treatment planning, and (4) providing a baseline for goal setting. An initial assessment, sometimes referred to as a screening assessment, can also assist in establishing rapport or referring to other team members or other health services.

Ongoing assessment helps identify rehabilitation progress. Ongoing assessment serves to monitor the effects of intervention and assists the clinical reasoning process as the MDT considers the way in which the patient is responding to the treatment plan. In a number of clinical areas, best practice guidelines and government policy recommend ongoing assessment as an essential component of medical management. The frequency of re-evaluation will depend on the rate of progress and anticipated length of service provision. With an increasing trend towards shorter hospital admissions, pre-discharge assessment plays an essential role in providing information about the patient's readiness for discharge, equipment needs and environmental supports, identifying necessary and available social supports, and any requirements for follow-up therapy.

Finally, *outcome assessment* should be undertaken at the time when a phase of rehabilitation ends. Outcome assessment provides an evaluation of the effectiveness of rehabilitation and may help to define future goals for post-discharge health services to strive for. In areas of rehabilitation medicine that lack strong evidence for intervention efficacy, the need for individualized outcome assessment is even greater to demonstrate treatment benefits and to justify support for ongoing intervention.

Types of assessment measures

When selecting a specific assessment, the MDT team members need to consider the purpose for which the assessment is being conducted and how the assessment results will be interpreted or used. When undertaking a critical appraisal of the intended assessment tool (➲ see 'Critical appraisal of assessment tools'), it is important to understand the utility, validity, reliability, and sensitivity of the assessment evaluated against the intended purpose and planned use of the collected information.

When considering clinical evaluation, assessments can be categorized based on four primary purposes: descriptive, discriminative, predictive, and evaluative. Some rehabilitation assessments have been developed to assess one of these main purposes, while others can be used for a combination of purposes.

Descriptive assessments are the most commonly used tools in rehabilitation medicine. These assessments provide information that describes the patient's current medical or functional status, problems, needs, or circumstances. Descriptive assessments often focus on a patient's strengths and limitations, describing the patient's current status such as ability to perform ADLs, available range of movement at a specific joint, or current level of care assistance required for transfers and mobility. When considering measurement properties of standardized descriptive assessments, content and construct validity should be well established.

Descriptive assessment provides a 'snap-shot' of the patient's ability at one time point, and are often used to provide a baseline for intervention planning and clinical decision-making. For example, the Modified Barthel Index indicates overall level of independence/dependence. One limitation to be aware of when selecting a descriptive assessment tool is the level of detail that can be obtained relative to the requirements for accurate intervention planning. Determining that a patient is dependent or requires assistance with ADLs does not provide data on the underlying reasons for activity restrictions or the reasons for observed performance deficits.

Discriminative assessments attempt to distinguish between individuals or groups on the basis of predetermined criteria or symptoms. Comparisons are usually made against a normative group or another diagnostic group. The purpose of a discriminative assessment may be to make a clinical diagnosis, to match a patient against referral criteria, to decide on appropriate placement, or to detect specific impairments or restrictions in a diagnostic group. As such, discriminative validity is the critical psychometric property of this form of assessment, to justify its validity in distinguishing between individuals or groups. For example, the MMSE is a screening tool to identify the presence of dementia in older adults.

Predictive assessments, otherwise referred to as prognostic assessments, make predictions about a patient's future performance or ability. Predictive assessments usually classify patients into predetermined levels or categories in an attempt to predict a specific outcome. For example, the American Spinal Injury Association (ASIA) Impairment Scale predicts degree of impairment based on motor and sensory deficits, level of spinal cord injury, and degree of injury completeness. When evaluating the psychometric properties of predictive assessments, the most critical measurement property is predictive validity, which is defined as the accuracy with which an assessment can predict a future event. More detailed evaluation of assessment sensitivity and specificity also provides additional information on an assessment tool's ability to correctly predict the occurrence of an event or outcome.

Predictive assessments can also be used to identify patients who are at risk of a particular outcome, for example, falls risk or pressure sore risk. The Ontario Modified STRATIFY tool provides a falls risk grading with high sensitivity and specificity. The Braden Scale for predicting pressure sore risk has high levels of sensitivity and specificity, particularly in the higher score range (indicating higher risk).

Evaluative assessments measure change in performance over time, usually in response to rehabilitation interventions. The purpose of an evaluative assessment is to quantify a patient's progress or to determine the effectiveness of an intervention. Evaluative assessments are also referred to as *outcome measures*. Evaluative assessments need to be specifically selected to measure the magnitude of longitudinal change on the targeted outcome of interest. As evaluative assessments are administered over time, this form of assessment requires high levels of test–retest reliability and ability to detect change, referred to as sensitivity. A commonly used outcome measure in various areas of rehabilitation medicine is the Functional Independence Measure (FIM™), used to measure a patient's functional disability and to indicate how much assistance is required for the person to carry out ADLs in the areas of self-care, transfers and mobility, bladder and bowel control, language, and cognitive abilities (http://ahsri.uow.edu.au/aroc/whatisfim/index.html (Australia), http://www.udsmr.org/WebModules/FIM/Fim_About.aspx (US).

Critical appraisal of assessment tools

An assessment tool should be clinically useful; that is, it should accurately measure what it is intended to measure (valid), with minimal measurement error (reliable), in a way that is responsive to the provided intervention (responsive), and is sustainable in clinical practice (acceptability).

The main forms of validity relevant to rehabilitation clinicians are content, construct, and criterion-related validity. These forms of validity are defined in Table 6.1. *Content validity* is often determined during the test development stage and relates to the rigour with which items for a test have been gathered, examined, and selected. Measures of expert agreement, content analysis, or descriptive methods can be used to report on *content validity*. In contrast, measures of *construct validity* include various statistical methods such as factor analysis and Rasch analysis. *Criterion validity* evaluates the effectiveness of a test against predetermined criteria, often for a specific purpose such as to discriminate between diagnostic groups (discriminative validity), to predict an outcome (predictive validity), or to determine level of agreement with a gold standard (referred to as concurrent, congruent, or convergent validity).

Reliability informs the clinician about how test performance may be affected by time or by the person administering the assessment. High levels of reliability indicate that clinicians can have a high level of confidence that the assessment scores reflect the patient's true performance. Terms such as agreement, concordance, repeatability, and reproducibility are sometimes used to describe different aspects of reliability. The main types of reliability relevant to rehabilitation clinicians are *internal consistency* (measured using Cronbach's alpha) and stability measured by *test–retest reliability* and *inter-rater reliability* (measured using intraclass correlation coefficients or Pearson's r). These forms of reliability are typically measured using correlational analysis, producing a reliability score between 0 ± 1. Different forms of reliability are defined in Table 6.1.

Test sensitivity determines the degree to which the assessment tool accurately identifies patients according to agreed diagnostic criteria. When using evaluative assessment tools, test responsiveness is critical, as this can indicate how well the assessment tool identifies both the type and amount of change in function that can be attributed to the intervention. It is important that evaluative assessments can identify clinically important change, even if that change if quite small. Sensitivity and responsiveness are defined in Table 6.1.

To ensure practice sustainability, assessment tools need to be acceptable to the MDT. Acceptability refers to the *respondent burden* and the *administrative burden*. These aspects influence the pragmatic reasoning aspects of assessment tool selection and are defined in Table 6.1.

Table 6.1 Definition of measurement properties relevant to rehabilitation assessment tools

Measurement property	Definition
Content validity	Assessment comprehensiveness and inclusion of items that fully represent the measured attribute
Construct validity	The extent to which an assessment measures a theoretical construct or constructs
Criterion validity: • Discriminative • Predictive • Concurrent	The ability of a test to distinguish between individuals or groups on a specific construct The degree to which a measure predicts a future event, outcome or categorization The extent to which the results on an assessment tool agree with another measure of the same or similar traits, abilities or behaviours
Test–retest reliability	Consistency of the assessment instrument over time measured by the correlation between scores on two test administrations on the same patient using the same assessment
Inter-rater reliability	Agreement between or among different clinicians (raters) measured by the correlation between scores recorded by two or more clinicians administering the assessment to the same patient at the same time
Internal consistency	The degree to which test items all measure the same behaviour or construct, measured by comparisons between test items intended to measure the same construct to determine if they produce a consistent result
Sensitivity	Ability of an assessment or screening test to identify patients who have a condition, calculated as a percentage of all cases with the condition who were judged by the test to have the condition: the 'true-positive' rate
Responsiveness	Efficiency with which an assessment measure can detect clinical change, often measured by the effect size associated with an intervention
Minimum clinically important difference (MCID)	The smallest difference in score in the domain of interest which patients perceive as beneficial. MCID values can be derived using distribution-based or anchor-based methods
Acceptability	*Respondent burden*—is the length and content acceptable to the intended respondent (patient)? *Administrative burden*—how easy is the tool to administer, score, and interpret? Cost implications?

Assessment within the ICF framework

In rehabilitation medicine, the focus of outcome measurement shifts from measuring the activity of a pathology or disease to measuring change due to the rehabilitation process, that is, the added value of the rehabilitation given to a patient over and above a spontaneous recovery or improvement following an injury or illness. However, the approach to outcome evaluation in rehabilitation medicine does not assume that a condition will improve. For example, rehabilitation may slow down the deterioration and improve quality of life in patients with progressive disability, for which outcomes measures used for static or improving conditions will be inappropriate. Measurement is thus important at an individual patient level to demonstrate a change in functioning, as well as at a health service level to assist in funding allocation.

The ICF (as described in ⊃ Chapter 2) provides a framework that describes a person's health status as the interaction between three domains: body functions and structures, limitations in activity execution or performance, and restriction of participation. Multidisciplinary team assessments can be planned to evaluate one or several areas of the ICF depending on the patient's health concerns and goals. Assessing the first domain, targeting impairment of body functions and structures, is common practice across all medical specialities (e.g. through assessment of blood pressure, muscle strength, pain, etc.). Assessing the ICF's second and third domains, activities and participation in the individual's life situations, is less common in medicine, but fundamental in rehabilitation. Furthermore, evaluation of environmental factors including physical, social, and attitudinal environments that inhibit activity and health is also critical to understanding the holistic effect of rehabilitation on patients. Finally, personal factors that influence the rehabilitation process such as coping style, personal characteristics, and behavioural patterns should be formally or informally evaluated to determine individual factors that may enable or inhibit the rehabilitation process.

Each ICF domain should be specifically assessed in order to obtain a comprehensive assessment of the patient. Discrete assessment of each ICF level is recommended as there is no causative relationship between different ICF domains. Multidimensional assessment tools that simultaneously assess several domains can be useful in some contexts, where interactions are of importance to understanding the disease process and/or functional implications. However, it has been noted that results of multidimensional assessments can be misleading. To make the ICF applicable in practice, the WHO in collaboration with the ICF Research Branch have created the ICF Core Sets to facilitate the description of functioning in clinical practice. The ICF Core Sets provide diagnostically linked lists of ICF categories that are relevant for specific health conditions and healthcare contexts. Core sets have been developed for a wide range of health conditions.

Rasch analysis applied to outcome measures

Functional observations of patient performance in rehabilitation are typically measured using 'ordinal'-level rating scales; for example, performs independently, requires assistance, or is dependent. The rating categories represent a decreasing hierarchy of independence but the difference between categories is not quantified. Rasch measurement models quantify the difference between ordinal categories using a logistic transformation of raw ordered data into equal-interval units expressed as logits. Equal interval scales enable more accurate measurement of a patient's ability over time, measurement between individuals or across groups. In addition, a logit scale has a mathematical advantage in the measurement of people with severe and mild disabilities, as log odds scales do not bias towards scores in the middle of the scale, or against people who score at the extremes.

In addition to producing interval-level measures, Rasch measurement techniques can be used for evaluating the construct validity of an assessment tool using an item fit analysis. Rasch measurement models answer questions of validity such as: How well does each assessment item or task fit with the underlying construct? How well do the set of assessment items or tasks define a single construct (unidimensionality)? How well do raters use the rating scale? In Rasch measurement, construct validity is supported when the recorded performances of patients and test items are true reflections of a single underlying construct. Fit analysis provides an indicator of how well each item and person fits with the underlying construct. Items that do not fit the unidimensional construct are those that diverge unacceptably from the expected ability/difficulty pattern. Several rehabilitation measures have undergone Rasch analysis as part of the development process or retrospectively to evaluate construct validity. For example, the ABILHAND was originally constructed using Rasch analysis, including 46 items rated by patients with rheumatoid arthritis on their perceived level of difficulty performing everyday tasks. Later Rasch analysis reduced the number of items to 23 and validated the ABILHAND across cultures and medical conditions (e.g. stroke). Rasch analysis of a 'generic' ABILHAND scale has been applied to 126 patients with various chronic upper limb impairments. To further facilitate clinical application, Rasch analysis was used to develop a normative cut-off value.

Goal setting and goal attainment

Rehabilitation is a complex intervention, involving multiple disciplines each focusing on different clinical outcomes. In this context, a goal-planning process should be used to ensure that all the people involved, especially the patient, agree on the goals of rehabilitation. Goal achievement at the end of the rehabilitation process is a measure of success, but the true value of goal setting and goal attainment depends on the skill of the MDT in defining realistic, achievable, and desirable goals in a partnership with the patient. If a goal is too easy, then the measure will have a ceiling effect, whereas if it is too difficult, the patient's achievements will not be sufficiently recognized. The goal setting process itself can be effective in achieving behavioural changes in some patients, particularly if the goals are relevant to the patient, are in accordance with their values, are challenging but realistic and achievable, and are measurable. Therefore, well-written rehabilitation goals are often abbreviated to the acronym SMART (specific, measurable, achievable, realistic/relevant, and timed). Defining the characteristics of a SMART goal can be challenging and writing SMART goals in rehabilitation is often perceived as time-consuming and difficult. However, well defined goals are particularly needed for goal attainment scaling which is sometimes used in rehabilitation as way of measuring success.

First introduced by for assessing outcomes in mental health settings, Goal Attainment Scaling (GAS) is now used in many areas of rehabilitation. A process to assist with writing GAS goals has been proposed by Bovend'Eerdt et al. to assist MDTs to define goals, identify target activity outcomes, specify required supports (e.g. equipment or assistance), identify measures to quantify performance (time, amount, distance, frequency), and the time required to achieve the goal. GAS tasks are individually identified to suit the patient and the levels of achievement are individually set around their current and expected levels of performance. A flowchart outlining this process is included (Fig. 6.1). GAS is a method of scoring the extent to which a patient's individual goals are achieved. Each patient is evaluated according to their own specific goals; however, scoring is standardized to allow statistical analysis. GAS goals can be selected from any or all domains of the ICF (activity, participation, quality of life, and environmental factors). This contrasts with traditional outcome measures discussed previously in this chapter, where a standard set of tasks are assessed according to pre-set 'levels' (e.g. the FIM).

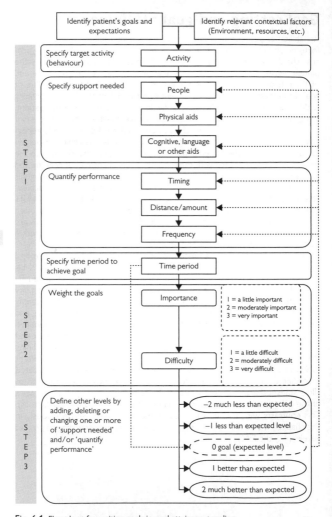

Fig. 6.1 Flowchart for writing goals in goal attainment scaling.

Reproduced with permission from Bovend'Eerdt T.J.H. et al. Writing SMART rehabilitation goals and achieving goal attainment scaling: a practical guide. *Clinical Rehabilitation*, 23(4): 352–361. Copyright © 2009 SAGE Publications. https://doi.org/10.1177/0269215508101741.

Further reading

Bond TG, Fox CM (2013). *Applying the Rasch Model Fundamental Measurement in the Human Sciences*, 2nd edn. Taylor and Francis, Hoboken, NJ.

Bovend'Eerdt TJH, Botell RE, Wade DT (2009). Writing SMART rehabilitation goals and achieving goal attainment scaling: a practical guide. *Clinical Rehabilitation* 23, 352–361.

Laver-Fawcett A (2013). *Principles of Assessment and Outcome Measurement for Occupational Therapists and Physiotherapists: Theory, Skills and Application*. Wiley, Hoboken, NJ.

Pynsent P, Fairbank J, Carr A (eds). *Outcome Measures in Orthopaedics and Orthopaedic Trauma*, 2nd edn. Arnold, London.

Turner-Stokes L (2009). Goal attainment scaling (GAS) in rehabilitation: a practical guide. *Clinical Rehabilitation* 23, 362–370.

Wade DT (1992). *Measurement in Neurological Rehabilitation*. Oxford University Press, Oxford.

Websites

ICF Core Sets: ℗ http://www.icf-core-sets.org/.

Rehabilitation Measures Database (Rehabilitation Institute of Chicago): ℗ http://www.rehabmeasures.org.

Webinar: Demystifying Rasch Analysis for Rehabilitation Clinicians (Retirement Research Foundation-funded webinar presented by Dr Jennifer Moore and Dr Chih-Hung Chang—requires Adobe Connect software): ℗ http://www.rehabmeasures.org/rehabweb/education.aspx.

WHO International Classification of Functioning, Disability and Health: ℗ http://www.who.int/classifications/icf/en/.

Cognition and behaviour

Cognition: general background

Cognition is the term that refers to all the processes involved in perceiving, learning, remembering, and thinking. Thus, cognitive problems are very common in any process that affects brain function. In this chapter, cognition is defined as an interaction of processes which involve all forms of awareness and knowing such as perceiving, conceiving, insight, remembering, questioning, reasoning, judging, problem-solving, and decision-making.[1] Simply put, cognition refers to the functions of the mind that result in thought and goal-directed action.

The processes involved in cognition have been defined using various models and theories. Pertinent to this chapter on cognition and behaviour is the model of information processing that describes a sequence of steps or stages through which information is manipulated to facilitate decision-making and action. As depicted in Fig. 7.1, information is initially sensed (from either the internal or external environment) then registered for sensory processing. Following this initial reception of information, a processing function occurs involving various short- and long-term memory structures. In situations that are novel or more complex, executive control processes may also be recruited to plan and evaluate the final output of the system, which can be in the form of thoughts or observable behaviours.

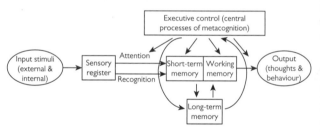

Fig. 7.1 Components of information processing.

From Lerner/Johns. *Learning Disabilities and Related Mild Disabilities*, 12E. © 2012 South-Western, a part of Cengage, Inc. Reproduced by permission. www.cengage.com/permissions.

Perception

Perception is the dynamic process of receiving sensory information from the environment and translating that information into meaning. Perceptual disorders occur as a result of acquired brain injury such as stroke, traumatic brain injury (TBI), brain tumour, or central nervous system (CNS) diseases including dementia. The disorders may result in difficulties organizing, processing, and interpreting information, and acting appropriately on the basis of this information. Perceptual impairments are related to reduced independence and safety in self-care activities and community living tasks, and subsequently affect rehabilitation prognosis and discharge options. These disorders may be evident through any of the senses but the most important are visual perception, auditory perception, and tactile perception. Perceptual deficits of taste and smell do exist, but in humans are of less functional significance.

The terminology used in cognitive and perceptual assessment and rehabilitation can be confusing and the following sections offer a simple guide to nomenclature. Where possible, alternative terms have been included for clarity.

Agnosia

Agnosia refers to the inability to recognize and classify objects, shapes, people, words, and colour in a variety of settings. Deficits cannot be explained by a primary sensory disorder. Each of the senses has a specific agnosia. *Visual agnosia* is the most important. (Visual agnosia may also be referred to as visuoperceptual or visual perceptual impairment, or visual discrimination.) Specific visual agnosias include:
- *object agnosia*—inability to recognize objects
- *form constancy*—inability to recognize shapes and objects as the same, when presented in different sizes or orientations
- *colour agnosia (achromatopsia)*—inability to recognize colours
- *prosopagnosia*—inability to recognize familiar faces
- *impaired visual analysis and synthesis*—associated with figure-ground discrimination, visual closure, and simultanagnosia (an inability to perceive all the elements of a scene simultaneously, i.e. recognition of parts of the scene but not the whole).

The other senses also have their own forms of agnosia, such as tactile agnosia and auditory agnosia.

Visuospatial impairments

Visuospatial skills involve the ability to relate oneself to the position, direction, or movement of objects, or points in space. Visuospatial impairments are also referred to as spatial disorientation, visuospatial agnosia, or spatial relations syndromes. Specific forms of visuospatial impairments can include:
- impaired depth perception
- impaired judgement of direction, distance, or position in space
- topographical disorientation.

Body scheme disorders

Body scheme is the knowledge of the position of the parts of the body and the spatial relationship between them. This knowledge is based on the integration of perceptual processing of the input from vision, proprioception, tactile sensation, and pressure sensation in all the parts of the body as we move around. Specific impairments can include the following:

- *Asomatognosia*—inability to recognize parts of the body and their relative position in space. Movements are inaccurate in the presence of normal proprioception.
- *Left–right discrimination*—inability to distinguish right and left in the symmetrical parts of the body, for example, Gerstmann syndrome after injury to the left inferior parietal lobe.
- *Anosognosia*—denial of the impairment of (or even the presence) of an affected body part, for example, Anton syndrome after occipital lobe injury where the person denies blindness.
- *Autopagnosia*—inability to identify parts of the body. Specifically, finger agnosia describes inability related to the fingers only.

Neglect

Neglect (often termed unilateral neglect) is the failure to attend to, respond to, or orient to stimuli from one side of space or body. Neglect can occur in the visual, tactile, and auditory modalities and in different spatial domains: personal, peri-personal, or extra-personal space. Individuals with *visual neglect*, for example, will commonly bump into things on the affected side or fail to see food on one side of the plate thinking they have finished the meal when in fact it has only been half eaten.

The diagnosis of neglect can only be made after screening for sensory loss, visual field loss, and primary motor deficits. Neglect is commonly a right hemisphere problem (affecting the left side/space) and is particularly common after stroke.

Apraxia

Apraxia is the inability to perform a purposeful function in the setting of preserved overall neurological function. The term *apraxia* usually relates to disorders in adults while the term *dyspraxia* is typically used in childhood developmental disorders. Apraxia is more common in left hemisphere injury. There are two main forms of apraxia—ideational apraxia relates to breakdown at the conceptual level and ideomotor apraxia refers to the production stage:

- *Ideational apraxia*—inability to perform purposeful movement due to the loss of conceptual knowledge about movement and objects. Patients are unable to produce an action on command or to pantomime a gesture (e.g. blowing out a match), but can imitate actions.
- *Ideomotor apraxia*—disorder in the selection, timing, and spatial organization of purposeful movement, causing inability to perform motor actions on command, to pantomime gestures, or to imitate. This differentiates ideational and ideomotor apraxia on assessment.

Attention

Attention is a cognitive process that occurs early in the information processing system. Attention enables the selection of important features/
stimuli in the environment and filters out the remaining, competing stimuli.
Attention processing can be thought of as a hierarchy. The basic level is
arousal and vigilance, or our state of readiness for action. Next is our ability
to select relevant information from the surrounding environment and to
shift attentional focus from one stimuli to another. The highest level is controlled processing, which is responsible for sustained attention, modulation,
and regulation of attention. In the early stages of rehabilitation, attention is
a priority because deficits impact all other cognitive functions.

Arousal

Level of arousal is determined by the ascending reticular activating system
running through the brainstem to the cerebral cortex. Sensory information
is modulated in the reticular formation and the thalamus to determine a
person's level of arousal. Tonic arousal changes with a person's sleep and
wake cycle, while phasic arousal occurs in response to activity demands.

Selective/focused attention

The brain is bombarded with sensory information from all over the body
and from the environment (refer back to Fig. 7.1). It is critical to filter out
some of this information to ensure the brain's capacity for information
processing is not exceeded. Selective attention facilitates this process of
attending to critical information while ignoring the rest. This process is effective for a range of sensory inputs such as visual, auditory, and tactile
sensory information.

Shifting attention

Our attentional focus frequently shifts or changes in line with the demands
of the task and the environment. Attention can be specifically directed
towards different locations, different people or objects, or to our own
bodies. Shifting attention requires redirection of attention from one point
of focus to another, in a multistep process: disengage, shift, and then engage with new target stimulus. Errors in attentional shifting can occur at
all three stages of this process. People with attentional impairments may
appear rigid or fixed, with the inability to respond to peripheral stimuli, for
example, someone calling their name or movement of a person into their
peripheral visual field.

Divided attention

Multitasking is a feature of several more complex everyday tasks, such as
driving a car. These tasks require the ability to divide attention between
multiple tasks or task components. Attentional errors occur when the combined demands of the two tasks exceed our attentional capacity. Factors
that impact divided attention are task similarity, practice, and task difficulty.

Memory

Memory includes the processes of encoding information (storage) and also retrieving information (recall). Memory impairments are probably the most commonly experienced (or reported) cognitive problem following brain injury and one that has a profound impact on daily function. The neuroanatomic circuitry that underpins memory is extensive, and involves sensory association areas, the limbic system, and its connections to the neocortex. This section will describe different aspects and functions of memory. Cognitive rehabilitation for memory impairments will be addressed later in this chapter (➲ see 'Cognitive rehabilitation approaches').

Different memory structure/systems

- *Short-term or working memory*—retains information over a period of seconds or minutes and has limited capacity. Information enters the working memory system from the sensory register or can be drawn in from long-term memory (refer back to Fig. 7.1). Information from the long-term memory is transferred back into working memory to assist with interpretation of the information coming in via the sensory register.
- *Long-term memory*—has an unlimited capacity and processes a variety of information that is being constantly updated. Information from the short-term or working memory enters long-term memory where it is processed for meaning and context. These processes enable retrieval at the required time in the future, for interpretation and reflection.

Different memory forms: 'How?', 'What?', and 'When?'

Information in the long-term memory is thought to be divided into subsystems:

- *Procedural memory*—memory for skills and procedures ('How?'). All motor and language skills are part of procedural memory. This aspect of memory is *implicit*, developed through repetition and practice, and is often preserved in brain injury when episodic and semantic memory are not.
- *Declarative memory*—memory for factual knowledge, people, objects, places, and events ('What?'). Declarative memory is *explicit* and is divided into *semantic memory* for knowledge of the world, organized by concepts and associations and retrieved without context (i.e. knowing that bananas are yellow), and *episodic memory* which relates to facts and events in context, therefore retrieval depends on the ability to recall the relevant contextual information of the time and place in which something occurs.
- *Prospective memory*—is the activation of stored plans at some time point in the future. Prospective memory is remembering what to do and 'When?' to do it. Everyday routines are mostly automatic and depend on implicit procedural memory, whereas non-routine activities require prospective memory to activate the plan at the right time.

Executive functions

The term executive functions refers to a range of high-level cognitive processes that combine together to set goals, problem-solve, make choices, and determine if behaviours are appropriate in context. These cognitive processes are initiated primarily in novel situations that require decisions about what to do and how to do it. The prefrontal cortex has been implicated in the operation of executive functions and the cluster of symptoms observed in patients with damage to the frontal lobe is known as the *dysexecutive syndrome*.

A major role of the executive system is to coordinate and monitor the cognitive system as a whole. Neuropsychologists have attempted to partition the executive system into independent components but thus far this approach has yielded limited success as this discounts the interaction required between different cognitive skills for optimal function. The different cognitive skills or processes consistently described as part of the executive system include the following:

- *Initiation and termination*—a task or activity can be initiated by an external or internal cue. Goal-directed activity includes multiple cognitive processes of initiation, termination, and suppression of non-task behaviour. In non-routine activities, this relies on the inhibition of automatic processing and the maintenance of sustained attention.
- *Goal setting*—realistic goal setting requires a degree of insight or awareness of our own strengths and weaknesses, with an estimate of task difficulty. Formulating a goal involves reasoning and also some abstract thinking, that is, beyond the here and now.
- *Planning and organizing*—effective planning and organizing involve the formation of strategies to achieve a desired goal. These strategies may include identifying the problem, the solution, and any obstacles to goal achievement; formulating a plan and activating strategies; and changing or modifying these strategies if the task or conditions change.
- *Adaptation and flexibility*—adaptations are the changes that people make in their task performance when they encounter an obstacle or challenge. Monitoring the environment and self-monitoring are important components of flexibility, as this enables the person to regularly check how the task is progressing and keeping track of the task sequence. People with frontal lobe damage are easily distracted and find it difficult to get back on track, particularly in prolonged tasks with multiple task steps.

Metacognition

Metacognition is our knowledge and beliefs about our own cognitive processes and capacities. This knowledge enables us to monitor our own thoughts, speech, and actions. Executive functions are inextricably linked with metacognition, without which we could not monitor our changing behaviour or evaluate strategies for change. Loss of awareness leads to inability to detect errors in performance or to anticipate problems or plan strategies, and is associated with reduced insight.

Cognitive rehabilitation approaches

Evidence relating to the effects of cognitive rehabilitation is rapidly evolving. The traditional approaches to cognitive rehabilitation tended to focus on a binary classification of treatment approaches as being either *remedial/ restorative* including tasks and activities aimed at decreasing impairments in basic cognitive functions or *compensatory/functional* including interventions aimed at maximizing function with or without changes to the underlying cognitive impairments.

Remedial training: using residual skills more effectively

There are a number of techniques in this area that have mainly been developed in the field of attention and memory. Techniques use mnemonics, acronyms, rhymes, and systematic cueing to enhance use of residual skills more efficiently. Generalization of these learned skills into everyday life has not been particularly effective and in patients with significant cognitive impairments, is highly dependent on family members and caregivers.

Compensatory training: finding a way around the problem

Compensatory devices, techniques, or strategies are designed according to the individual problem, and may include assistive equipment such as external memory aids (diaries, lists, alarm clocks, timers, and tape recorders). Reminders on mobile phones are also useful. However, these methods are not always successful as people need some residual memory in order to remember what they are being reminded about.

A different approach to compensation is to modify or adapt the surrounding environment in order to reduce cognitive load. For example, clear use of signage and colour differentiation between spaces can assist with recognition and recall in rehabilitation ward environments. In dementia-specific rehabilitation, environmental adaptation aims to decrease agitation, increase well-being, provide safety, reduce exiting behaviours, improve privacy and dignity, and increase participation and engagement. As such, the recommended environmental interventions target everyday functional behaviour and decrease environmental complexity by minimizing distractions for residents, increasing orientation and awareness through the use of sensory stimuli and cues, and through creation of a low-stimulation and comfortable environment for residents. Adaptation may also involve a rigid organization of daily life so that limited planning and organizational skills are required. A very structured day, with diaries and prompts from caregivers, can often assist someone with aspects of the dysexecutive syndrome.

Cognitive or metacognitive strategy training

Contemporary cognitive rehabilitation practice also includes a third approach using *cognitive or metacognitive strategy training*.[2] Utilization of this approach does not yet appear to be widely reported in surveys of current practice, even though evidence supporting the effectiveness of this approach is increasingly available. For example, Cicerone et al.'s update of evidence-based cognitive rehabilitation[3] recommends a combination of direct attention training and metacognitive training to promote generalization to real-world tasks. Memory strategy training is recommended for mild memory impairments, while use of external compensation strategies and errorless learning with direct application to functional activities is recommended for people with severe memory deficits after TBI or stroke. These are examples of *domain-specific* cognitive strategies.

More general or *global metacognitive strategy instruction* (including self-monitoring and self-regulation) is recommended for executive deficits.[3] This reinforces the earlier level A recommendation by the Academy of Neurologic Communication Disorders and Sciences that metacognitive strategy instruction is recommended for adults with TBI experiencing difficulties with executive functions such as problem-solving, planning, organizing, and multitasking.[4] This recommendation has also been recently supported by the INCOG recommendations for management of cognition in adults with TBI stating that incorporation of metacognitive strategy instruction in cognitive rehabilitation has a solid evidence base.[5]

Behaviour: general background

Behaviour can be thought of as the observable output from the information processing system described in Fig. 7.1. Cognitive processes underpin thoughts and behaviour and changes to behaviour can be achieved through changes to cognition. There are many theories and approaches to understanding behaviour in the context of rehabilitation. This section will focus on two approaches used in current practice: cognitive behaviour approaches and behavioural management/modification based on learning theories.

Problems with behaviour, also termed *challenging behaviours* or *behaviours of concern* are observed in rehabilitation wards or units, particularly those managing adults with CNS disorders such as TBI or dementia. Some behaviours are of short duration and are associated with specific stages of recovery, such as the period of confusion during post-traumatic amnesia that follows a TBI. However other forms of challenging behaviour are evident long term and require a MDT approach, including a clinical/neuropsychologist to inform the assessment and management process.

Behavioural problems can be grouped into two broad categories: inappropriate *excessive* behaviour and inappropriate *lack of* behaviour.

The former can present with a variety of difficulties:
• Verbal aggression: usually targeted at others.
• Physical aggression: targeted at others, self or objects.
• Aggressive refusal to cooperate with the rehabilitation programme.
• Impulsivity.
• Inappropriate sexual behaviour.

At the other end of the spectrum, inappropriate lack of behaviour can include:
• apathy
• lack of initiation.

In these circumstances, individuals are often labelled as lacking in motivation. This label should be avoided, as it can imply that the observed 'lack of motivation or laziness' is the fault of the individual and that little can be done to correct the problem. This is particularly unhelpful in rehabilitation settings.

Learning theory

Behavioural management or modification techniques are typically based on various classical learning theories. A detailed overview of learning theory is beyond the scope of this chapter. Presented in the following sections is a clinically applicable summary of learning theory and behaviour modification.

Classical conditioning

Several perspectives exist on how humans learn. In common, most theories recognize that learning occurs through repeated exposure to a stimulus of some form, which results in a repeatable and predicable outcome. For example, *classical conditioning* describes a learning process whereby a specific (conditional) response is trained to occur following a specific (conditional) stimulus. This form of learning has been made famous by classical Pavlovian experiments that trained a dog to salivate on presentation of a stimulus, such as a bell or light, when on previous occasions this stimulus had been associated with the presentation of food. The bell or light is known as the *conditional stimulus* and the salivation as the *conditional response*. This association can be broken if one stimulus becomes disassociated with the other—known as extinction.

Operant conditioning

A different perspective on learning is *operant or instrumental conditioning*, which occurs when individuals learn the association between their own actions or behaviours and an environmental consequence. This can include the delivery of rewards such as praise, benefits, and food. Procedures adapted from operant conditioning studies form the majority of behavioural modification techniques.

Classical and operant conditioning are both forms of associative learning. In other words, the individual learns a link between one experience and another. There is now good evidence showing that associative learning abilities are retained even in the presence of severe brain impairment.

Behaviour observation and analysis

The basis of most behaviour management or modification programmes is clear identification of the behaviour to be changed and the circumstances in which the behaviour tends to occur. A useful approach to structure behaviour observation and analysis is termed ABC: Antecedent, Behaviour, and Consequence. Charts are regularly used to identify and monitor behaviours. An example is shown in Fig. 7.2.

The *antecedent* determines what seems to occur immediately prior to, or triggers the inappropriate behaviour. Using the information processing model depicted in Fig. 7.1, this is represented by the left-hand side processes of sensory input and registration. Sensory input can be internal, for example, hunger or pain, or external, for example, a specific noise in the surrounding environment or location on the rehabilitation ward such as the physiotherapy gym. Different questions can be asked to clearly identify the behavioural antecedent:

• What appears to trigger it?
• In what circumstances does it occur?
• Is it situation specific?
• Is it environment specific?
• Is it person specific?
• Are there instances when it is not triggered?

Next, the *behaviour* itself requires close analysis:

• What are the characteristics of the behaviour?
• What form does it take?
• To whom or what is it directed?
• How long does it last (duration)?
• How often does it occur (frequency)?

Using the information processing model depicted in Fig. 7.1, this is represented by the right-hand side processes of output—thoughts or behaviours. Information processing breakdowns can occur anywhere along the cognitive processes that link the antecedent to the behaviour output, such as misattributions based on memory impairment, or reduced executive control resulting in dysregulated behaviour. This information processing model enables the link between cognition and behaviour to be more explicit.

Finally, ABC analysis focuses on what are the *consequences* of the behaviour? Analysis should include the following:

• Is there an observed benefit?
• Does it lead to reward or another form of positive reinforcement?
• Does the individual calm down quickly or slowly?

After a period of close behavioural observation, a pattern usually emerges. It is unusual for behavioural disturbance not to be triggered by anything and to have no pattern at all. Once a pattern is identified, a behavioural modification programme can be developed in consultation with the MDT and a clinical psychologist.

DATE	SETTING EVENTS (events that could possibly contribute to problem behaviour, even if there is extended time between event and behaviour)	ANTECEDENT (what happened immediately before the behaviour)	BEHAVIOUR (what does the behaviour look like, be specific)	CONSEQUENCE (what happened directly following the behaviour)

Fig. 7.2 Example of an ABC chart.
http://www.playwithjoy.com/2013/06/abcs-of-behavior.html.

Behaviour management/modification

After definition and analysis of the specific behaviour to be changed, a modification plan with specific goals can be set. As with all rehabilitation processes, a measuring instrument or process can be used to monitor achievement or progress towards the defined goal. Non-specific goals such as 'patient will be less aggressive' are inadequate (ℒ see SMART goals, described in Chapter 1). Specific goals are required, such as how many times the patient is aggressive over a given period of time or during a specific activity.

Treatment approaches to increase desirable behaviours

The most common method for increasing desirable behaviours is by *positive reinforcement*. A positive reinforcement is something which is delivered immediately following the occurrence of a behaviour which will increase the probability of that behaviour being repeated again in the future. The reinforcement can be tangible, such as food, or in some settings, additional permissions, such as visits off the ward area. Reinforcers can also be less tangible, such as praise or task participation/achievement. Natural reinforcers, such as praise, are typically more effective long term than artificial reinforcers, such as food. Whatever the reinforcer, all members of the rehabilitation team must know the behavioural modification being implemented so that every time a particular behaviour occurs it can be appropriately reinforced in a consistent and clear manner. *Shaping* is a related technique, also used to increase desirable behaviour that involves reinforcement of the small steps towards an eventual desired behaviour. For example, if a patient refuses to dress in the mornings they could be initially rewarded for just looking at or touching their clothes, and then rewarded step by step over a period of time for each item of clothing that is correctly put on. Eventually, the small reinforcers are withdrawn and larger steps, such as dressing the top half of the body without prompts, are reinforced until finally positive reinforcement is only given after completion of the entire task. Other techniques used to increase desirable behaviours include:
• *modelling* of the desired behaviour by a member of staff
• *environmental restructuring* to reduce the likelihood that a situation occurs in which the behaviour can be triggered.

Treatment approaches to decrease undesirable behaviours

There are two basic methods to decrease undesirable behaviours:
• *Extinction*—which occurs when the reinforcer is no longer delivered to a previously reinforced response.
• *Punishment*—which involves the presentation of an aversive stimulus or removal of a positive stimulus immediately following the inappropriate behaviour.

These approaches are not used widely in contemporary practice, which tends to focus on increasing desirable behaviours in preference to decreasing undesirable behaviours.

Cognitive behavioural approach

In contrast to the learning-based approaches that emphasize changing behaviours through changing external stimuli and reinforcement, the cognitive behavioural approach focuses on the relationship between thoughts and behaviour. The cognitive behavioural approach asserts that thoughts, feelings, and behaviours are linked: that behaviour arises as a result of a person's thoughts, that is, behaviour is dependent upon thought, therefore negative or irrational thoughts can lead to behaviours that are maladaptive. The cognitive behaviour approach forms the foundation of cognitive behaviour therapy (CBT), used widely in contemporary behaviour management practice. Important components of CBT include a focus on helping patients solve problems; become behaviourally activated; and identify, evaluate, and respond to their own thinking, especially to negative thoughts about themselves, their worlds, and their future. CBT is individually tailored; however, there are several underlying principles. These include establishing a therapeutic alliance, being goal oriented and problem focused, and taking an educative approach. Contemporary CBT uses a variety of techniques or core principles to change thinking and mood. Several of these are listed in Box 7.1.[6]

Studies of CBT efficacy have demonstrated efficacy with a wide range of conditions including substance use disorder, schizophrenia and other psychotic disorders, depression, bipolar disorder, anxiety disorders, somatoform disorders, eating disorders, insomnia, personality disorders, anger and aggression, criminal behaviours, general stress, distress due to general medical conditions, chronic pain and fatigue, distress related to pregnancy complications, and female hormonal conditions. A recent review[7] of over 100 meta-analyses examining CBT efficacy reports a very strong evidence base for CBT with the greatest clinical benefit observed in studies involving people with anxiety disorders, somatoform disorders, bulimia, anger control problems, and general stress.

Box 7.1 CBT techniques/core principles

- Functional analysis and contingency management
- Skills training
- Exposure
- Relaxation
- Cognitive restructuring
- Problem-solving
- Self-regulation
- Behavioural activation
- Social skills
- Emotional regulation
- Communication
- Positive psychology
- Acceptance

Pharmacological management of behaviour

While the emphasis for behavioural management is on psychological evaluation and intervention, a subgroup of people will benefit from the use of sedative, anxiolytic, or psychotropic medication. It needs to be noted that medications by themselves are a poor substitute for a behavioural management programme. In some cases, idiosyncratic reactions to these drugs can exacerbate problem behaviours. Other drugs, in particular haloperidol, have been reported to permanently impair brain recovery and should be avoided.

That being said, pharmacological management is justified where there is real risk to the patient, staff, or other patients, for example, in patients with explosive dyscontrol. People with acute psychosis or other acute thought disorders (e.g. delirium, drug withdrawal, and so on) are more likely to be able to benefit from psychological intervention once medication has been initiated. The key purpose of using medication in this scenario is to allow the person to process behavioural cues and show consistency when engaging with others.

For this reason, many pharmaceutical options can be considered. For some situations, 'mood stabilizers' (e.g. propranolol, carbamazepine, lithium, and lamotrigine) can be advantageous. Medications that decrease arousal and/or anxiety include the newer atypical antipsychotics (e.g. olanzapine and quetiapine), pregabalin/gabapentin, and many of the antidepressants (e.g. sertraline, trazodone, and buspirone). Individuals with behavioural disturbance resulting from decreased arousal/poor concentration or inadequate attention may respond to dopamine agonists or central stimulants such as dexamphetamine or methylphenidate.

All such medication should be used with caution. ⅋ See Chapter 26 for more information.

References

1. VandenBos GR (2015). *APA Dictionary of Psychology*, 2nd edn. American Psychological Association, Washington, DC.
2. Sohlberg MM, Turkstra LS (2011). *Optimizing Cognitive Rehabilitation Effective Instructional Methods*. Guilford Publications, New York.
3. Cicerone KD, Langenbahn DM, Braden C, et al. (2011). Evidence-based cognitive rehabilitation: updated review of the literature from 2003 through 2008. *Archives of Physical Medicine and Rehabilitation* 92, 519–530.
4. Kennedy MRT, Coehlo C, Turkstra L, et al. (2008). Intervention for executive functions after traumatic brain injury: a systematic review, meta-analysis and clinical recommendations. *Neuropsychological Rehabilitation* 18, 257–299.
5. Tate R, Kennedy M, Ponsford J, et al. (2014). INCOG recommendations for management of cognition following traumatic brain injury, part III: executive function and self-awareness. *Journal of Head Trauma Rehabilitation* 29, 338–352.
6. Fisher JE, O'Donohue WT (2012). *Cognitive Behavior Therapy*. Wiley, Hoboken, NJ.
7. Hofmann SG, Asnaani A, Vonk IJJ, et al. (2012). The efficacy of cognitive behavioral therapy: a review of meta-analyses. *Cognitive Therapy and Research* 36, 427–440.

Communication

Introduction

The concept of communication encompasses speech and language alongside our ability to understand non-verbal communication. While communication appears effortless in normal circumstances, large amounts of unconscious processing are required from widely distributed brain regions. The traditional cortical language areas (Broca's and Wernicke's areas) are situated in the posterior inferior frontal cortex and the superior temporal cortex respectively. Other accessory language centres have become apparent with functional magnetic resonance imaging scanning techniques (Fig. 8.1). Language function is left dominant in 96% of right-handed people, compared with 75% of strongly left-handed people. A small proportion of people have mixed dominance (i.e. bilateral language centres), a potentially important site for language function recovery in people experiencing global dysphasia.

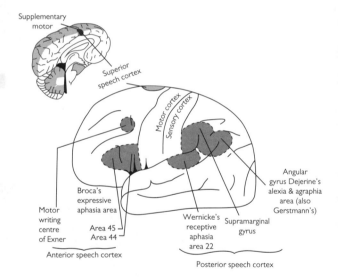

Fig. 8.1 Traditional cortical speech areas of the dominant hemisphere.

Reproduced with permission from Marcus E.M. et al. 'Speech, Language, Cerebral Dominance, and the Aphasias' in *Integrated Neuroscience and Neurology: A Clinical Case History Problem Solving Approach* (2 ed.). Oxford, UK: Oxford University Press. © 2014 Oxford University Press. Reproduced with permission of Oxford University Press through PLSclear. http://oxfordmedicine.com/view/10.1093/med/9780199744435.001.0001/med-9780199744435-chapter-24.

In addition to the classical cortical centres, two broad sets of white matter pathways (the dorsal and ventral language tracts) are vital for language processing. Debate remains about the functional and anatomical details of these systems in humans. Interconnections with biographical memory and other brain regions are also necessary to interpret the meaning of language as it relates to personal memories and contexts.

Non-verbal communication incorporates additional neurological systems including visual pathways, occipital lobes, mirror neurons, and so on. The signals require processing through emotional circuitry and are integrated with verbal communication to determine the finer nuances of communication (such as the use of sarcasm).

These observations mean that language function can be impaired from a much wider range of brain injuries than the relatively focal lesions that were traditionally considered. Speech pathologists play a major role in the assessment of communication and in the treatment of its various disorders. Early referral of patients with communication disorders can assist the whole rehabilitation team in adopting the most effective and sensitive way to communicate with patients.

Acquired speech and language disorders

Dysphasia/aphasia

Dysphasia or aphasia is a communication disorder characterized by deficits in language modalities: expression (understanding speech and writing) and comprehension (understanding spoken language and what is read). The pattern and severity of deficits depends on the location and severity of the brain lesion or damage. Dysphasia is seen following cortical damage in conditions such as stroke, TBI, and brain tumours.

Fluent dysphasias

These dysphasias comprise fluent speech with normal prosody but containing unintended, incorrect, and nonsense words, thus making the language empty of meaning. Written language often reflects this impairment. Patients have difficulty in understanding others language and are often not aware of their own errors.

Example: Wernicke's dysphasia
When the individual is asked 'Why have you been admitted to hospital', the individual says 'I am fine, thank you, husband area evening'.

Non-fluent dysphasia

These dysphasias are characterized by slow and laboured speaking, with difficulty in retrieving words, naming objects, and forming sentences. Written language can be similarly affected. Comprehension may be relatively unimpaired. There may be a correspondingly high level of awareness of errors in the patient's own language, often producing a significant degree of frustration.

Example: Broca's dysphasia
When the individual is asked 'Why have you been admitted to hospital', the individual says 'Broke ... stroke'.

Global dysphasia

A global dysphasia affects both the expression and comprehension of language, whether the written or the spoken word. When severe, global dysphasias may also limit a person's ability to understand and use non-verbal communication.

Dysarthria

Dysarthria is a speech disorder resulting from neurologically based impairments to speech musculature control such as weakness, spasticity, incoordination, involuntary movements, and variable muscle tone. It is seen in damage to the CNS and/or peripheral nervous system including cerebrum, cerebellum, basal ganglia, brainstem, or cranial nerves. Different types of dysarthria are recognized including flaccid, spastic, ataxic, hypokinetic, hyperkinetic, mixed, unilateral UMN, or undetermined. The patterns of dysarthic speech depend on the muscles affected as shown in Table 8.1.

Table 8.1 Patterns of dysarthic speech

Muscles affected	Examples
Respiratory muscles (e.g. diaphragm, intercostals)	The patient may run out of breath when speaking or their voice may lack intensity/volume
Phonatory muscles (e.g. vocal cords)	The vocal folds may not move properly causing breathy voice quality, dysphonia, or vocal tremor
Resonatory muscles (e.g. soft palate)	The soft palate may not function properly causing nasal airflow during speech
Articulatory muscles (e.g. lips and tongue)	The tongue, lips, and facial and jaw muscle movements may be impaired causing slurred speech

Apraxia of speech

Apraxias constitute a group of acquired disorders of motor planning with an impaired ability to perform sequential and coordinated muscle movements for speech. The deficit is not due to paralysis, weakness, or incoordination of muscles. Similarly, respiration, resonance, and voice are not impaired in this condition. The presentation of this condition is either significant deficits in articulation and rhythm or significant difficulty in initiating speech (sometimes the person may not be able to speak at all). Differentiating between dysarthria and apraxia is important because treatments for each can be very different.

Neurogenic stuttering

Neurogenic stuttering is an acquired fluency disorder characterized by repetition of parts of words, whole words, and phrases. There might be hesitations, pausing, and getting 'stuck' on a word. There can be extra movements of the lips, tongue, face, etc., while attempting to speak. Stuttering often co-occurs with other acquired speech and language disorders.

Assessment

As effective communication is essential for all interactions in the patient's life, early speech pathology referral is mandatory. Speech and language disorders are analysed with a view to how best to assist patients in communicating with those around them. Because neurological conditions can result in a variety of speech and language disorders which require different management, early differential diagnosis is important. All aspects of communication, including non-verbal communication, are assessed by the speech pathologist. Identification of the underlying aetiology of the speech and language disorder is critical. Therapy goals and expectations vary: a patient with an acute disabling process (e.g. cerebrovascular accident or TBI) will be expected to improve with therapy. A patient with a progressive degenerative neurological condition (Parkinson's disease, dementia) may have different management strategies implemented. Considering the various aspects of the individual patient's language disorder allows appropriate treatment and management strategies to be determined to manage the communication disorder.

Therapy and management

Depending on the cause and type of communication disorder and the wishes of the patient and their families/caregivers, speech pathologists will utilize a combination of impairment-based therapy and communication-based management techniques. Therapy for very mild communication disorders is likely to differ from therapy and management for a very severe impairment. Management and therapy techniques may change over time as the underlying cause of the disorder improves or worsens.

The multidisciplinary rehabilitation team should be aware of and adopt the management strategies recommended by the speech pathologist. The team approach maximizes gains for the patient as they generalize skills to new environments and it helps to minimize their frustration if there is one set of rules required to make the patient more easily understood.

Impairment-based therapy

Impairment-based therapy focuses on improving the disordered aspects of speech and language. It involves specific speech pathology therapy interventions such as:
- semantic-based tasks to stimulate word retrieval
- exercises using writing and reading skills to support comprehension of sentences
- exercises focused on improving the prosody (rhythm and pace) of speech
- vocal exercises aimed at reducing breathy phonation (voice).

Communication-based management

Communication-based management focuses on improving overall communication through the use of alternate approaches. Communication aids are most suitable for people with severe dysarthria and/or expressive dysphasia. They tend to be less helpful in the presence of significant receptive language disorders. Examples of communication-based management include the following:
- Conversational techniques taught to caregivers and staff to improve communication. For example, with patients who have difficulty comprehending language, carers and staff can be encouraged to converse in short, simple sentences, giving the patient time to process the information. Conversations can also be supported by the use of photographs and other visual information to assist with comprehension.
- Communication board—these are easily made, utilizing a customized combination of letters, words, phrases, and/or symbols which are placed in front of the patient to point to.
- Electronic communication aids include devices such as speech-generating devices (➔ see also Chapter 23). These may be operated by touching keys in the same style as a keyboard or through use of visual scanning in the case of people with severe physical disabilities. Stock phrases can be nested to allow for more fluent communication.

Further reading

Duffy JR (2013). *Motor Speech Disorders: Substrates, Differential Diagnosis and Management*, 3rd edn. Elsevier Mosby, St. Louis, MO.

Webb WG (2017). *Neurology for the Speech-Language Pathologist*, 6th edn. Elsevier Inc, St. Louis, MO.

Swallowing

Introduction

Dysphagia is the over-arching term referring to disorders of swallowing. Dysphagia is a common complication of many acute and chronic neurological conditions. In acute neurological conditions such as TBI and stroke, symptoms and signs are often worst immediately post event and show improvement over time. In contrast, in degenerative neurological diseases (e.g. MS, MND, and Parkinson's disease), a deterioration in swallowing can be expected as the disease progresses. Other causes of dysphagia include those with changes to anatomical structures (e.g. laryngeal and oral cancers and patients with tracheostomies). In addition, cognitive communication and behavioural issues can also affect swallowing (e.g. impulsively putting too much food into the mouth creating a choking risk). Dysphagia is important in the rehabilitation setting as it can produce common and potentially avoidable complications, morbidity, and death.

The normal swallow

Before reviewing abnormalities of swallowing, it is advantageous to under-stand normal physiology. Swallowing is divided into four phases:

Phase 1: oral preparation phase
- Food entering the mouth is masticated, combined with saliva, and aggregated into a bolus.
- This process requires proper coordination, strength, and speed of movement of the lips, tongue, and jaw (Fig. 9.1a).

Phase 2: oral phase
- This phase is under voluntary muscle control and involves transferring the food/fluid bolus backwards towards the pharynx.
- The tongue moves the bolus up and backwards to contact with the hard palate.
- The swallowing reflex is initiated when the bolus reaches the anterior faucial arch (Fig. 9.1b, c).

Phase 3: pharyngeal phase
- This phase is reflexive rather than being under voluntary control (Fig. 9.1d, e).
- The velopharynx closes to prevent food and fluid regurgitating out of the nose.
- The larynx closes to prevent food or fluid entering the larynx and airway. This is achieved via laryngeal elevation and anterior movement which also stretches and opens the cricopharyngeal sphincter.
- Pharyngeal peristalsis helps move the bolus towards the oesophagus.
- The opening of the cricopharyngeal sphincter allows passage of the bolus into the oesophagus.

Phase 4: oesophageal phase
- This is another reflexive phase.
- The bolus passes from the relaxed cricopharyngeal sphincter down into the oesophagus.
- Oesophageal peristalsis pushes food along the oesophagus to enter the stomach through the relaxed gastro-oesophageal/cardiac sphincter (Fig. 9.1f).

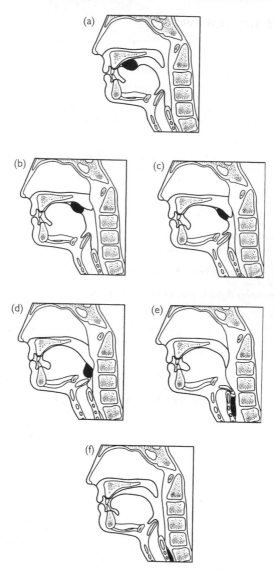

Fig. 9.1 Phases of swallowing.

Dysphagia

While the causes of dysphagia can be multifactorial in any given individual, dysphagia occurs because of impairment to any or all of the first three phases of swallowing (the oral preparatory, the oral, and the pharyngeal phases). The severity of dysphagia occurs across a spectrum from minimal (difficulty chewing certain foods when distracted) to severe (often necessitating enteral feeding). Furthermore, the severity of dysphagia can also vary across the day, depending on additional contributing factor/s, such as fatigue or reduced level of arousal.

Assessment

The clinical assessment of dysphagia is a multidisciplinary process. Speech and language therapists specialize in dysphagia assessment and management and work in conjunction with dieticians, occupational therapists, psychologists, and physicians.

The multifactorial nature of dysphagia means that a comprehensive assessment of the patient is required. A detailed history, cognitive communication screening, behavioural observation, oromotor assessment, bedside swallowing assessment (including a blue dye test for patients with tracheostomies), instrumental assessment of swallowing (where indicated), and nutritional assessment all comprise a thorough clinical assessment of swallowing.

Clinical indicators

While dysphagia can sometimes be observed from the end of the bed, it is more common for its presence to be less obvious. This requires the clinician to engage a reasonable index of suspicion in clinical problem-solving. The common symptoms and signs of dysphagia include:

- taking excessive time to eat meals or drink
- difficulty chewing food
- food residue in the mouth after eating
- excessive secretions
- wet or hoarse voice after eating or drinking
- coughing or choking during or after eating or drinking
- wheezing or difficulty breathing during or after meals or drinks
- complaints of a sensation of food being stuck in the throat
- increased throat clearing
- reflux or regurgitation of food or fluid
- aspiration (silent or overt) of food or fluid
- recurrent chest infections
- weight loss
- malnutrition and/or dehydration.

Medical and background history

Once alerted to the possibility of dysphagia, the nature and severity of any structural anatomical or neurological factors causing or contributing to the dysphagia should be noted. For example, the site and severity of stroke, the progression of neurological disease, or any relevant head and neck surgery or radiotherapy should be noted. The patient's level of alertness, positioning, need for enteral feeding, and respiratory status (e.g. oxygen via nasal prongs or ventilation via tracheostomy) should also be observed.

Informal cognitive communication and behavioural assessment

The patient's cognitive communication skills and behaviour can be informally assessed. Information about a patient's ability to express themselves or understand instructions, as well as memory and orientation deficits can be gained by taking the history from the patient (when possible). Issues such as agitation, combativeness, and distractibility should also be noted.

Oromotor assessment

This involves the speech and language therapist observing the oral structures and their functions (e.g. symmetry and speed of movement), oral hygiene, state of dentition, and assessing the cranial nerves involved in swallowing (Table 9.1). These factors will help determine whether a bedside swallowing assessment is appropriate.

Bedside swallowing assessment

The patient is observed by the speech and language therapist to eat or drink food and/or fluid of varying consistencies, depending on the deficits noted in the above-mentioned assessments. The patient should be able to maintain alertness and be seated upright and symmetrically. The speech and language therapist observes the three phases of the patient's swallow and may trial thickened fluids or foods of easier consistency (e.g. pureed fruit) with the patient. If the patient is able to feed themselves, the speech and language therapist observes eating and drinking behaviours such as speed of intake, amount taken per mouthful, and the patient's awareness of their eating and drinking behaviours. If a carer or family member typically feeds the patient, then the feeding behaviours of the carer as well as the patient should be observed and critically assessed.

In patients where dysphagia is suspected to involve the pharyngeal phase of the swallow (e.g. coughing and choking frequently during or even many hours after swallowing), then further instrumental assessments, such as a videofluoroscopic swallow study (VFSS) or a fibreoptic endoscopic evaluation of swallowing (FEES) will be ordered.

Blue dye test in patients with tracheostomies

A blue dye test is a rudimentary method of determining whether patients are aspirating their secretions or food and fluid that can be performed in most clinical situations. Blue dye is either placed on the patient's tongue (if assessing secretions) or mixed into food or fluid and swallowed by the patient. Tracheal suctioning is performed to check for the presence of

Table 9.1 Cranial nerves involved in the swallowing process

Cranial nerve	Function
V	Muscles of mastication and sensation to the anterior two-thirds of the tongue and buccal cavity
VII	Nerve to supply the orbicularis oris muscle required for lip closure and taste to the anterior two-thirds of the tongue
IX	Taste and sensation to the posterior third of the tongue and buccal cavity and sensation to the tonsils, laryngeal mucosa, and soft palate and involvement of the gag and cough reflexes
X	Similar to cranial nerve IX but also involved with phonation and vocal cord closure in the larynx and sensation and motility of the oesophagus
XII	Movement of the tongue

blue-stained secretions or food and fluid which may be suggestive of aspiration. It is sometimes used as a test procedure to help determine the safety and timing of changing from a cuffed to an uncuffed tracheostomy tube.

VFSS and FEES

The VFSS is a radiological assessment that provides information on the speed and coordination of movements during the three phases of swallowing and is the gold standard for determining whether the patient is aspirating or not. The VFSS is performed by mixing liquid or powdered barium into food and fluids of varying consistencies. The speech and language therapist gives the food or fluid to the patient to consume and the radiologist screens the patient's swallow. VFSS is also very useful for assessing the effectiveness of management strategies such as thickened fluids, postural adjustments and swallowing manoeuvres.

FEES involves passing an endoscope through the patient's nose and observing the patient swallow food and fluid. A major benefit of FEES is that the patient is not exposed to X-ray radiation and barium is not required. However, only the pharyngeal phase of the swallow can be observed, meaning that this investigation will not be able to identify all causes of dysphagia. VFSS and FEES may not be appropriate for patients who have behavioural issues such as agitation, combativeness, or cognitive communicative issues to the extent that the patient cannot follow simple instructions.

Nutritional assessment

The dietician typically determines the patient's nutritional status, collecting height, weight, and body mass index (BMI) information. Blood tests can be ordered to confirm dietary deficiencies. The diet of the patient can then be optimized with regard to their caloric requirements, protein intake, and appropriate supplementation of trace vitamins and minerals. Education of the patient, the patient's family, and/or nursing staff regarding the amount and type of food/fluid to be consumed is often important.

The management of dysphagia

The strategies selected to manage a patient's dysphagia depend on the causal and/or contributory factors of the dysphagia. For instance, a patient with unilateral paralysis of oral structures following a stroke, but without behavioural impairments, may benefit from a modified diet or swallowing manoeuvres.

Strategies

Impaired swallowing physiology and anatomy

- Modifying the consistency of food and viscosity of fluid to reduce the risk of aspiration.
- Changing sensory aspects of the bolus (e.g. temperature, taste) to promote the reflexive phases of swallow.
- Postural adjustments during swallowing (e.g. chin-down position or head turned to the weakened side) to redirect the bolus and reduce the risk of aspiration.
- Compensatory swallowing manoeuvres (e.g. supraglottic swallow) which aim to improve airway closure during swallowing.

Behavioural and/or cognitive communication issues

- Smaller meals more frequently, so the patient does not have to maintain attention for long periods of time.
- Minimize environmental stimuli during meal times (e.g. turn off the television) to improve attention.
- Identify and remove potential triggers that may elicit behavioural outbursts during mealtimes.
- Provide verbal cues to assist implementation of mealtime strategies.

Maintaining good oral hygiene

- Poor oral hygiene and dentition in people with dysphagia can provide a source of bacteria that can seed recurrent respiratory infections, as well as being linked with an increased risk of stroke and myocardial infarction. Implementation of an oral hygiene programme along with referral to dental services can be beneficial.

Team-based approach

- In the longer term, education of the patient, family, and/or carers maximizes the chance of producing sustained behavioural change appropriate to different settings (e.g. hospital vs home).
- Involvement from occupational therapy is essential in all patients who are having difficulties feeding themselves.
- Social workers or psychologists may assist with counselling patients regarding grief surrounding lost abilities.
- Dieticians provide invaluable assistance regarding the patient's nutritional and hydration needs.

Non-oral feeding options
- These options are necessary if the patient is aspirating and/or unable to obtain sufficient nutrition orally.
- Nasogastric (NG) feeding is a good short-term option for non-oral feeding.
- Percutaneous endoscopic gastrostomy (PEG) is more appropriate for patients with long-term dysphagia.

Further reading

Logemann JA (1998). *Evaluation and Treatment of Swallowing Disorders*, 2nd edn. Pro-Ed, Austin, TX.

Spasticity and contractures

Introduction

Disruption of the upper motor neuron (UMN) pathways following acquired brain injury (ABI) leads to the characteristic clinical features of the UMN syndrome. This syndrome has many components, often conceptualized as consisting of both positive and negative features. Negative UMN features are considered an underexpression or loss of muscle activity, comprising muscle weakness, reduced motor control or dexterity, muscle fatiguability, and learned non-use. Conversely, positive UMN features are considered to be present when there is an overexpression or exaggeration of muscle activity. Clinical terms incorporating this concept include muscle overactivity, spasticity, co-contraction, dystonia, clonus, associated reactions, hyperactive reflexes, flexor or extensor spasm, hypertonicity, and overactive flexor withdrawal reflex. Other factors also contribute to the functional limitations that a person with an UMN syndrome may experience including sensorimotor dysfunction, cognitive changes, motor planning problems, and pain. This chapter focuses on the positive UMN feature of spasticity and the associated problem of contracture following UMN injury, regardless of whether the onset is acute or degenerative in nature.

Definition of spasticity

Spasticity is one positive UMN feature that can be a primary source of disability after neurological impairment. The traditional definition of spasticity derived from electrophysiological studies and states 'Spasticity is a motor disorder characterised by a velocity-dependent increase in tonic stretch reflexes (muscle tone) with exaggerated tendon jerks, resulting from hyperexcitability of the stretch reflex, as one component of the upper motor neuron syndrome'. This definition focuses entirely on the phasic (i.e. movement-based) component of spasticity and does not acknowledge the persistent tonic aspects of motor overactivity. The traditional definition is of limited utility for clinicians when considering the impact of spasticity on an individual's function. More recently, the EU-SPASM group have incorporated both motor and sensory aspects into a definition of spasticity, being 'disordered sensorimotor control, resulting from an upper motor neurone lesion, presenting as intermittent or sustained involuntary activation of muscles'. By considering both phasic and tonic aspects of motor overactivity, the EU-SPASM definition has greater clinically relevance.

Spasticity may be further described by its clinical expression as being focal, regional or generalized in nature. Focal or regional spasticity presents in defined areas of the body, for example, in a single limb. Interventions for focal spasticity can be targeted at the site of spasticity such as with botulinum neurotoxin A (BoNT-A) injection. In contrast, generalized spasticity affects the patient's whole body, with a broader range of interventions often being more useful.

In contrast to spasticity, which is an active/dynamic process, muscle contracture is identified as physical 'shortening and reduced extensibility of the soft tissue including muscles, tendons, ligaments, joint capsules, skin, vessels, and nerves'. Muscle contracture is addressed via mechanical/physical-based interventions aimed at lengthening muscles (described later). Soft tissue changes commence very quickly post event, with altered protein synthesis being recorded within 6 hours of initial immobilization. Within weeks, an immobilized muscle will demonstrate changes in force production, contraction and relaxation times, and electromyographic (EMG) output. Commonly, muscles lose functional length and collagenous tissue develops. These changes combine to make a less elastic muscle, adding to the difficulty with muscle control that is already compromised by the imbalance in muscle activity and weakness, or poor positioning and immobilization.

Spastic dystonia, or spastic hypertonia as it is known in some countries, produces a greater functional impact than spasticity alone. Spastic dystonia implies a persisting, stimulus-dependent increase in involuntary motor activity that continues well after the stimulus has been withdrawn. The stimulus maybe externally applied (e.g. in performing tendon reflexes) or be initiated by the person voluntarily moving a limb. The prolonged muscle contraction limits function by impairing the fine motor control and coordination required for successful task-specific movement. Spastic dystonias can occur focally (e.g. with persisting quadriceps overactivity on testing knee reflexes) or regionally across multiple muscles. Stereotypical, non-voluntary limb movements are often described by terms such as 'associated reaction' or 'action dystonia' and commonly occur with yawning or walking.

Prevalence of spasticity

The available literature base regarding the incidence and prevalence of post-event spasticity is incomplete, with values differing based on the underlying aetiology. For example, the presence of post-stroke spasticity has been reported to range anywhere between 4% and 46%, with values increasing over the course of the first year. In adult TBI, spasticity has been reported in approximately 10–75% of patients. The reported incidence of spasticity in people with MS is approximately 84%. Following spinal cord injury (SCI), approximately 65–78% of patients experience spasticity. Taken together, the prevalence of spasticity in people with neurological impairment is high.

Impact of spasticity on function

Spasticity often affects the upper limb (UL) more than the lower limb (LL). While LL spasticity may be functionally useful, spasticity in the UL rarely assists the arm and/or hand during everyday function, a consequence of restricting movement quality required for dexterity. However, spasticity is not the sole contributor to reduced function post ABI. Clinically, it is the balance between the expression of negative and positive UMN features which results in the wide range of difficulties experienced with motor function. In addition to the positive and negative UMN features, which are considered the neural or reflex components of the UMN syndrome, the non-neural, biomechanical components also play a role in altering movement patterns following an ABI.

Measurement of spasticity

Outcomes of rehabilitation following ABI are increasingly being framed in the context of the WHO ICF domains (➜ see Chapter 1). Measures in adult spasticity management focus on evaluating the impact of spasticity at either the body function and structure or the activity domains, with extremely limited assessment of spasticity within the participation domain.

Outcome measures used in spasticity evaluation are primarily observational or self-report in nature. Common observational clinical measures can be divided into those that require either passive (e.g. Modified Ashworth/Tardieu Scale) (Table 10.1) or active movement (kinematic analysis) by the patient. Measures of passive movement are commonly used; however, they ignore the consequences of how the affected person's self-directed 'dynamic' movement modulates expression of the UMN syndrome. This limitation is significant as passive movements do not reveal the extent of the functional limitation experienced by the patient in everyday life. Assessing the impact of spasticity during patient-directed movement is also problematic as measurement requires specialized equipment. These limitations make it difficult for clinicians to objectively measure the impact of the UMN syndrome on everyday function.

Assessing a patient's function within the ICF 'activity' domain can be performed using standardized tasks, through patient self-report or activity monitoring, and can examine both positive and negative UMN features. For example, a patient with a predominance of positive features may benefit from interventions reducing positive UMN features (e.g. BoNT-A injection, or casting and/or splinting). Conversely, patients with predominantly negative UMN features are more likely to benefit from interventions such as strengthening, electrical stimulation, and task-specific retraining. In clinical practice, many patients will present with a mix of positive and negative features necessitating an individualized approach to assessment and choice of intervention/s. Further, observed behaviours may be influenced by cognitive, motor planning, and/or sensory limitations that are not assessed by standardized assessment tasks or in self-report or activity monitoring. These factors also require consideration in assessment and planning for interventions.

Table 10.1 Modified Ashworth Scale

0	No increase in muscle tone
1	Slight increase in muscle tone, manifested by a catch and release or by minimal resistance at the end range of motion when the affected parts moved in flexion or extension
1+	Slight increase in muscle tone, manifested by a catch, followed by minimal resistance throughout the remainder (less than half) of the range of motion
2	More marked increase in muscle tone through most of the range of motion, but the affected part is easily moved
3	Considerable increase in muscle tone, passive movement is difficult
4	Affected part is rigid in flexion or extension

Goal setting in spasticity management

Adult spasticity management aims to improve the patient's ability to engage in everyday function with or without the assistance of a carer. Patients present to spasticity management services with varying degrees of functional limitations (from mild to severe) and expectations/hopes for outcomes from interventions. An individual's clinical presentation may vary due to a number of factors including diagnosis (e.g. stroke, TBI, SCI, MS, or cerebral palsy, etc.), severity of injury/disease, time post injury or progression of disease, and the aforementioned complexity of motor control.

Furthermore, individual goal setting is a critical element in identifying an optimal spasticity intervention programme for the patient (Table 10.2). Each individual with spasticity is likely to have multiple goals that they would like to achieve. However, using the available interventions to achieve one goal may prevent another from being realized. Such mutually incompatible goals are a direct consequence of neurological damage and limitations in how the interventions work. This necessitates an individualized approach during all stages of the spasticity management cycle from assessment, goal setting, intervention selection and delivery, and post-intervention evaluation. For these reasons, a 'prescriptive model' of spasticity management is not possible. However, clinical decision-making can be enhanced by referencing common goal categories, including active and passive function, impairment, involuntary movements, mobility, and pain. Interestingly, adults with longstanding ABI-related UL spasticity continue to focus on the achievement of 'self-care' (passive function) type goals such as UL dressing, caring for the UL, and eating/drinking.

Table 10.2 Common goals of spasticity management

Domains	Common goal areas in spasticity management
Symptoms and impairments	Pain
	Involuntary movements (associated reactions/spasms)
	Range of motion (contracture prevention; splint tolerance)
Activities/functions	Passive UL function (caring for the UL)
	Active function (active participation of affected UL in the task)
	Mobility

Management of spasticity

Recommendations for spasticity management suggest that it be delivered via a dedicated MDT. The health professional members of different MDTs will vary depending on the needs of the patient and the service. Commonly, MDTs include a rehabilitation physician, physiotherapist, occupational therapist, and/or nurse. Spasticity management should focus on patient-centred goals. Ideally, patient goals for intervention should be set collaboratively with the patient and/or carer/family member and the MDT. The specialist skills of the MDT are required to provide guidance and direction for realistic patient expectations and goal setting. Patient goals for intervention should be communicated within the MDT to ensure a focused team approach to goal achievement. This is particularly important for focal interventions such as BoNT-A injection where specific patient goals will influence the injection strategy selected.

Spasticity management may be categorized as comprising physical, pharmacological, and/or surgical interventions. Physical interventions include stretching, casting, and splinting, and are traditionally supported by physiotherapists and occupational therapists. Pharmacological interventions for generalized spasticity include oral antispastic medications, intrathecal medications such as baclofen, and injectables such as BoNT-A or phenol for focal spasticity. Permanent surgical interventions are potentially under-utilized interventions for focal UL spasticity. Most often, effective patient management of spasticity requires a combination of interventions to optimize individual patient outcomes such as BoNT-A injection as an adjunct to casting combined with a follow-up splint.

Alleviation of exacerbating factors

The impact of spasticity can be exacerbated by increased sensory stimulation, particularly any form of noxious stimuli. Sources of such stimuli should be sought whenever there is a sudden increase in spasticity. Common causes include:

- urinary retention or infection
- constipation
- skin irritations, such as in-growing toenails and pressure sores
- pain, for example, from undiagnosed limb fracture or occult intra-abdominal sources
- increased external sensory stimuli, including ill-fitting orthotic appliances, catheter leg bags, and tight clothing or footwear
- inappropriate seating or bad positioning in a wheelchair.

Sometimes attention to these details can be sufficient to treat the spasticity without the need for other interventions.

Physical interventions

Physiotherapy/occupational therapy intervention

The role of the physiotherapist and/or occupational therapist is to assess the implications of spasticity and the other UMN features on an individual's everyday function.

Assessment process may include:

- the identification and assessment of muscle activity (voluntary and involuntary activation)
- identification and measurement of an achievable range of motion (active and passive)
- assessment of the impact of the UMN syndrome (i.e. both positive and negative UMN features) on everyday function, including the difficulty carers may have with assisting a patient's function.
- assessment of pain, during rest, sleep, or during active movement.

Intervention in adult spasticity management aims to address the neural and non-neural components of the UMN syndrome, ultimately aiming to positively influence an individual's everyday function. Selection of appropriate intervention strategies will be determined primarily by the clinically identified goal of intervention agreed with the patient. However, as a general guide, the balance of positive and negative UMN features may give an indication of interventions that are more appropriate. Simplistically, a patient presenting with predominantly positive UMN features is more likely to benefit from interventions that reduce these positive features, for example, through referral for BoNT-A injection with follow-up casting, splinting, positioning, or stretching. In contrast, patients presenting with primarily negative UMN features, who have potential to improve motor control, may be offered interventions including task-specific retraining, functional electrical stimulation, strengthening, functional splinting, or constraint-induced movement therapy. As discussed, however, individuals with primarily positive features may still benefit from task training and strengthening if motor control is an achievable goal.

Interventions to manage paresis

Postural and physical management

Bed positioning programmes

These can be instigated following baseline assessment to ascertain current position and current tonal and musculoskeletal problems, and to implement change. To be effective, the MDT needs to provide for 24-hour postural management to provide prolonged low-load stretch. There is a wide selection of positioning equipment available to facilitate postural change (e.g. sleep systems, T-rolls, and wedge cushions).

Seating systems

These systems should be seen as a tool to apply a specific stimulus intended for corrective purposes such as normalizing alignment and/or reducing abnormal tone while providing pressure area relief in people with poor voluntary movement. Considerations when seating clients should be made such as pelvic stabilization, trunk alignment, and alignment of the head and neck.

Stretching programmes

Current evidence varies regarding the optimum length of time for a muscle to be stretched, ranging from 6 hours per day to more recent evidence (in 2005) of 30 minutes per day. Even at the minimum of 30 minutes per muscle, manual stretch of individual muscles becomes impossible to carry out, necessitating the use of tilt tabling, serial casting, splinting, and positional programmes.

Serial casting

This is used to increase or maintain muscle length and joint range. Application of serial casts made of plaster of Paris or soft and scotch cast have been shown to increase the number of sarcomeres and muscle length. They can be changed every 3–5 days in a series over several weeks to gradually increase ROM and joint position until the desired range is achieved. As with positioning programmes, serial casting is applied to provide prolonged low load stretch with the aim of increasing muscle length. Serial casting is most commonly used for elbows, knees, and ankles. Casting may also be completed as part of functional retraining to allow a patient to be positioned in an optimal way to learn to reuse another joint optimally for example—casting forearm and wrist in optimal position for grasp and then engaging patient in a programme of active grasp and release activities to encourage optimal wrist, finger and thumb position during grasp and release. This type of cast often will come after a series of castings to increase ROM. Serial casting must be approached with a clear plan and follow-up after the last cast is removed, to assist with maintaining gains achieved.

Orthotic management

Orthotic management including thermoplastic splinting is often required following serial casting to enhance the capacity to maintain the gains in ROM achieved by the series of casts. Orthotic management including splinting is required immediately following the final cast in a series. Thermoplastic splinting may be used to maintain a patient's UL or LL positioning without the need for casting. Often splints are recommended to be worn by patients for varying periods of time dependent on the purpose of the splint. Wear length will often be longer (e.g. 24 hours/overnight wear) if maintaining ROM and joint alignment are primary goals of the intervention. Shorter wear times may be selected for splints that are provided to improve capacity to move the limb to improve function, such as typing splints or an ankle–foot orthosis (AFO). Splints may also be used to stabilize a joint to facilitate improved movement or training of movement of another joint (e.g. using a wrist cock-up splint to stabilize the wrist while training improved grasp and release with the fingers and thumb).

Interventions to develop motor control

Electrical stimulation

This is used as an intervention for impairments of spasticity, weakness, and pain. Specifically following BoNT-A, ES has been shown to enhance the effect of and improve the reduction of spasticity in targeted muscles. Further, ES has been used to facilitate and strengthen the agonist following injection of an overactive antagonist muscle.

Targeted strengthening programmes

Systematic review of the impact of strength training in various forms (EMG biofeedback, ES, muscle re-education, progressive resistance exercise, robot-assisted movement) has found that improvement in strength can improve activity performance without producing a detrimental effect on spasticity.

*Task practice and constraint-induced therapy in combination
with botulinum toxin*

Repetitive task training involves the repeated practice of functional tasks, combining elements of practice intensity and functional relevance. Repetitive task training improves lower limb function. It has also been shown to improve upper limb function when delivered at a high dose (involving at least 20 hours of practice). In a small study, task practice in combination with BoNT-A was reported to improve arm function compared to baseline. Repetitive task training should be included as an element of rehabilitation programmes to improve active function.

General interventions which aim to influence the UMN syndrome

Home exercise and stretching programmes

Traditional home exercise/stretching programmes are individualized programmes which may include a combination of self or assisted stretching and/or splinting, with or without targeted UL strengthening or task specific retraining. These programmes are typically prescribed by therapists with advice and instruction and are followed and modified as required over time. Guided self-rehabilitation contracts have recently been reported as a potentially useful methodology for engaging patients with spasticity in long-term UL rehabilitation for spasticity. Contracts are made between therapists and patients for daily practice of 'prolonged self-administered stretch' and 'intensive motor training' involving repetitive maximal rapid alternating movements of the affected UL. Guided self-rehabilitation contracts are reported to increase patient and therapist motivation during rehabilitation.

Pharmacological interventions

Early intervention in spasticity management appears to reduce the incidence of problematic muscle shortening and contractures. Medications with the potential to decrease spasticity have been available for many decades, but have only become widely used in the last decade or so. Many medications are poorly tolerated and it is necessary to carefully weigh up the potential benefits and risks prior to commencing a medication trial. Medications are often used in combination with physical therapies, with the selection of agents depending on the severity and distribution of spasticity (generalized or focal) and whether the spasticity exerts any benefit to the patient.

Oral medication

The main limitation of oral medications is that they produce generalized 'whole-person' effects. While exerting their antispastic effects at the spinal cord level, common adverse reactions (such as balance disturbance, dizziness, sedation, and fatigability) result from cerebral penetration of the drug. The sensation of weakness that sometimes goes along with oral medications is multifactorial in nature. Some agents may produce this effect centrally, others by weakening the muscle, and yet others by decreasing the involuntary muscle contraction that the person has learnt to use functionally. For some people, the lack of specificity of effect of the oral medications can be more troublesome than the spasticity they are trying to treat. As a result, all drugs should be used with care and constant monitoring. Available drugs include the following:

- Baclofen: a highly polar gamma-aminobutyric acid type B ($GABA_B$) receptor agonist. Beneficial antispastic effects occur from the activation of inhibitory spinal interneurons (Fig. 10.1). Side effects are common, potentiated through central effects at areas where the brain lacks a blood–brain barrier, such as the area postrema. These areas allow high cerebral baclofen levels despite potentially subtherapeutic levels in the spinal cord. Side effects are dose dependent and there is often only a narrow therapeutic window between benefit and unacceptable side effects. Common doses are between 50 and 100 mg of oral baclofen daily in divided doses.
- Dantrolene sodium: a ryanodine receptor antagonist whose predominant effect is to reduce calcium efflux in skeletal muscle following neural activation. This produces partial uncoupling of muscle contraction from the action potential, thereby weakening the muscle (Fig. 10.1). Due to this alternative mechanism of action, dantrolene can be used synergistically with other medications. While generally considered not to have central effects, intravenous dantrolene can produce dizziness and other cognitive side effects. Furthermore, dantrolene produces hepatotoxicity in around 2% of patients, a third of which are potentially fatal. The likelihood of toxicity is greater in higher doses and over longer treatment intervals (months to years). This necessitates regular liver function monitoring and cessation of the drug if hepatotoxicity is identified. Doses start at around 25 mg daily and can be titrated upwards over several weeks to a maximum of around 400 mg daily in divided doses.

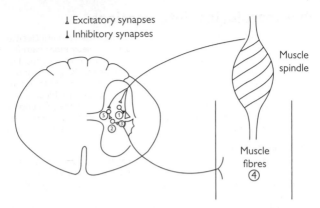

↓ Excitatory synapses
↓ Inhibitory synapses

Muscle
spindle

Muscle
fibres
④

Fig. 10.1 Presumed site of action of drugs with antispastic effects. (1) Diazepam facilitates presynaptic inhibition; (2) baclofen inhibits polysynaptic reflexes activation; (3) tizanidine acts on α_2-adrenergic receptors; (4) dantrolene weakens muscle contraction; (5) pregabalin decreases excitatory synapse formation.

- Tizanidine: an α_2 adrenergic agonist with similar efficacy and side effects to diazepam and baclofen (Fig. 10.1). It has significant drug interactions, particularly with fluvoxamine and fluoroquinolone antibiotics. Some people may develop clinically significant hypotension on commencing the medication; 5% of people may develop reversible hepatotoxicity, and liver function tests need regular monitoring. Tizanidine is titrated in an individualized fashion over a period of 2–4 weeks. It is usually initiated at 2 mg twice daily and increased in 4 mg increments every 4–7 days to a maximum of 36 mg per day, divided into three or four daily doses.
- Gabapentin/pregabalin: these drugs act at the $\alpha_2\delta$ subunit of a voltage-gated calcium channel to inhibit excitatory synaptogenesis (Fig. 10.1). While these agents are commonly used for neuropathic pain, they also show promise as antispastic agents. Both agents have good penetration through the blood–brain barrier. Pregabalin is becoming the medication of choice due to its more consistent pharmacokinetics at higher doses. Dosages of pregabalin normally start at 75 mg nocte and are titrated upwards to a maximum dose of 600 mg per day in divided doses, depending on the degree of benefit and the presence of any adverse reactions (commonly sedation, dizziness, and minor cognitive dysfunction). Antispastic effects will usually be evident at doses less than 300 mg per day if the medication is going to be effective. Gabapentin doses are usually a multiple of six times larger than pregabalin doses and the medication can be directly substituted without a washout period.

- Diazepam: the first antispastic agent to be used, working as a GABA$_A$ receptor agonist, diazepam exerts central effects while increasing inhibitory interneuron activation in the spinal cord (Fig. 10.1). While producing antispastic effects, the agent can induce unacceptable weakness, sedation, and fatigue and is now rarely used. Starting dose is 2 mg twice daily and then slowly increased by 2 mg increments up to a maximum dose of 20 mg per day in divided doses.

Other antispastic drugs

Other oral medications have been reported anecdotally or in randomized controlled trials. These include:

- cannabinoids—medical cannabinoids have been approved (or are in the process of being approved) for use in spasticity management in many countries; while there is evidence of efficacy, the role that medical cannabinoids may have as compared to other spasticity interventions remains unproven.
- clonazepam
- clonidine
- levodopa
- cyproheptadine.

Intrathecal medication

Intrathecal baclofen

The highly polar nature of the baclofen molecule prevents adequate penetration of the drug through the blood–brain barrier and into the spinal cord. An effective way to overcome this limitation is to inject baclofen directly into the cerebrospinal fluid. Intrathecal baclofen (ITB) is the single most effective agent in terms of reducing generalized spasticity and spasms. It also has the advantage of treating some neuropathic pain states occurring at the spinal cord level. ITB involves subcutaneous insertion of a programmable pump connected to a catheter that delivers baclofen solution directly into the cerebrospinal fluid (CSF) space.

The assessment process for ITB requires a rehabilitation physician-led MDT who will first plan a test dose (via lumbar puncture) of baclofen to assess the patient's response in terms of spasticity, spasms, and pain levels. This allows the team and the patient to decide whether ITB pump insertion is indicated and to refer to a surgeon with expertise in this area. ITB is more effective for LL conditions, as an average 4:1 ratio between lumbar and cervical drug levels has been reported.

A substantial minority of people with ITB pumps report complications, most commonly minor in nature. ITB therapy requires close monitoring and frequent refills of the subcutaneous pump to prevent baclofen withdrawal, a potentially life-threatening complication needing intensive care management. Similarly, an overdosage of ITB can produce potentially fatal respiratory suppression. It is therefore important to only offer this treatment to people with reliable cognition and/or adequate family and carer support to enable monitoring and supervision. ITB treatment requires a high degree of experience on the part of the clinician and MDT, in particular with problem-solving any issues that may arise. The patient needs to have 24-hour access

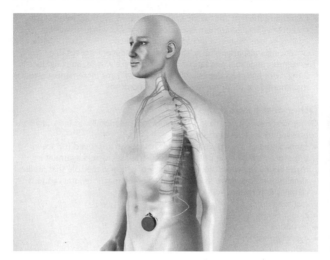

Fig. 10.2 Intrathecal baclofen pump and catheter placement.
Reproduced with permission of Medtronic, Inc.

to a physician with experience in ITB therapy who is able to interrogate the pump with the programmer and make changes to the dose in case of emergencies.

Intrathecal phenol
In carefully selected patients, intrathecal phenol may also be a valuable treatment approach. Phenol is a chemical neurolytic agent and will therefore produce more long-lasting, semi-permanent effects, particularly for LL spasticity. It does not require pump insertion or refilling and therefore ongoing management complications are less likely, particularly for very dependent patients. However, due to its destructive nature, there is a potential risk to bladder and bowel function following the procedure. For this reason intrathecal phenol is only appropriate for those patients with bowel and bladder incontinence (such as people with late-stage MS).

Injectables
Injectable medication has the major advantage of targeting focal or regional spasticity. This helps to avoid the non-specific effects of oral medication, both in terms of side effects but also avoiding a reduction in 'useful' spasticity that may be supporting function in other body regions. These agents have revolutionized the treatment of spasticity in many people and have become the treatment of choice for focal spasticity.

Botulinum toxin
The BoNTs are potent neurotoxins that block the release of acetylcholine from nerve endings. BoNT produces multiple effects on muscle including

'chemodenervation' at the neuromuscular junction, thereby producing muscle weakness. More importantly for spasticity management, it also decreases overactivity in muscle spindles and in unmyelinated C fibres, which both assist by decreasing overactivity of spinally mediated reflex arcs. Two toxin serotypes are commercially available; however, BoNT-A has a far wider role than BoNT-B. Commercial preparations of BoNT-A (Dysport®, Botox®, and Xeomin®) are not bioequivalent and caution needs to be exercised in determining the appropriate dose. The effect of BoNT-A is transient with an average period of effect of approximately 3 months, although shorter and longer periods of action are not uncommon. Adverse drug reactions are rare but include a flu-like illness, generalized weakness, and swallowing problems.

Nerve and motor point blocks

These two approaches remain useful modalities in spasticity management. In general, three agents are used—local anaesthetic, phenol, and alcohol—with procedures usually undertaken by rehabilitation physicians or anaesthetists, depending on training and availability. The approach to nerve blocks and motor point blocks are quite different. In both (as with intrathecal phenol described previously), local anaesthetic can be used to provide a short-duration effect as 'proof of concept', thereby identifying whether the predominant issue is spasticity/muscle tone or soft tissue contracture. This can be useful before undertaking longer-acting and potentially riskier procedures such as phenol and alcohol injection. However, these agents all have the advantage of being much cheaper and longer-lasting than BoNT-A.

Peripheral nerve blocks involve injection of the active agent into the vicinity of a peripheral nerve. The most common targets include:
- obturator nerve for adductor spasticity
- posterior tibial nerve for calf spasticity
- sciatic nerve for hamstring spasticity
- musculocutaneous nerve for elbow flexor spasticity

The technique involves injection of the medication through a needle electrode. The tip of the needle is manoeuvred as close as possible to the nerve and its position is confirmed by ultrasonography and/or ES. A small volume of phenol or alcohol is then injected down the same needle. This produces an immediate nerve block with relaxation of the muscle supplied by that nerve. The duration of effect is usually 2–6 months, but can be permanent. For this reason, these long-duration blocks are best avoided when early recovery in the affected muscles remains possible. The injection technique can be more time-consuming and technically demanding than BoNT-A. Injection of mixed motor/sensory nerves can produce painful dysaesthesia that may need treatment with neuropathic medications.

Motor point blocks are similar to nerve blocks in approach; however, the target injection site is the motor endplate/s of the muscle. In this case, the endplate is identified with the needle electrode as being the site requiring the lowest amplitude of ES to produce muscle contraction. Motor point injections with alcohol or phenol are cheaper than BoNT-A, but require a greater degree of technical knowledge and are more time consuming to perform. They have the advantage over injections along mixed sensory/ motor nerves in that they do not produce dysaesthesias.

Surgical and orthopaedic procedures

A proportion of people with spasticity will warrant consideration for surgical intervention. In some cases this may be due to inadequate or failed physical and/or pharmacological spasticity interventions; however, some degree of soft tissue change is probably unavoidable in those with UMN syndromes. The main strength of surgery is its permanence and capacity to assist people with fixed contractures that are not amenable to other interventions. However, the permanent nature of the correction is also a potential failing, in that poorly planned surgery can increase disability and pain, and any potential surgical procedures are probably best undertaken when recovery has plateaued. Surgical interventions fall into three main categories: those that interfere with neural feedback arcs, lengthening procedures, and those that rebalance forces across a joint.

Neural feedback arcs

There are again two main interventions in this group: rhizotomies and surgical division of motor nerve branches. Both procedures interrupt part of the reflex arc, decreasing the muscle's capacity to respond to stimuli that would otherwise contribute to the expression of spasticity. Rhizotomies have largely fallen out of current practice and are only available in some services. Partial motor neurotomies are simpler surgical procedures but share difficulties in terms of the availability of surgical expertise.

Lengthening procedures

Surgically repositioning joints and limbs can be necessary to facilitate proper seating in severe spasticity, to ease positioning, to apply orthoses, and reduce the likelihood of further complications such as pressure areas. The commonest orthopaedic interventions include tenotomies, Z-plasty of tendons, capsular releases, and surgical migration of muscles to more distal locations. These procedures can be accompanied by surgical fusion of joints in the case of joint subluxation. The success of these procedures is dependent on the expertise of the surgeon, their awareness of the dominant patterns of spasticity, and the post-surgical rehabilitation plan, for example, provision of an orthotic. Fixed contractures are generally easier to treat surgically and have more predictable outcomes than in people with variable spasticity and/or dystonias.

Rebalancing procedures

Tendon transfer procedures are most commonly undertaken for weakness, for example, following SCI. However, tendon transfers can also be used to rebalance forces across a joint in patients with spasticity. For example, a person with a plantarflexed and varus foot deformity will commonly have an overactive tibialis posterior muscle. Tunnelling the tibialis posterior tendon through the interosseous membrane to the anterolateral compartment allows the overactive muscle to generate dorsiflexion and eversion, turning problematic spasticity into a functional benefit.

Further reading

Ada L, O'Dwyer N, O'Neill E (2006). Relation between spasticity, weakness and contracture of the elbow flexors and upper limb activity after stroke: an observational study. *Disability and Rehabilitation* 28, 891–897.

Brashear A (2010). *Spasticity: Diagnosis and Management*. Demos Medical Publishing, New York.

College of Occupational Therapists and Association of Chartered Physiotherapists in Neurology (2015). *Splinting for the Prevention and Correction of Contractures in Adults with Neurological Dysfunction: Practice Guidelines for Occupational Therapists and Physiotherapists*. College of Occupational Therapists Ltd, London.

Copley J, Kuipers K (2014). *Neurorehabilitation of the Upper Limb Across the Lifespan: Managing Hypertonicity for Optimal Function*. Wiley-Blackwell, Hoboken, NJ.

Esquenazi A, Albanese A, Chancellor MB, et al. (2013). Evidence-based review and assessment of botulinum neurotoxin for the treatment of adult spasticity in the upper motor neuron syndrome. *Toxicon* 67, 115–128.

Lance JW (1980). Symposium synopsis. In: Feldman RG, Young RR, Koella WP (eds), *Spasticity: Disordered Motor Control*, p. 485–494. Syposia Specialists, Miami, FL.

Mayer NH, Esquenazi A (2003). Muscle overactivity and movement dysfunction in the upper motorneuron syndrome. *Physical Medicine and Rehabilitation Clinics of North America* 14, 855–883.

Pandyan AD, Gregoric M, Barnes MP, et al. (2005). Spasticity: clinical perceptions, neurological realities and meaningful measurement. *Disability and Rehabilitation* 27, 2–6.

Pollock A, Farmer SE, Brady MC, et al. (2014). Interventions for improving upper limb function after stroke. *Cochrane Database of Systematic Reviews* 11, CD010820.

Royal College of Physicians (2018). *Spasticity in Adults: Management Using Botulinum Toxin*. Royal College of Physicians, London.

Sheean G, Lannin NA, Turner-Stokes L, et al. (2010). Botulinum toxin assessment, intervention and after-care for upper limb hypertonicity in adults: international consensus statement. *European Journal of Neurology* 17 Suppl 2, 74–93.

Turner-Stokes L, Fheodoroff K, Jacinto J, et al. (2013). Results from the Upper Limb International Spasticity Study-II (ULIS-II): a large, international, prospective cohort study investigating practice and goal attainment following treatment with botulinum toxin A in real-life clinical management. *BMJ Open* 3, e002771.

Yelnik AP, Simon O, Parratte B, et al. (2010). How to clinically assess and treat muscle overactivity in spastic paresis. *Journal of Rehabilitation Medicine* 42, 801–807.

Chronic pain

Definition of acute and chronic pain

The International Association for the Study of Pain (IASP) defines pain as 'an unpleasant sensory and emotional experience associated with actual or potential tissue damage or described in terms of such damage'. It is a subjective experience influenced by a complex dynamic interplay of the noxious stimulus and neuronal networks in the peripheral nerves, spinal cord, and brain.

Acute pain is the pain associated with ongoing tissue injury and the healing process. Chronic or persistent pain continues beyond the normal expected healing time, generally considered as pain of more than 3 months' duration. Typical examples of chronic pain are arthritis pain, phantom limb pain, neuropathic pain in brain injury and SCI, spinal pain, fibromyalgia, and chronic widespread pain.

Inadequately treated acute pain can lead to the development of chronic pain. Therefore, in acute settings there is an emphasis on adequately treating pain, for example, postoperative pain or polytrauma pain. The presence of personal, psychological, and social factors can contribute to the persistence and refractory nature of chronic pain. Chronic pain is common in developed countries and has significant implications for healthcare budgets and lost work productivity. It is associated with a disturbed sleep pattern, declining function, mood alterations, and a poorer health-related quality of life. The reported suicide rate in chronic pain individuals is double that of controls.

Chronic pain needs to be recognized as a complex, multidimensional biopsychosocial phenomenon, and management of chronic pain needs a multifaceted and multidisciplinary rehabilitation approach. To provide an effective management for the individual with chronic pain, the treating rehabilitation or pain physician requires a thorough understanding of the physiological, psychological, personal, and socioeconomic factors involved. Some common terminology used in pain literature is listed in Table 11.1.

Table 11.1 Terminology used in pain literature

Allodynia	Pain due to a stimuli that does not normally provoke pain
Analgesia	Absence of pain in response to stimulation that normally provokes pain
Causalgia	A burning pain associated with neurological impairment
Central pain	Pain initiated or caused by dysfunction in the CNS
Dysaesthesia	Abnormal sensation (spontaneous or evoked) that is unpleasant
Hyperalgesia	An increased response to a stimulus that is normally painful
Hyperaesthesia	Increased sensitivity to non-painful stimulus, excluding the special senses
Hyperpathia	Repeated innocuous stimulation triggers pain
Neurogenic/neuropathic pain	Pain initiated or caused by dysfunction in the CNS or peripheral nervous system
Nociceptor	A receptor preferentially sensitive to a noxious stimuli or to a stimulus that would become noxious if prolonged
Paraesthesia	Abnormal sensation (spontaneous or evoked), need not be unpleasant
Psychogenic pain	Pain not due to an identifiable, somatic origin and that may reflect psychological factors

Epidemiology of chronic pain

Prevalence rates for chronic pain worldwide vary widely in the literature, with estimates between 2% and 55% of population reported. This wide variation is due to study design, for example, from different definitions (3 months vs 6 months as cut-off criteria for chronicity) and different aetiologies of pain. In the US, one-third of the population is estimated to be suffering from chronic pain with a cost of US$100 billion to the economy (including healthcare, compensation, and litigation costs).

Common chronic pain conditions are listed in Box 11.1. A pan-European epidemiological systematic review of non-cancer chronic pain (i.e. including musculoskeletal pain, neuropathic pain, fibromyalgia, osteoarthritis, and rheumatoid arthritis) estimated the point prevalence to be 17% of the population.[1] This study also showed a significant correlation between chronic pain and reduced functioning and well-being. The mean number of workdays lost in this meta-analysis was 7.8 days in 6 months. These conditions identified in this review (i.e. non-cancer chronic pain) are the focus of this chapter and this handbook.

Box 11.1 Common chronic pain conditions

- Chronic back pain, chronic neck pain
- Arthritis (osteoarthritis, rheumatoid arthritis)
- Fibromyalgia
- Neuropathic pain (trigeminal neuralgia, phantom pain, post-herpetic neuralgia)
- Migraine, chronic headache
- Cancer pain
- Cardiac pain
- Pain associated with other conditions (MS, stroke, etc.)
- Complex regional pain syndrome (CRPS)

Pathophysiology of pain

Nociception is a protective safety mechanism that enables initiation of avoidance behaviour from the noxious stimulus. Four processes are involved in the pain pathway: transduction, transmission, modulation, and perception (Fig. 11.1).

Transduction is the process of a noxious stimulus stimulating the nociceptors to initiate a nerve impulse in the primary afferent neurons. The primary afferent neurons have their cell bodies in the dorsal root ganglia (spinal cord) or trigeminal ganglion and nerve endings in skin, muscles, and joints. Inflammatory mediators (prostaglandins and leukotrienes), substance P, and other neuropeptides play a key role in this process.

Transmission is the process whereby nociceptive information travels along the primary afferent neurons to the spinal cord dorsal horn, brainstem, thalamus, and higher cortical structures. The fibres in primary afferent neurons are of three types: Aβ, Aδ, and C. Aβ fibres are large diameter, myelinated nerve fibres that conduct innocuous mechanical stimulation rapidly. Aδ fibres are medium diameter and thinly myelinated, while C fibres have a small diameter and are unmyelinated; these fibre groups transmit noxious thermal, mechanical, and chemical stimuli.

Modulation involves modification of incoming signals within the dorsal horn of the spinal cord and is influenced by brain-mediated descending inhibition and facilitation. The axons of primary afferents terminate in the dorsal horn of the spinal cord and are divided into parallel laminae, numbered I–VI. Lamina I neurons are the nociceptive-specific neurons and lamina V has dynamic range neurons responding to wide stimulus intensities. Aδ and C fibres convey nociceptive information to superficial laminae (I and II) and deep laminae (V and VI), whereas Aβ fibres transmit innocuous mechanical stimuli to deeper lamina (III–VI). The process of modulation is influenced by sodium and calcium channels and release of neurotransmitters (such as glutamate).

Perception refers to the activation of the sensory cortex and related areas in brain. The projection neurons in laminae I and V relay via the spinothalamic and spinoreticular tracts to various brain regions implicated in pain processing, including the periaqueductal grey, thalamus, parabrachial region, reticular formation of medulla, the thalamus, hypothalamus, and amygdala. From these areas, nociceptive information is projected to (1) areas involved in sensory–discriminatory pain perception (somatosensory cortex; referred to as lateral pain system), (2) areas involved in affective–motivational pain perception (insula and anterior cingulate cortex; referred to as medial pain system), and (3) areas involved in descending modulation of spinal cord neurons (rostral ventromedial medulla).

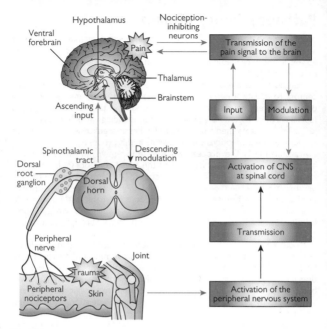

Fig. 11.1 Pain pathways.

Reproduced with permission from Bingham B et al. The molecular basis of pain and its clinical implications in rheumatology. *Nat Clin Pract Rheumatol*, 5: 28–37. Copyright © 2009, Springer Nature. doi:10.1038/ncprheum0972.

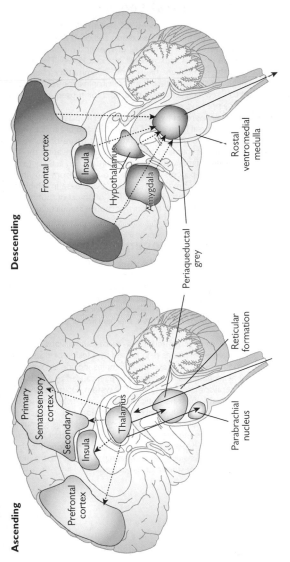

Descending

Frontal cortex

Insula

Hypothalamus

Amygdala

Periaqueductal grey

Rostral ventromedial medulla

Ascending

Primary Sematosensory cortex

Secondary

Insula

Prefrontal cortex

Thalamus

Reticular formation

Parabrachial nucleus

Periaqueductal grey

Fig. 11.1 (Contd.)

Peripheral and central sensitization

Two mechanisms that underlie the process of sensitization that leads to chronic persistent pain are peripheral sensitization and central sensitization. Peripheral sensitization results from a release of chemical mediators (such as prostaglandins, thromboxanes, leukotrienes, and cytokines). This inflammatory cascade and the subsequent neurogenic inflammatory mediators (such as serotonin, glutamate, substance P, and calcitonin gene-related peptide (CGRP)) lead to a reduced activation threshold for subsequent stimuli (that would previously not have elicited pain).

Central sensitization is a process whereby long-term plasticity changes occur in the neurons of dorsal horn of the spinal cord and brain as a result of the increased peripheral activation associated with tissue or nerve injury. In the spinal cord, this is characterized by decreased activation thresholds (mediated by calcium influx) and increased spontaneous activity (even to non-noxious input). This process is believed to result from Aδ fibres forming synaptic links with C fibres. There is also a decrease in inhibitory inputs to spinal cord neurons and facilitatory effect of spinal output, which enhances pain perception in response to non-nociceptive stimuli (allodynia).

Nociceptive and neurogenic pain

Nociceptive pain is the pain generated by tissue damage (noxious stimuli) via the peripheral nociceptors and an intact nervous system of the pain pathway. Nociceptive pain is often described as sharp, aching, or throbbing pain and is often exacerbated by movement or load bearing. Examples are burns, ligament sprain, or muscle strain. Chronic nociceptive pain can develop aspects of neuropathic pain due to the mechanisms of peripheral and central sensitization.

Neuropathic pain is pain generated by a damaged nervous system. Central neuropathic pain is defined as pain caused by a lesion or disease of the central somatosensory nervous system. Examples include stroke, SCI, and MS. Peripheral neuropathic pain is defined as pain caused by a lesion or disease of the peripheral somatosensory nervous system. Examples include painful diabetic neuropathy, post-herpetic neuralgia, and trigeminal neuralgia (TN). Neuropathic pain has a variable presentation and is described by affected individuals as either shooting, stabbing, burning, tingling, numb, itching, or a sensation of 'pins and needles'. The positive signs that are commonly present are allodynia, hyperalgesia, hyperpathia, or autonomic signs (changes in skin temperature, swelling, and sweating); however, there might also be negative signs of hypoaesthesia or hypoalgesia.

Common pain syndromes

Table 11.2 provides a summary of the mechanisms of common pain syndromes. Many pain syndromes are difficult to discretely categorize as there is considerable overlap of mechanisms across conditions. Current evidence supports the argument that chronic conditions such as arthritis and low back pain that were previously considered as purely nociceptive pain syndromes also involve central pain mechanisms.

Table 11.2 Examples of pain syndromes

	Nociceptive	Neurogenic		Visceral	Combined (± psychogenic)
		Peripheral	Central		
Acute	Sprain Strains Burns Post-operative	Nerve injury		Calculi pain Ulcer	
Intermittent	Headache Migraine Acute arthritis	Trigeminal		Dysmen-orrhoea Dyspepsia	Cancer Migraine Endometriosis IBS
Chronic		Nerve injury Neuropathy	Brain injury SCI MS Parkinson's Stroke	Pelvic pain	Low back pain Whiplash Chr. arthritis Fibromyalgia Cancer PLP CRPS

CRPS, complex regional pain syndrome; IBS, irritable bowel syndrome; MS, multiple sclerosis; PLP, phantom limb pain; SCI, spinal cord injury.

Examination of a patient with pain

Pain is a subjective phenomenon without confirmatory laboratory tests or radiological investigations that can quantify pain. The rehabilitation physician must undertake a thorough biopsychosocial history and perform a comprehensive neuromusculoskeletal examination.

The pain history should establish the nature of pain, site, onset, duration of the pain (hours/days/weeks/months), nature of pain (dull/burning/ stabbing/throbbing etc.), radiation of pain, intensity of pain (using numerical rating scale of 0–10 or mild/moderate/severe), fluctuations (pain at rest/activity, diurnal variations, seasonal variations), provoking factors, relieving factors, associated symptoms, and presence of abnormal sensation or paraesthesia (pins and needles, allodynia).

The impact of pain on sleep/mood/behaviour/ADLs/extended daily activities/sex life/social life and vocation needs to be established. An in-depth history of any psychosocial problems (psychological problems, drug/addiction problems, psychiatric illness, family circumstances, relationships, social support system, litigation, culture, and spirituality) will prove useful for the physician to make a comprehensive biopsychosocial assessment. The potential barriers to improvement (sometimes referred to as yellow flags) need to be addressed when a management plan is formulated (Box 11.2).

Some patients are unable to give a complete or coherent history due to problems in speech and language, psychological, or mental function. The physician can obtain useful information from family members, carers, and other healthcare professionals in the team.

An examination of the painful area (look, feel, move) and relevant neuromusculoskeletal examination needs to be performed as summarized in ➲ Chapter 5. Positive Waddell's non-organic signs (tenderness, simulation, distraction, regional sensory and regional motor impairments) can indicate psychological distress. Findings benefit from a structured approach to documentation and a management plan formulated that needs to be discussed with the patient.

> **Box 11.2 Yellow flags: psychosocial predictors of chronicity**
> - A negative belief that pain is harmful or potentially severely disabling
> - Fear avoidance behaviour and reducing activity levels
> - An expectation that passive rather than active treatment will be beneficial
> - Tendency to depression, low mood, and social withdrawal
> - Social or financial problems

Measurement of pain

The multidimensional influence of pain in domains of physical health, mental health, activities, and participation in societal roles implies the measurement of pain should aim to capture these various aspects of health status. The physician has the choice to use a multidimensional tool or a combination of tools to ensure that all important domains are covered.

Pain intensity can be measured using a numerical rating scale (0–10 or 0–100), a visual analogue scale (0–10 cm line), or a verbal rating scale (no pain, slight pain, moderate pain, severe pain, extreme pain). Anxiety can be measured using the Pain Anxiety Symptoms Scale (PASS) or the Spielberger State-Trait Anxiety Inventory (STAI). The Hospital Anxiety and Depression Scale (HADS) is a generic scale used to capture anxiety and depression, and may be useful in the context of chronic pain. Depression can also be captured using Zung self-rating depression or Beck Depression Inventory (BDI). The Coping Strategies Questionnaire (CSQ) or the Survey of Pain Attitudes (SOPA) can assess the style of cognitive and behavioural coping strategies used by the individual in pain, and to facilitate early identification of potential yellow flags.

Multidimensional scales such as Brief Pain Inventory (BPI), McGill Pain Questionnaire (MPQ), Sickness Impact Profile (SIP), 36-item Short-Form Health Survey (SF-36), or Multidimensional Pain Inventory (MPI) can measure functional capacity and activity interference. The Oswestry Disability Index (ODI) is specifically used in chronic low back pain to capture functional status.

Neuropathic pain can be measured by either using purely subjective scales, such as the Neuropathic Pain Questionnaire (NPQ), or combination scales such as the Leeds Assessment of Neuropathic Symptoms and Signs (LANSS) that incorporates a combination of subjective symptoms and objective physical tests.

Management of chronic pain

The goals of treatment are to reduce (not eliminate) pain, maximize the activity/function, reduce the misuse of dependency-producing medications, reduce maladaptive pain behaviours, introduce strategies around acceptance of pain, and assist the individual to maintain their chosen vocation. A MDT comprising a physician, physiotherapist, occupational therapist, psychologist, vocational rehabilitation specialist, specialist nurses, and social worker can facilitate the multimodal approach to effectively managing chronic pain.

Pharmacological management

The WHO analgesic ladder (Fig. 11.2), originally developed for management of cancer pain, is also a useful guide for medication use in the management of acute and chronic pain. The analgesic effect of any medication may differ between individuals, due to a variety of personal factors including genetic make-up. There can also be variability in efficacy of different medications of the same class within the same individual.

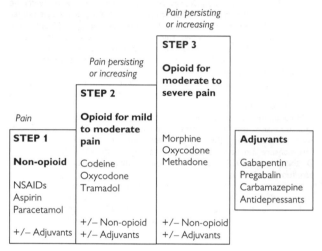

Fig. 11.2 The WHO analgesic ladder.

Non-opioid analgesics

Non-steroidal anti-inflammatory drugs

Non-steroidal anti-inflammatory drugs (NSAIDs) inhibit the cyclooxygenase (COX) enzyme of the prostaglandin synthesis pathway, having anti-inflammatory, analgesic, and antipyretic effects. NSAIDs can be used effectively for management of flare-ups in inflammatory arthritis, osteoarthritis, and chronic non-specific low back pain. There is no convincing evidence to suggest superior efficacy between different NSAIDs (e.g. ibuprofen/naproxen/diclofenac). NSAIDs are not recommended for treatment of neuropathic pain. They can cause gastrointestinal (GI) side effects, with 60% of users experiencing dyspepsia/heartburn and 20–30% developing GI ulcers. They need to be used with caution in individuals on anticoagulants or corticosteroids, individuals with a history of dyspepsia, and the elderly. Selective COX-2 inhibitors (e.g. meloxicam) have fewer GI adverse effects. Alternatively, GI toxicity can be reduced by concomitant use of a proton pump inhibitor. NSAIDS also tend to increase cardiovascular risk and can cause renal impairment, and therefore need to be used with caution in people with cardiac or renal impairment, hypertension, diabetes or those on medications that decrease renal perfusion (e.g. angiotensin-converting enzyme (ACE) inhibitors or diuretics).

Paracetamol

Paracetamol acts by selective COX inhibition in the CNS and has analgesic and antipyretic properties with no anti-inflammatory action. It is recommended for use either alone (1 4 g/day) or in combination with NSAIDs for pain in hip or knee osteoarthritis and chronic low back pain.

Opioids

Opioids bind to three different opioid receptor types: mu (supraspinal analgesia and euphoria), delta (dysphoria, psychomimetic effects), and kappa (spinal analgesia and sedation). Opioids can be classified as weak (i.e. showing limited potency at the mu receptor) or strong opioids (greater potency at mu receptors). The division is somewhat arbitrary, as large doses of weaker opioids can exhibit the side effects of strong opioids, and a low dose of a stronger opioid can be used as a weak opioid. Weak opioids include codeine, dihydrocodeine, and tramadol. Stronger opioids are morphine, diamorphine, hydromorphone, oxycodone, fentanyl, buprenorphine, and methadone. The approximate equivalent doses of commonly used opioid medications are shown in Table 11.3. This concept of relative potency is inaccurate but does provide a rough guide for physicians when switching medications.

Opioids have been shown to be effective in chronic low back pain, osteoarthritis, and neuropathic pain. However, doses need to be regularly reviewed and be advocated only as part of a multimodal pain management/rehabilitation plan. It is preferable to use regular sustained-release formulations (oral or transdermal) with short-acting oral preparations for breakthrough or rescue analgesia. Opioid response can be variable in every individual due to variations in metabolism, mediated by the cytochrome P450 enzyme. If the individual is not responding to a reasonable dose of a particular opioid (or developing side effects), the physician must consider providing the patient with information on an alternative opioid based on equianalgesic dose tables (Table 11.3) and then try opioid rotation if the patient is willing to try.

Adverse effects are common with opioids, and can occur in up to 80% of individuals. Commonly observed are GI effects (nausea, vomiting, and constipation) and cognitive impairment (fatigue, lethargy, somnolence, and impaired concentration). Serious adverse effects such as sedation and respiratory depression can occur, particularly with parenteral opioids. Chronic opioid use has been shown to cause tolerance, cognitive dysfunction, hypothalamic–pituitary–adrenal/gonadal axis abnormalities, immune suppression, and potentially opioid-induced hyperalgesia.

Table 11.3 Approximate equivalent doses of opioid analgesics for adult use

	Opioid	Dose	Equivalent oral morphine dose
Weak opioids	Codeine	30 mg	4.5 mg
	Dihydrocodeine	10 mg	1 mg
	Tramadol	50 mg	5 mg
Strong opioids	Oxycodone	10 mg	20 mg
	Fentanyl patch	25 mcg/hour	60–90 mg/24 hours
	Buprenorphine patch	52.5 mcg/hour	95–145 mg/24 hours

Adjuvants

Gabapentin

Gabapentin acts via the $\alpha2\delta$ subunit of the voltage-gated calcium channel. It is thought to reduce presynaptic calcium influx, thereby inhibiting the polysynaptic reflex in the dorsal horn. However, it has recently been shown to inhibit the construction of new excitatory synapses via an effect on thrombospondin receptors. Gabapentin shows efficacy in the management of neuropathic pain (CNS injury, peripheral neuropathy, post-herpetic neuralgia) in divided doses between 900 and 3600 mg/day. The pharmacokinetics of gabapentin is non-linear at higher doses, in that saturation of intestinal absorption disrupts the relationship between dosage and serum concentration. This necessitates a significant increase in dosage for a relative increase in response. Side effects at higher doses include somnolence and dizziness.

Pregabalin

Pregabalin is structurally related and acts in a neurologically similar manner to gabapentin. It is effective for neuropathic pain management in doses between 150 and 600 mg/day. It also has an anxiolytic effect and can also be used in fibromyalgia. In comparison to gabapentin, it has a quicker onset of action and linear pharmacokinetics (i.e. has stable bioavailability independent of dose). Side effects of dizziness and cognitive impairment have been reported. Tolerance can be improved with flexible dosing (e.g. using a lower dose in morning and a higher dose at night).

Carbamazepine

Carbamazepine acts by blocking sodium channels and can be used in the management of neuropathic pain and TN. It induces the hepatic microsomal enzyme system that can influence the metabolism of several drugs. Other side effects are dizziness, sedation, skin toxicity, and hyponatraemia. Oxcarbazepine has a better tolerability and can be tried in individuals who experience undesirable side effects.

Lamotrigine, tiagabine, topiramate, and zonisamide are other agents being considered for the management of chronic pain.

Antidepressants

Amitriptyline and other tricyclic antidepressants (imipramine, nortriptyline) inhibit the reuptake of noradrenaline and serotonin (alongside cholinergic and histaminergic effects). They have shown to be effective in a variety of chronic pain conditions (neuropathic, nociceptive, inflammatory, CNS injury, fibromyalgia, headache). They also improve mood and sleep. The analgesic effect is observed in lower doses and earlier (typical onset of action is 1 week) than the antidepressant effect (observed at higher doses and later onset of 3–5 weeks). Common side effects are dizziness, sedation, dry mouth, constipation, and orthostatic hypotension. They are contraindicated in individuals with cardiac conduction disturbances, prostatic hypertrophy, or glaucoma.

Serotonin and noradrenaline reuptake inhibitors such as venlafaxine, duloxetine, and milnacipran have no cholinergic and histaminergic effect (hence fewer side effects than tricyclics antidepressants). They can be used in chronic pain syndromes such as neuropathic pain and fibromyalgia. Duloxetine is the drug of choice for diabetic neuropathy. Side effects include nausea and they must be used with caution in individuals with cardiac abnormalities and epilepsy. Mirtazapine is an enhancer of noradrenaline and serotonin neurotransmission and is used for depression and improving sleep. It is yet to be recommended for use in neuropathic pain.

Topical agents

Topical NSAIDs can be considered for chronic pain in musculoskeletal conditions. This has the advantage of fewer GI side effects but with a small chance of local reactions (itching, burning, rash). Topical diclofenac gel has supportive evidence for use in knee osteoarthritis. Topical capsaicin (the compound in chilli peppers) patches (8%) or topical lidocaine patches (5%) have been shown to be effective in peripheral neuropathic pain (e.g. post-herpetic neuralgia). These options can be considered when first-line pharmacological agents have not been effective or were poorly tolerated.

Sleep and chronic pain

Sleep is considered essential for survival and 8 hours is restorative in adults. Sleep comprises cycles of alternating non-rapid eye movement (NREM) and REM stages. Each sleep cycle has four stages of NREM sleep (1–4) followed by REM sleep, with three to six complete sleep cycles in a typical 8-hour sleep period. About 50–90% of chronic pain patients have a disturbed sleep pattern. They have frequent sleep fragmentation, non-restorative sleep pattern, and feel fatigued and sleepy during the day. Medications can help initiate sleep, decrease sleep fragmentation, and increase NREM sleep.

Benzodiazepines such as diazepam were popular agents used until the introduction of non-benzodiazepine agents such as zopiclone/zolpidem. They have a shorter half-life and are devoid of the muscle relaxant, anxiolytic, and anticonvulsant effect of benzodiazepines. Eszopiclone has a greater half-life (5–5.8 hours) when compared to the relatively shorter half-life of zopiclone/zolpidem. Medications such as trazadone or tricyclic antidepressants can be used in patients with concurrent anxiety, depression, and neuropathic pain. Anticonvulsants generally increase sleep time and slow-wave sleep. All medications for insomnia must be used with caution as they have side effects and may not be as effective if used long term. Chronic benzodiazepine use can cause cognitive impairment, falls, rebound insomnia, and have an abuse potential. Chronic opiate use can increase sleep fragmentation and decrease NREM and REM sleep. Nicotine delays sleep onset. Alcohol may facilitate sleep by increasing slow waves but can also cause rebound increased sleep fragmentation in later stages of the sleep cycle. Medications that decrease REM sleep, while being withdrawn, can lead to rebound increased REM sleep with some individuals experiencing vivid unpleasant dreams. This is classically seen with benzodiazepines. Therefore, these medications must be weaned down gradually.

Multidisciplinary pain management programmes

There is substantial evidence to support a biopsychosocial assessment and treatment approach in the effective management of chronic pain. A multidisciplinary pain management programme is delivered by a team of professionals led by a pain or rehabilitation physician. The team members work in an interdisciplinary fashion with the common goal of minimizing pain and maximizing function of the individual. Such programmes have demonstrated significant improvements in return to work, daily function, reduced healthcare utilization, and reduced disability claims.

In chronic low back pain, such programmes (functional restoration programme) have led to a significant reduction in spinal fusion surgeries in most developed countries. Studies also suggest that such programmes can be as effective as disc replacement surgeries. The essential components of a multidisciplinary pain management programme are shown in the Table 11.4. It is worth noting that some of the individual components (CBT, operant behavioural therapy, brief education, meditation, manual therapy, exercise therapy) have also been shown to be effective as a unidisciplinary programme in the management of chronic pain. Referral to a multidisciplinary pain management programme should perhaps be tried once unidisciplinary programmes have failed to restore function and quality of life.

Table 11.4 Components of a multidisciplinary pain management programme

Medical therapy	Responsible for a patient's physical well-being
	Manage medications
	Educational component (e.g. neurophysiology, diagnosis, prognosis)
	Co-morbidity management
Cognitive therapy	Responsible for psychological aspects of a patient's care
	Cognitive behavioural therapy (CBT)—graded exposure therapy, cognitive restructuring, problem-solving, relapse prevention, refuting fear expectations
	Operant behavioural therapy (OBT)—reducing pain behaviours (kinesophobia) and establishing wellness behaviours
	Mind–body techniques (biofeedback, relaxation therapy, meditation, guided imagery)
	Co-morbid psychological conditions management
	Educational component
Physical and occupational therapy	Physical therapy and/or occupational therapy
	Stretching, strengthening and aerobic conditioning—graded therapeutic exercises (flexibility, ROM, posture, body mechanics, ambulation, gait training, core strength/stability, cardiovascular fitness, pacing)
	Functional activities—ADLs, leisure activities, pacing (energy conservation)
	Flare-up management
	Passive physical treatments (ultrasonography, electrical stimulation, massage) generally avoided in multidisciplinary pain management programmes
	Job analysis, postural training, ergonomics, and vocational rehabilitation
	Educational component
Education	Improved self-management
	Educational component of medical, behavioural, and physical components
	Home exercise training
	Support from carers, family, and employers
	Diet and nutrition
	Re-engagement in leisure activities
	Stress management training, and wellness therapies
	Address nicotine, alcohol, and drug use
	Sleep hygiene

Intrathecal drug therapy

Intrathecal and epidural drug delivery systems are used for patients with pain and spasms that are non-responsive to oral or parental pharmacological therapy, or those who experienced intolerable side effects. The rationale is to deliver a higher concentration of the drug to the spinal cord receptors and avoid the side effects of high-dose systemic therapy. They are predominantly used for painful limb spasms, cancer pain, or chronic non-malignant pain. The medications used are morphine, baclofen, or ziconotide. The system comprises an intrathecal catheter placed subcutaneously and connected to an implanted pump that delivers the drug at a fixed or variable rate. The complications include surgical complications and catheter-related complications that can lead to life-threatening overdose or withdrawal states. Individuals undergoing this therapy must have access to 24-hour on-call services and close monitoring by their pain physicians.

Neuromodulation and neuroablation procedures

Neuromodulation refers to iatrogenic modification of signal transmission in the pain pathway in order to achieve pain alteration. The various modalities available are spinal cord stimulation, deep brain stimulation, or motor cortex stimulation. Neuroablation refers to iatrogenic damage to the pathway structures to achieve analgesia, either in the CNS or the peripheral nervous system.

Spinal cord stimulation involves electrical stimulation of the dorsal column of the spinal cord by impulses from small wires placed on the spinal cord. The wires are connected to an implanted or external pulse generator that is rechargeable and programmable. A trial period is undertaken before deciding on long-term use of the device. The electric signals from the device suppress the hyperexcitability of the dorsal horn and activate the central inhibitory mechanisms. Spinal cord stimulation reduces rather than eliminates the pain, making the pain manageable for the individual. A National Institute for Health and Care Excellence (NICE) approved indication for spinal cord stimulation is refractory neuropathic pain (>6 months and must have tried other conservative treatments). Trials suggest efficacy particularly in failed back surgery and complex regional pain syndrome (CRPS). Contraindications for this treatment are the presence of significant psychological issues and/or drug-seeking behaviour. Individuals need to be thoroughly assessed by a MDT prior to the procedure. Complications are reported in around 30–35% with hardware complications of lead migration and battery failure being the commonest problems.

Deep brain stimulation treatment for chronic pain remains experimental without conclusive evidence of efficacy. Neurostimulation of the thalamus and periaqueductal grey matter activates the descending inhibitory pain pathways to provide pain relief. The stimulating electrodes are accurately placed using stereotactic neurosurgery and an externalized trial is undertaken before implantation of the generator. Some patients with refractory chronic pain in TBI, post-stroke pain, thalamic syndrome, and cranial nerve pain have been offered deep brain stimulation provided there is an understanding of the risks involved. A 4% risk of intracranial haemorrhage (including one death) was reported in one series. Other complications are related to hardware complications such as those of spinal cord stimulation.

Motor cortex stimulation is done by placing electrodes on the surface of the brain (motor cortex) through burr holes or craniotomy. Stimulation of the motor cortex is believed to inhibit thalamic hyperactivity and also reduce the emotional component of chronic pain by activating the anterior cingulate cortex and insula. Relative preservation of the pyramidal tract and somatosensory pathway is essential for a favourable result. A trial of an external system is undertaken before implantation of the generator. It can be used for refractory neuropathic pain syndromes, particularly TN. A large cortical stroke with encephalomalacia is a contraindication for the procedure. Complications include extradural/subdural haematoma, seizures, and paraesthesia/dysaesthesia.

Neuroablation surgeries include sectioning of: (1) peripheral nerve—peripheral neurectomy (stump neuroma, meralgia paraesthetica), dorsal rhizotomy (occipital neuralgia), sympathectomy (causalgia, CRPS); (2) spinal cord—dorsal root entry zone lesioning (spinal cord injury pain, brachial plexus injury), cordotomy (cancer pain, spinal cord injury pain), myelotomy (cancer pain); (3) brainstem—mesencephalotomy (post-stroke pain); or (4) intracranial—thalamotomy (cancer pain, central pain), cingulotomy (cancer pain, failed back surgery, chronic pain with severe depressive illness).

These procedures lack level I evidence and are mostly supported by case series only (level III evidence). The surgical ablation procedures at spinal cord or brain level have mainly being used in terminal cancer pain utilizing a palliative approach.

Specific chronic pain conditions

Trigeminal neuralgia

TN is a rare pain syndrome is characterized by paroxysmal pain in the distribution of thtrigeminal nerve. Typical TN episodes comprise unilateral, intense, sharp/shooting/stabbing pain without pain between episodes. Episodes can be triggered by facial stimulation, eating, talking, or cleaning of teeth. Atypical TN has sensory loss in the fifth nerve distribution area and background facial pain in between episodes. The natural history of the condition is unclear, but 70% of patients have further episodes after the first attack. Magnetic resonance imaging (MRI) and magnetic resonance angiography can help identify compression of the nerve by vessels (80–90% of classical TNs) or neoplasm/other structural abnormalities.

NICE recommends carbamazepine (or oxcarbazepine) as first-line management for the syndrome. For non-responders, microvascular decompression provides dramatic relief of symptoms (two-thirds of patients achieve immediate complete pain relief and among those, two-thirds remain pain free at 10–20 years after surgery). Surgical advancements include stereotactic radiosurgery such as Gamma Knife®. Other alternative options are percutaneous radiofrequency thermocoagulation or glycerol rhizolysis.

Complex regional pain syndrome

CRPS is a syndrome characterized by pain, sensorimotor changes, vasomotor, sudomotor, and trophic changes, motor dysfunction, and psychological distress. CRPS is commonly seen in the limbs and there is often a history of injury to the limb. The syndrome was previously known by several names: reflex sympathetic dystrophy, Sudek's atrophy, causalgia, and post-traumatic arthritis. The common type is CRPS type I where there is no damage to a major nerve, whereas type II is less common and seen after nerve damage. The diagnostic criteria are shown in Table 11.5.

There is no medical cure for the condition. Early identification and prompt diagnosis is required to direct the patient to an appropriate multidisciplinary rehabilitation programme that focuses on education, prevention of further disuse of the limb, and management of the associated psychological distress in the condition. There is no convincing level I evidence to support the use of any of the pharmacological agents or interventional procedures. The medications that can be considered in the management are neuropathic pain medications and pamidronate (60 mg intravenous single dose if symptoms <6 months). Spinal cord stimulation can be tried for refractory cases (symptoms >6 months) that have not responded to other conservative multidisciplinary rehabilitation measures. There is no evidence in support of amputation having a beneficial effect for the pain syndrome.

Table 11.5 Budapest diagnostic criteria for CRPS

All of the following statements must be met:
- Presence of continuing pain that is disproportionate to any inciting event
- Presence of at least one sign in two or more of the following categories
- Presence of at least one symptom in three or more of the following categories
- No other diagnosis that can better explain the signs and symptoms

Category	Sign/symptom
1. Sensory	Allodynia
	Hyperaesthesia
2. Vasomotor	Temperature asymmetry
	Skin colour changes
	Skin colour asymmetry
3. Sudomotor/oedema	Oedema
	Sweating changes
	Sweating asymmetry
4. Motor/trophic	Decreased range of motion
	Motor dysfunction (weakness, tremor, dystonia)
	Trophic changes (hair/nail/skin)

Chronic pain conditions covered elsewhere
- Headache (➜ see Chapter 26)
- Chronic low back pain (➜ see Chapter 37)
- Fibromyalgia (➜ see Chapter 37)
- Chronic fatigue syndrome/myalgic encephalopathy (➜ see Chapter 37)
- Cancer pain (➜ see Chapter 38)
- Phantom pain/stump pain (➜ see Chapter 41).

Reference

1. Reid KJ, Harker J, Bala MM (2011). Epidemiology of chronic non-cancer pain in Europe: narrative review of prevalence, pain treatments and pain impact. *Current Medical Research and Opinion* 27, 449–462

Further reading

Brook P, Connell J, Pickering T (2011). *Oxford Handbook of Pain Management*. Oxford University Press, Oxford.

Goebel A, Barker CH, Turner-Stokes L, et al. (2012). *Complex Regional Pain Syndrome in Adults: UK Guidelines for Diagnosis, Referral and Management in Primary and Secondary Care*. Royal College of Physicians, London.

Lynch ME, Craig KD, Peng PWH (2011). *Clinical Pain Management: A Practical Guide*. Blackwell Publishing Ltd, West Sussex.

National Institute for Health and Care Excellence (NICE) (2009). *Rheumatoid Arthritis: National Clinical Guideline for Management and Treatment in Adults*. Clinical Guideline [CG79]. NICE, London. ℞ http://www.nice.org.uk/guidance/cg79.

National Institute for Health and Care Excellence (NICE) (2013). *Neuropathic Pain in Adults: Pharmacological Management in Non-Specialist Settings*. Clinical Guideline [CG173]. NICE, London. ℞ http://www.nice.org.uk/guidance/cg173.

National Institute for Health and Care Excellence (NICE) (2014). *Osteoarthritis: The Care and Management of Osteoarthritis in Adults*. Clinical Guideline [CG177]. NICE, London. ℞ http://www.nice.org.uk/guidance/cg177.

Scottish Intercollegiate Guidelines Network (SIGN) (2013). *Management of Chronic Pain*. SIGN Publication No. 136. SIGN, Edinburgh. ℞ http://www.sign.ac.uk.

Stanos SP, Tyburski MD, Harden RN (2011). Management of chronic pain. In Braddom RL (ed), *Physical Medicine and Rehabilitation*, pp. 935–970. Saunders, Philadelphia, PA.

Neurogenic bladder and bowel

Introduction

Most people never consider the impact of bowel or bladder incontinence unless or until they experience problems. Young children usually develop an awareness of bladder fullness in their first 1–2 years; however, 'toilet training' (i.e. social continence) isn't common until around the age of 3. Thereafter, 3–5% of children aged 5–15 will have an intermittent daytime wetting problem and around 1–3% will experience soiling (faecal incontinence). Once a person has attained continence, however, each of us expects to stay that way.

It is therefore unsurprising that even the most intermittent or minor loss of social continence is very embarrassing. Even the *fear of incontinence* has the capacity to modify a person's behaviour, adversely affect their quality of life, as well as having a potentially significant financial impact. But while social continence is important to each of us, it is not just the *lack of incontinence* that is important. The absence of symptoms and/or medical complications from disordered bladder or bowel function is just as necessary for maintaining good health. For example, renal failure was historically a major cause of mortality in neurologically impaired patients, particularly after SCI. Appropriate and timely attention through rehabilitation and urological assessment can prevent this, so that renal compromise and death are now rare, and death by renal failure implies a failure of adequate care.

Bladder and bowel anatomy and physiology are complex, with continence being dependent on both intact anatomical structures and normal peripheral, autonomic, and CNS function. Damage to anatomical or neurological function impacts the control of continence in predictable ways, and by inference, assists in determining appropriate intervention to minimize any adverse effects. This chapter will focus on continence and incontinence, but with an emphasis towards the neurological substrates.

Physiological considerations of normal bladder and bowel function

The neural control of bladder and bowel extends from the frontal lobes down into the sacral cord, with multiple feedback loops providing information that helps to provide optimal function. Damage to these structures can produce incontinence, irrespective of damage to the anatomical structures. Bladder and bowel physiology will be discussed in turn.

Normal bladder function

The anatomy and physiology of the urine collecting system is complex (Fig. 12.1). From the renal calyces, the ureters transport urine to the bladder. The acutely angled entry of the ureter into the bladder, the pelviureteric junction, provides a defence against pressure being exerted back up the ureter towards the kidney. The bladder itself is composed of the detrusor muscle, which relaxes to allow urine to be collected without a rise in pressure. The internal sphincter at the base of the bladder is comprised of smooth muscle and does much of the work in maintaining continence. The muscles of the pelvic floor provide an external sphincter that is under voluntary control.

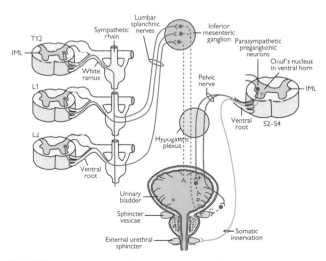

Fig. 12.1 Neural control of the bladder. Purple = sympathetic nervous system; dark grey = parasympathetic nervous system. Solid lines = preganglionic fibres, dotted lines = postganglionic fibres. The light grey line represents somatic innervation. IML, intermediolateral cell column; L, lumbar; S, sacral; T, thoracic spinal segment.

http://what-when-how.com/neuroscience/the-autonomic-nervous-system-integrative-systems-part-3/.

The bladder receives innervation from both branches of the autonomic nervous system. The main nerve supply to the detrusor is cholinergic from parasympathetic neurons arising from the S2–S4 level. The internal sphincter is innervated by adrenergic postganglionic sympathetic fibres from the thoracolumbar sympathetic chain. In males, the prostate (and ejaculation) is also sympathetically innervated, providing an integrated mechanism to prevent retro-ejaculation of semen into the bladder. While other neurotransmitters are involved, this simple classification is useful when considering treatment rationales. Bladder sensation is mostly conveyed via the pelvic and pudendal nerves to the spinal cord and rostrally via the lateral spinothalamic tract. Afferent fibres also synapse within Onuf's nucleus in the ventral horn at the S2–S4 level.

In normal situations, filling of the bladder is associated with detrusor relaxation and tonic contraction of the internal and external sphincters via inputs from the pontine micturition centre. As bladder volume increases, sensory inputs into the pontine micturition centre increase the likelihood of reflexive bladder emptying via bladder smooth muscle contraction and sphincter relaxation. This is the process that dominates bladder emptying until 'toilet training' is achieved. In adults, this will normally occur at a volume of around 150 mL.

To fill the bladder further requires inhibitory drivers from the anteromedial frontal lobes to the pontine micturition centre. While this is associated with the conscious awareness of bladder fullness, there is also a behavioural/stress response driving the person to seek an appropriate voiding opportunity. Increasing bladder volumes increase the amount of conscious attention required to control micturition. At an individualized volume, the higher centres will no longer be able to suppress voiding and the detrusor will contract irrespective of the individual's societal preferences. When toileting is appropriate, conscious removal of inhibition of the pontine micturition centre allows the voiding reflex to fire, with coordinated detrusor activation and urinary sphincter relaxation.

Normal bowel function

The large bowel is extremely richly innervated. In addition to autonomic and somatic nervous inputs, the bowel has its own enteric nervous system comprising the submucosal (Meissner) and the myenteric (Auerbach) plexuses that control segmental function. These plexuses are partially responsible for bowel transit time through reflexes such as the gastrocolic reflex (where stomach filling increases peristalsis). Reflex control of the bowel occurs through spinal reflex arcs (such as the rectoanal contractile reflex, where rectal fullness proportionately contracts the internal sphincter) which are essential for maintaining continence and are again under highercentre control. Parasympathetic innervation (S2–S4) of the rectum is inhibitory, while sympathetic is excitatory (as any nervous student could tell you before exams!).

With similarity to the bladder, the anal sphincter has two components: an internal smooth muscle part under sympathetic control and a skeletal muscle component under voluntary control. While the internal anal sphincter provides most of the resting anal pressure, it can be voluntarily reinforced by the external sphincter. The anal mucosal folds and the anal endovascular cushions combine with the sphincters to produce resistance to prevent the inadvertent leakage of flatus or other material. Additionally, continence is assisted by the puborectalis muscle which loops around the rectum, maintaining the anorectal angle.

Controlled defecation is dependent on the integrity of the anorectal mechanism. Continence is easiest to maintain when the bowel motion is of at least a semisolid consistency. Emptying the rectum requires relaxation of both internal and external sphincters coupled with a Valsalva manoeuvre. Defecation occurs when the internal abdominal pressure is greater than the resistance at the sphincters.

Urinary incontinence

The likelihood of incontinence increases with age in both sexes, with urinary incontinence considerably more frequent than faecal incontinence. The prevalence of incontinence is much higher in females, estimated at a 10:1 ratio compared to males, with damage caused during childbirth and postmenopausal changes being significant risk factors. It is estimated that 70% of people self-manage incontinence without medical assistance, and that only people severely affected by incontinence approach the medical profession. It is further estimated that around 5% of middle-aged people have 'intolerable' incontinence, a figure that rises to 15% in older groups.

Any neurological pathology can give rise to problems in micturition and defecation, such as urgency, urge incontinence, loss of bladder sensation, and urinary retention. Frontal lobe lesions may produce social disinhibition or unawareness of bladder filling leading to voiding at inappropriate times and places, even though the voiding mechanism is normal.

Urinary incontinence is commonly divided into various categories whose likelihood differs between the sexes (Table 12.1):

- Stress incontinence: an involuntary leakage of urine associated with increased intra-abdominal pressure, such as on effort or exertion, or from coughing. Stress incontinence commonly arises from conditions that damage the pelvic floor, its peripheral nervous supply, or in males following prostatectomy.
- Urge incontinence: the involuntary leakage of urine associated with a sudden/strong desire to urinate before being able to reach a toilet. The sensation of urgency, along with frequency and nocturia, can affect quality of life even in the absence of actual leakage. The aetiology of urge incontinence is commonly neurological in nature.
- Mixed incontinence: combines features consistent with both stress and urge incontinence. Often, one of the two forms of incontinence is predominant.
- Overflow incontinence: a bladder with little or no detrusor tone will fill until it reaches the point where its internal pressure overcomes sphincter pressure, resulting in leakage of urine. This is most common following injury to peripheral nerves from surgical or postpartum complications.

A number of conditions can temporarily increase the likelihood of developing incontinence, such as urinary tract infection (UTI), certain medications (particularly those affecting autonomic function or arousal),

Table 12.1 Approximate percentage of types of urinary incontinence by sex

	Female (%)	Male (%)
Stress	45	<10
Urge	10	65
Mixed	45	25

prolonged immobility, recent childbirth, or temporary cognitive impairment. Nocturia can be exacerbated by conditions that reduce the release of antidiuretic hormone from the pituitary that would otherwise produce small volumes of concentrated urine at night.

Pathophysiology

Bladder and bowel disorders are consistently associated with the level of interruption within the nervous system (Table 12.2). For urinary function, these can be divided into three levels:
- Suprapontine
- Suprasacral
- LMN.

Detrusor sphincter dyssynergia

Detrusor sphincter dyssynergia (DSD) describes an incoordination of normal voiding, whereby the detrusor contracts, the internal sphincter relaxes, but the external urinary sphincter remains contracted. Detrusor pressure may be sufficient to produce interrupted bursts of urinary flow but with high residual volumes. Depending on the anatomy of the pelviureteric junction, the raised intravesical pressure may cause back pressure on kidneys with consequent upper tract dilatation and renal damage.

DSD results from SCI between the pontine micturition and sacral spine centres. Incidence and prevalence data is poor, although it is suggested that around 75% of patients with suprasacral SCI and 25–50% of patients with

Table 12.2 Pathophysiology of bladder and bowel disorders

Lesion	Disease examples	Functional change	Outcome
Suprapontine	TBI MS Stroke Parkinson's disease Hydrocephalus Dementia	Interruption of frontal lobe pathways to the pons	Disinhibited micturition Normal voiding reflex Low-volume bladder Rarely urinary retention
Suprasacral	SCI Transverse myelitis MS	In/complete spinal cord lesions leads to incoordination of external sphincter and detrusor activation	Hyperreflexic bladder (urgency, frequency, urge incontinence) Detrusor sphincter dyssynergia (see below)
Lower motor neuron	Lumbar disc prolapse Pelvic trauma Intraspinal lesions	S2–S4 damage produces external sphincter and detrusor hypoactivity, reduced bladder sensation/activity, with loss of bulbocavernosus reflex	Hypotonic bladder Urinary retention and leakage High residual volumes Stress incontinence

MS and spinal dysraphism have DSD. Untreated, there is a tendency for DSD to worsen over time, and half of patients with DSD may develop serious urological complications. In people with an SCI above T7, DSD also provides a powerful stimulus for autonomic dysreflexia, with a consequent risk of secondary medical complications (➔ see Chapter 27).

Management of urinary problems
See Table 12.3 and Figure 12.2.

Table 12.3 Management of urinary problems

Problem	Action	Reason/details
Impaired renal function	Investigation (biochemical screen, ultrasonography, intravenous pyelogram) and medical management	Need to preserve renal function to reduce comorbidity
Impaired bladder emptying	Assess post-void residual volume by catheter drainage or ultrasonography <100 mL considered insignificant UTI risk increases >300 mL	Residual urine stone formation, infection, renal dysfunction
	Frequency/volume chart	Defines the pattern of incontinence for medical team or continence adviser
	Catheterization: Intermittent Indwelling	Urinary incontinence, urinary retention, structural abnormality (prostatectomy/pelvic floor damage)
	Monitor/treat for urinary infections	Protect renal function and general health
	Urinary retention due to poor detrusor contraction (rare)	Cholinergic, anticholinesterase, or selective α_1 blocker medication
Detrusor hyperreflexia	Urodynamic studies/ cystometrogram (± video)	Assess intravesical pressure and detrusor hyperreflexia
	Bladder training	Reduce intravesical pressure
	Anticholinergic medication to reduce detrusor activity	Oxybutynin, tolterodine, solifenacin, fesoterodine
	Reduce urine production	Desmopressin
	BoNT to relax the detrusor muscle	Good efficacy and lasts 6–9 months.
	Catheter and condom drainage. Absorbent pads, napkins, etc.	Protection against urinary leaking

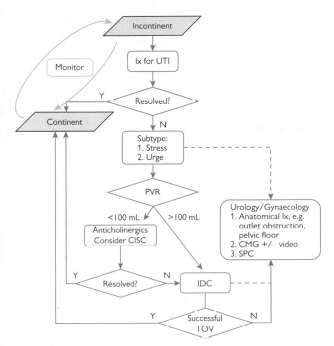

Fig. 12.2 Bladder management flowchart. Note: dotted line implies that referral may be considered at this point. CISC, clean intermittent self-catheterization; IDC, indwelling catheter; Ix, investigation; PVR, post-void residual; SPC, suprapubic catheter; TOV, trial of void; UTI, urinary tract infection.

Catheters

Catheters are a practical solution for some people with urinary incontinence, irrespective of type. Catheterization can either be undertaken on an intermittent or indwelling basis. Clean intermittent self-catheterization (CISC) is best suited for people without detrusor overactivity and with functioning sphincters. In this scenario, the person can continue to use their bladder as a low-pressure storage vesicle with minimal risk of leakage. CISC can be performed by the individual or a carer using an 8 or 10 F catheter on a regular, at least twice daily basis. While safe, CISC requires patient or carer education, sufficient upper limb positioning, and dexterity to perform the procedure and good compliance.

Where an indwelling catheter is required, a 14–16 F silastic catheter can be inserted using a sterile technique. Using larger catheters against leakage is unhelpful, as they increase detrusor irritability and can promote further leakage. Instead, use of a small balloon and avoiding traction on the catheter minimizes nociceptive irritation of the trigone that is a cause of bladder spasms. Anticholinergic medication can be used to suppress detrusor over-activity and to maintain bladder capacity. Potential complications include leakage, blockage, stone formation, and infection.

Suprapubic catheters are preferred when catheterization is likely to be necessary for the long term. While the procedure is more invasive and has recognized morbidity and mortality rates, they are generally well tolerated. Suprapubic catheters also avoid some local complications (such as urethral damage and hypospadias) and have less impact on sexual function compared to an indwelling catheter.

Botulinum toxin A

Many of the oral medications used to treat neurogenic bladder abnormalities have significant adverse drug effects. It is estimated that only 30% of people whose bladder management benefited from oral medications continue taking those medications a year after commencement. As a consequence, focal injection of BoNT-A into the detrusor muscle has become the treatment of choice for detrusor overactivity. BoNT has multiple targets relevant to the bladder, the dominant one being the cholinergic nerve endings of the detrusor. For this reason, around 1 in 20 people will have transient urinary retention of less than 150 mL for a few weeks post procedure and an increased risk of early UTI has been seen in studies. In addition, BoNT-A has effects on reducing the number of cell surface receptors associated with pain sensitization (specifically TRPV and CGRP) which could secondarily reduce neural excitability in neural pathways.

The procedure for BoNT-A injection is performed by cystoscopy under general or local anaesthesia, with a duration of effect of around 6–9 months.

Surgery

The introduction of BoNT-A has meant that the role of surgery has become a second-line intervention in most incontinence management plans. There are a number of recognized procedures, summarized in Table 12.4. Please refer to a urology text for a description of the indications and details of individual surgical procedures.

Table 12.4 Surgical procedures

Procedure	Description
Sphincter ablation	Sphincterotomy now rare outside some spinal injuries units. The need for this procedure has dramatically declined following the introduction of BoNT-A injections into the detrusor
Urinary diversions: • Mitrofanoff procedure • Ileal conduit	Allow continence while protecting against renal impairment
Other procedures: • Clam cystoplasty • Stimulators	Artificial urethral sphincters and sacral stimulators depend on an intact LMN. Are effective, but require patient compliance

Bowel incontinence

Faecal incontinence is the involuntary loss of bowel contents, including flatus, liquid stool elements, mucous, and/or solid faeces. It is estimated that around 2% of adults living in the community have some degree of faecal incontinence, half of these being severe. Faecal incontinence is most commonly transient and associated with infection. In chronic forms it tends to be a multifactorial problem, as any change in anatomy, physiology, or consistency of bowel contents can interact to cause symptoms. The incidence rises in the frail aged population (>85 years of age), with estimates of between 3% and 8%. Common contributors include the following:

- Anatomy:
  - Disruption or weakness of the pelvic floor muscles (particularly puborectalis and the external sphincter).
  - Damage following anorectal surgery (especially relating to anal sphincters or the haemorrhoidal vascular cushions).
  - Following obstetric trauma, with either immediate or delayed symptoms. A woman who sustains anorectal damage during childbirth may not develop symptoms until after she reaches menopause.
- Neurology:
  - Areflexic (LMN) bowel: cauda equina/pudendal nerve damage can impair rectal sensation and/or puborectalis function. This can lead to disruption of rectal reflexes (with faecal impaction, mega-rectum, and faecal overflow) or to reduced control of defecation.
  - Reflex (UMN) bowel: due to lesions above the sacral spinal cord or to cerebral centres influencing rectal reflexes with intact anal reflexes.
- Stool consistency:
  - Diarrhoea-associated faecal incontinence or diarrhoea.
  - Constipation with overflow diarrhoea.
  - Altered bowel habits (e.g. caused by irritable bowel syndrome, Crohn's disease, ulcerative colitis, food intolerances, etc.).

There are few medical consequences from faecal incontinence. It can be associated with secondary health effects including perianal skin irritation/maceration and an increased risk of decubitus ulcers and, potentially, UTIs. Rather than managing health risks, however, the management of faecal incontinence aims to reduce its devastating impact on socialization.

Faecal incontinence is generally managed via a combination of interventions. The first arm of management is dietary modification, with or without aperients, to reach and maintain a stool consistency of type 3 or 4 on the Bristol Stool Chart. Intercurrently, the reflexes of the enteric nervous system mean that the bowel can be trained to open along a timetable convenient to care needs, even in complete SCI. For example, eating a meal increases peristalsis via the gastrocolic reflex, while digital stimulation (or insertion of a rectal suppository or enema) will stimulate reflexive bowel opening (Table 12.5). In other situations, surgical measures such as a defunctioning colostomy can provide continence at the cost of additional care requirements.

Table 12.5 Bowel management programmes for neurogenic bowel

	Reflex bowel	Areflexic bowel
Target frequency	Daily or alternate days	Once or more daily
Target consistency	Bristol scale 4	Bristol scale 3
Step 1	Stimulant laxative 8–12 hours before planned movement (senna/bisacodyl)	Stimulant laxative 8–12 hours before planned movement (senna/bisacodyl)
Step 2	Gastrocolic reflex	Gastrocolic reflex
Step 3	Rectal stimulant—suppository (glycerine) or microenema (phosphate)	Abdominal massage ± digital removal of faeces
Step 4	Digital removal of faeces ± digital check to ensure complete evacuation	Digital check to ensure complete evacuation

Further reading

Bacsu C, Chan L, Tse V (2012). Diagnosing detrusor sphincter dyssynergia in the neurological patient. *BJU International* 109 Suppl 3, 31–34.

Multidisciplinary Association of Spinal Cord Injured Professionals (2012). *Guidelines for Management of Neurogenic Bowel Dysfunction in Individuals with Central Neurological Conditions.* ℘ http://www.mascip.co.uk/wp-content/uploads/2015/02/CV653N-Neurogenic-Guidelines-Sept-2012.

Nitti VW (2001). The prevalence of urinary incontinence. *Reviews in Urology* 3 Suppl 1, S2–S6.

Panicker JN, de Seze M, Fowler CJ (2010). Neurogenic lower urinary tract dysfunction and its management. *Clinical Rehabilitation* 24, 579–589.

Rao SS (2004). Pathophysiology of adult fecal incontinence. *Gastroenterology* 126 Suppl 1, S14–S22.

Stoffel JT (2016). Detrusor sphincter dyssynergia: a review of physiology, diagnosis, and treatment strategies. *Translational Andrology and Urology* 5, 127–135.

What-When-How. *The Autonomic Nervous System (Integrative Systems) Part 4.* ℘ http://what-when-how.com/neuroscience/the-autonomic-nervous-system-integrative-systems-part-4/.

Sexual function

General issues

Sex and sexuality in people with recent or chronic disability are among the least well-managed issues within rehabilitation. Even in the absence of disability, the complexity surrounding the expression of sexuality is considerable: the presence of disability only serves to make these complexities greater. The prevalence of people reporting sexual dysfunction among the disabled population is unknown, but figures ranging from 40% to 70% have been suggested (against a background of 25–50% in the general community). For some clinicians, the issue of sexuality for people living with disabilities is deemed too embarrassing, irrelevant, or is otherwise not mentioned. There remains a degree of stigma associated with elderly or disabled people having sexual feelings or participating in sex. As an added barrier, many rehabilitation services manage acute disability, with the goal being to return the person to a level of functional independence to go home. Most often, the issue of altered sexual functioning only becomes pertinent to the person with disability after their return home. Community rehabilitation is often of lower intensity, and the person's involvement with rehabilitation services more limited, thereby minimizing opportunities for the issues of sex and sexuality to be addressed.

However, the desires and wishes for emotional and personal attachments among people with disabilities are often no different from that of the rest of the population. Most people will want to engage in some form of sexual relationship. Therefore, the importance of sex and sexuality, issues around the emotional needs of individuals with disability, and how these interactions affect families and carers, are integral to the rehabilitation of the whole person in the attempt to maximize their quality of life.

Definitions

- *Sexual function*, at its most basic level, can be taken to mean the person's ability to perform the physical act of sex, taken outside of the context of emotional needs.
- *Sexual orientation* indicates which gender/s a person is attracted to, an important determinant of sexual interest in other people.
- *Sexuality* covers how sexual function may be experienced or expressed, incorporating fantasy, desires, and behaviours and is intrinsic to the formation of relationships. The expression of sexuality can be further modified by questions of self-esteem, personal appearance, and perceived attractiveness to potential partners. Sexuality plays a full part in the lives of almost everyone in the community, irrespective of disability.
- *Sexual health* is 'a state of physical, emotional, mental and social well-being in relation to sexuality; it is not merely the absence of disease, dysfunction or infirmity. Sexual health requires a positive and respectful approach to sexuality and sexual relationships, as well as the possibility of having pleasurable and safe sexual experiences, free of coercion, discrimination and violence' (WHO's working definition).

A biopsychosocial model of sexual function

Appropriately expressing one's sexuality, whether alone, within a relationship, or in society as a whole, can present many challenges. The reasons that people want to participate in sex vary widely, partly based on gender and personality type. These differences can lead to the background tensions between peers and across society itself. Given the complexity and nature of the various influences that affect an individual's sexual function, referencing a theoretical framework enhances our capacity to address issues in the rehabilitation of sexual function. A useful model can be borrowed from the biopsychosocial model used in chronic pain management (Fig. 13.1). This structure will be used to consider different aspects of sexual rehabilitation, evaluating each domain from the centre outwards.

Physiology

In this context, physiology refers to the variety of 'plumbing and wiring' processes that are required for sexual function. The basic anatomical and neurological systems for males and females are provided in Fig. 13.2 (● see 'Male sexual function and fertility') and Fig. 13.3 (● see 'Female sexual function and fertility'). Beyond the peripheral nervous system, however, lie multiple spinal cord centres that integrate response patterns for erection, ejaculation, vaginal lubrication, orgasm, and so on. In animal studies, ascending sensory information from the spinal cord is integrated in areas of

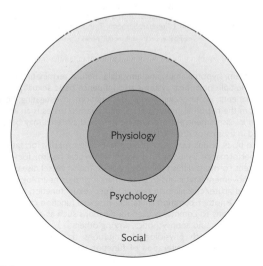

Fig. 13.1 The 'biopsychosocial' model of sexuality.

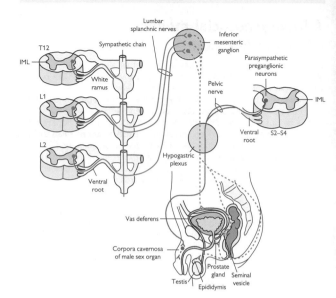

Fig. 13.2 Autonomic innervation of the male reproductive system.
Purple = sympathetic nervous system; dark grey = parasympathetic nervous
system. Solid lines = preganglionic fibres; dotted lines = postganglionic fibres. IML,
intermediolateral cell column; L, lumbar; S, sacral; T, thoracic spinal segment.
http://what-when-how.com/neuroscience/the-autonomic-nervous-system-integrative-systems-
part-4/.

the brainstem, hypothalamus, and amygdala, before terminating in cortical
regions. Multiple hormonal systems also influence basic sexual physiology,
and in patients experiencing sexual dysfunction, investigating hormone
levels from the hypothalamus, pituitary, and ovaries/testes is an important
first step in assessment. All of these neurological systems may be directly
damaged in trauma or disease states.

Whole-body issues may also affect a person's capacity for satisfactory
sexual performance including their general physical health, for example,
pre-existent co-morbidities (diabetes mellitus, major vessel disease), other
physical movement limitations (e.g. rheumatological or neurological impairments), and acute/chronic pain may all affect sexual function at a physiological level. Another common limitation in sexual function can stem from
adverse reactions to commonly used medications such as antidepressants,
antihypertensives, and antipsychotics, among others.

Any individual with physiological limitations to sexual function will
of necessity experience alteration of function within the other levels of
the model.

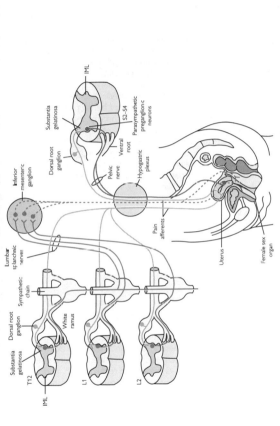

Fig. 13.3 Autonomic innervation of the female reproductive system. Purple = sympathetic nervous system; dark grey = parasympathetic nervous system; light grey = pain afferents. Solid lines = preganglionic fibres; dotted lines = postganglionic fibres. IML, intermediolateral cell column; L, Lumbar; S, sacral; T, thoracic spinal segment.

http://what-when-how.com/neuroscience/the-autonomic-nervous-system-intergrative-systems-part-4/.

Psychology

It is often said that the largest sex organ in the human body is the brain, for it is here that an individual's sexuality is created. However, there is a poor understanding of the interactions of the various supraspinal pathways. For rehabilitation purposes, it can be useful to divide the psychology domain into three major components; personality, learnt behaviour, and mood/emotional state:

- Personality traits intrinsic to an individual will influence the expression of sexuality, for example, traits such as novelty seeking, risk avoidance, extraversion, bonding, antisocial behaviours, and so on.
- Learnt behaviours: the extent to which personality variables are modifiable by experience is debatable, but certainly learnt behaviours modify sexuality and sexual behaviour. Any previous experience (whether good or bad) will tend to shape future behaviour. People who have experienced an ABI may experience personality changes that limit their ability to behave appropriately for the society in which they live.
- Mood/emotional state: at any period following a disabling event, altered feelings of self-worth, self-esteem, and/or depression may adversely affect a person's capacity to engage in sexual behaviour. Where identified, these secondary impacts may also require psychological or pharmacoactive intervention, while keeping in mind that many of the neuroactive medications can also impair sexual function.

The age of disability onset is another important modifying factor. People who experience disability prior to becoming sexually active may have never received education on contraception, for example, or had discussion of their own sexuality. Another person with a disability may be aware of their own sexual needs but lack the opportunity to discuss/act on their sexual desires due to a degree of isolation from peers.

Social

Beyond a person's individual needs and wants lie the complex rules and expectations imposed by the individual's society. Some societal rules appear to have an inheritable component, for example, the universally held taboo on incest. Many other rules exist that attempt to prevent the abuse of power or experience of one person over another, such as the age of consent. In other situations, religious edicts determine how one's sexuality should be expressed. These religio-cultural rules regarding what constitutes appropriate sexual expression are generally learned during adolescence, and it can be difficult for people migrating from one culture to another to recognize or adapt to the expectations of the culture they have moved to.

Investigating rehabilitation needs

The most commonly reported sexual dysfunctions include decreased or absent libido, decreased arousal, genital pain, impaired sex organ function, and difficulty in achieving orgasm. The impact of these problems are complicated by secondary issues such as bladder and bowel control, cognitive impairment, fatigue, reduced bed mobility, spasticity, medication use, and so on.

The clinician should consider whether a patient may have altered sexual function following a disabling event. Many people with disability will not broach the subject themselves, for fear of over-stepping social boundaries. Many clinicians avoid discussions around sexual rehabilitation from a fear of their own embarrassment or a lack of knowledge of the technicalities of sexual function. As an individual, if you are not comfortable with your own sexuality, you are at a disadvantage in assisting people who have experienced changes in theirs. An embarrassed, abrupt answer may prevent the person from asking further questions; an inappropriate outcome for the client! It is therefore important for the rehabilitation physician and other members of the team to address the subject of sexuality in an open and frank way, encouraging issues and questions to be discussed freely.

The PLISSIT model

With the wide potential impacts of disability on expressing sexuality, rehabilitation clinicians may be asked all sorts of questions. Will it work? How do we get physically close enough to each other? How do you undertake intercourse with a catheter *in situ*? What happens if I have an episode of incontinence during intercourse? What will my partner think?

Often, these questions cannot be answered generically; details will vary from one person to the next. Answering these questions also requires an approach that is sensitive to the psychosocial context of the person. A useful conceptual model for exploring and managing sexual problems is the 'PLISSIT' model. First proposed in 1976, the PLISSIT acronym stands for:

P   permission
LI limited information
SS specific suggestions
IT intensive therapy.

Seeking *permission* prior to commencing the conversation is vital to determine the person's comfort level before investigating any particular issues they wish to discuss. Often, permission will need to be requested on multiple occasions during a consultation. For example, discussing the mechanics of erection may be within a given person's comfort zone, but a discussion of oral sex may not. It is often better to approach issues regarding sex and sexuality once a rapport has been established between the clinician and the client over the course of previous consultations.

Providing *limited information* requires the clinician to have both a working knowledge of the physiology and mechanics of sex, as well as the psychological and cultural contributions. It is necessary to explore the person's understanding of what is normal, and how they feel they differ from that.

Making *specific suggestions* appropriate to the situation being discussed forms the next level of interaction. At this point, it is important for the interaction to stay relevant and be contained within the confines of negotiated permissions. This stage of the process can extend beyond the 'patient' to include other individuals. For this reason it may be relevant to seek permission to refer the issue to a third person, whether it be their partner, their urologist, psychologist, or other rehabilitation team members. The use of a specific suggestion requires a greater degree of knowledge and sensitivity from the clinician. This can be quite confronting, as relatively simple questions can overreach the knowledge base or emotional confidence of the clinician, making it hard to give advice. It is important (and appropriate) for clinicians to recognize their own limitations in these areas, and to feel comfortable saying 'I don't know, but I will help you find out' to the most difficult problems. This may mean that the specific suggestion may be as simple as providing a referral to a sexual health (genitourinary medicine) physician.

Intensive therapy often involves a 'hands-on' approach that will almost always be beyond the capacities of rehabilitation clinicians, or indeed many sexual health physicians, to offer. While 'sexologists' do exist, their services can be difficult to locate or access. Some psychosexual clinics have been established, but these are still relatively uncommon.

Using the PLISSIT approach, a useful first step is to ask about basic sexual function while considering the need for hormone testing. Depending on circumstances, medical interventions can be considered, acknowledging that there are more options for men than for women in this regard. In the absence of medical interventions, education and psychological counselling of the patient and partner plays a more primary role. This may include consideration of positioning, altering roles and expectations from lovemaking, and so on. An important issue to address is whether the individual's goals are for procreation or recreation, as procreation is dependent on fertility, a quite different goal than the ability to participate in sexual intimacy. Non-surprisingly, the approaches to fulfilling these goals may be quite different. Issues regarding contraception, risk of sexual abuse, and the person's capacity to provide consent for sex are also important considerations.

Male sexual function and fertility

The autonomic innervation of male reproductive system appears in Fig. 13.2. Simplistically, erection lies under parasympathetic control, whereas ejaculation is sympathetically mediated. In addition, somatic sensory nerve fibres ascend from the penis to spinal cord centres and rostrally to the brain. Other central fibres innervate the spinal cord centres, providing mechanisms for erection through psychological as well as physical stimulation.

Erectile dysfunction is common, resulting from impaired vasocongestion of the corpora cavernosa and spongiosa, in turn due to alterations in physiological and psychological drivers, singly or in combination. Purely psychogenic causes are estimated to account for 10–20% of erectile dysfunction, although psychological causes can be present in any organic cause as well. At the physiological level, erectile problems are more likely to occur in conditions involving vascular disease or injuries to the spinal cord. The blood supply of the penis often mirrors that of the body in general, making men with vascular diseases more likely to have erectile problems. Neurological impotence is associated with lesions of the autonomic and sensory pathways in the spinal cord or cauda equina. Men with an intact sacral portion of the spinal cord are likely to achieve reflex erection, although this may be inadequate for intercourse. Other conditions that adversely impact libido, such as depression, anxiety, post-traumatic stress disorder, hormonal imbalance, and so on, can also play a causative role. In addition, erectile dysfunction and other non-specific changes in sexual function can follow conditions such as TBI and severe MS.

Peripheral causes of erectile dysfunction can be amenable to a variety of approaches. Among the most common interventions are drugs such as sildenafil, tadalafil, and vardenafil. Sildenafil, taken an hour or so before intercourse, is useful in producing penile vasocongestion adequate for penetration in response to sensory or psychological stimulation. There is a dose-related response, but most people find that between 25 and 100 mg is sufficient, with 50 mg being the standard dose. Common side effects include headache and heartburn, and care should be exercised in men taking nitrates for coronary artery disease. It remains worth considering these agents in men with sacral or peripheral nerve injury as an aid to satisfaction with sex and erectile function.

Prostaglandin E1 (trade name Alprostadil®) has been of interest in producing penile rigidity by local stimulation of the glans penis for men unable to take sildenafil. The drug is applied with an applicator and an erection may be expected within 10–15 minutes. Older agents that can be injected directly into the penis exist but their use has decreased substantially in more recent years. Mechanical devices (e.g. pumps and penile rings), perineal electrostimulation, surgical prosthetic implants, and sacral anterior stimulator implants can also be used to achieve erection in men otherwise unresponsive to pharmaceutical approaches. A review of medication and counselling for adverse psychological states should be offered to any man where these issues are present.

Ejaculatory function is more commonly affected than erectile function in spinal cord-injured men. Only 5% of men with a complete UMN lesion and 18% with a complete LMN lesion report any persistence of the ability to achieve ejaculation. Ejaculatory function can also be affected by prostatic surgery, with retrograde ejaculation being a commonly reported problem. This is also a problem seen with older techniques such as sphincterotomy.

Premature ejaculation (PE) is another common difficulty with sexual function. The prevalence in males is estimated around 30%, irrespective of age. It is often defined as ejaculation before the man and/or his partner feels ready for this to happen. To be considered problematic, PE must be associated with distress, to either or both partners. Some men will experience PE from their first sexual experiences, whereas others develop secondary PE in later life. A number of approaches have been proposed including desensitization, anxiety management, and use of the squeeze technique. Medications that have been promoted as treatments for PE include the selective serotonin reuptake inhibitors (SSRIs) (e.g. dapoxetine which has a rapid onset and short half-life), tramadol, and topical anaesthetic spray. A daily dose of the tricyclic antidepressant clomipramine has greater efficacy than older SSRIs, but with a greater risk of side effects.

Male fertility is determined by the number, motility, and quality of sperm. Aside from genetic abnormalities, effective spermatogenesis can be impaired by low testosterone levels, elevated testicular temperatures, and decreased frequency of ejaculation. Where ejaculation is problematic, vibration applied to the penis can promote ejaculation for semen collection, as can electrical stimulation in the clinic. Vibro-ejaculation can be undertaken at home, but care is required in patients with SCIs above T6 due to the likelihood of autonomic dysreflexia.

With adequate sperm quality, any issues of sperm delivery can be bypassed by the variety of techniques used in in vitro fertilization.

Female sexual function and fertility

The autonomic innervation of the female reproductive system appears in Fig. 13.3. While obvious structural differences are evident, there remains a high degree of homology between male and female anatomy and neurology. Simplistically, clitoral and labial swelling lies under parasympathetic control. Vaginal lubrication requires an intact arterial blood supply and is under parasympathetic control, but with a strong influence from oestrogen. Vaginal and clitoral smooth muscle contraction result from sympathetic nerve activation, while the pelvic floor has both autonomic and somatic innervation. The nerves providing ascending somatic and autonomic innervation are equivalent between the sexes.

The most common forms of female sexual dysfunction include reduced or absent libido, decreased sensation, inadequate lubrication, vaginismus, dyspareunia, and/or orgasmic dysfunction. Normal female sexual function is dependent on oestrogen and testosterone, and levels should be tested in anyone with a disabling condition that could adversely affect levels. Psychogenic sexual dysfunction is also common, with libido affected by conditions such as depression, anxiety, post-traumatic stress disorder, and SSRIs. Cognitive change and fatigue can impact sexual capacity and satisfaction.

Interventions for sexual dysfunction are far more limited for women compared to men. Where deficient, hormone replacement may be needed in some patients with amenorrhoea following TBI, where pan-endocrine abnormalities are well recognized. In this context, the value of hormonal replacement has been shown for oestrogen but not testosterone per se. Vaginal lubricating agents are widely available and provide a non-pharmacological means of managing dryness. Reviewing medication with a view to changing antidepressants may be indicated. While considerable research has been undertaken into medications such as sildenafil, there is no clear role for these medications in women.

Female fertility is often preserved after disabling conditions, although there are many situations where pregnancy and delivery increase risks. The impact of structural damage, such as with pelvic fractures, requires antenatal planning to determine whether vaginal or caesarean delivery is optimal. Pregnancy carries increased risks in physically immobile women of, for instance, pressure sores and infections, particularly of the urinary tract. In the third trimester, many women may need greater assistance with transfers and bed mobility. Spinally injured women require special consideration, as those with injuries at the T10 level or above are at risk of premature delivery, and T6 and above of autonomic dysreflexia. Epidural anaesthesia or caesarean section should be considered as appropriate interventions for affected women.

Other issues in sexual rehabilitation

While clinicians can often vividly recall patients with sexual disinhibition and/or increased sexual drive, the literature reports that a reduction in the self-perceived quality or capacity for sex is by far the most common change to sexuality after a disabling incident. Individuals with such hyposexuality may report a significant reduction in quality of life as a result; however, the impact is often hidden as its effect tends to be limited to the individual and any intimate partner/s. In contrast, while the impact of hypersexuality can be profound for the person exhibiting the problem, the associated behaviour can also have a significant and sometimes devastating impact on other individuals within society.

People with disabilities (like most of the able-bodied population) may well fail to be satisfied by their initial forays into sex. Encouraging open communication between the two partners in a sexual relationship may assist relearning how to be intimate, without fear of being overwhelmed by failing to meet perceived 'expectations'. Techniques can be employed to assist function in the physical act and ensure satisfaction for the individual and for his/her partner. For those without a partner, the use of sexual surrogates is legal in some jurisdictions. For those with cardiac conditions, the general advice is that anyone who can climb a flight of stairs has the necessary cardiac reserve for intercourse.

However, the physical act of sex is only one aspect of the sexual rehabilitation paradigm. The promotion of quality of life in an open and full relationship can be more rewarding than the simple ability to perform sexual intercourse. Disabled young people may be actively hindered in expressing their own sexual feelings, or lack the freedom among their peers, in the same way that able-bodied young people may have. Very often, and particularly for young people, personal comfort with sexuality is as much a question of belonging to society as it an expression of what people want. Sexuality issues for people with acquired disabilities may be intermingled with their self-perception and self-esteem.

It is important to remember that many clinicians will not be in a place to offer sought-after advice. In this situation, the clinician's duty of care requires referral to an appropriate provider.

Further reading

Lombardi G, Musco S, Kessler TM, et al. (2015). Management of sexual dysfunction due to central nervous system disorders: a systematic review. *BJU International* 115 Suppl 6, 47–56.

Rees PM, Fowler CJ, Maas CP (2007). Sexual function in men and women with neurological disorders. *Lancet* 369, 512–525.

Scott KM, Fitzgerald CM (2011). Sexuality function and disability. In: Braddom RL (ed), *Physical Medicine and Rehabilitation*, 4th edn, pp. 661–682. Elsevier, Philadelphia, PA.

Simpson GK, Baguley IJ (2012). Prevalence, correlates, mechanisms, and treatment of sexual health problems after traumatic brain injury: a scoping review. *Critical Reviews in Physical and Rehabilitation Medicine* 23, 215–250.

Useful websites

British Society for Sexual Medicine: ℰ http://bssm.org.uk/resources.

Sexual Health Rehabilitation (British Columbia Institute of Technology): ℰ http://www.bcit.ca/health/industry/sexualrehab.shtml.

Wikipedia—'Sexual dysfunction': ℰ https://en.wikipedia.org/wiki/Sexual_dysfunction.

Skin problems

Introduction

Skin is the largest organ of the human body, measuring around 2 square metres and 16% of body weight in adults. The two main layers of skin are a superficial epidermis and a deep dermis that is four times the thickness of epidermis. The dermis has loose connective tissue along with blood vessels and nerves supplying the skin. Subcutaneous tissue is between the dermis and underlying muscle and bone. In tissue injury, normal wound healing is a complex and dynamic process with four main phases (Fig. 14.1).

This chapter will include some of the common skin-related problems encountered in rehabilitation settings, such as pressure ulcers, chronic venous ulcers, ischaemic ulcers, mixed ulcers, and osteomyelitis as a complication of chronic ulcers. The management of skin problems in amputees is described in more detail in ⮞ Chapter 41.

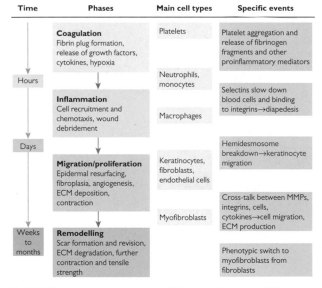

Fig. 14.1 Phases in normal wound healing. ECM, extracellular matrix; MMPs, matrix metalloproteinases.

Pressure ulcers

Definition

A pressure ulcer is an area of localized damage to the skin and underlying tissue caused by pressure, shear, and friction, either individually or in combination. It is usually observed over a bony prominence such as the occiput, sacrum, ischium, greater trochanter, or calcaneum. The risk of pressure ulcers is highest in patients with critical illness, neurological impairments, immobility, and/or malnutrition.

Applied pressure relates to compression forces that act on the soft tissues equally along all axes. This normally causes no tissue damage, but when applied over a prolonged period of time can occlude blood flow and lead to tissue ischaemia and damage. Shear force refers to the tangential force acting parallel to the plane and causes damage when combined with applied pressure. When there is slip between two surfaces, it is referred to as friction, which increases the risk of tissue damage.

Features

- The prevalence in hospitalized patients varies between 4% and 60% depending on healthcare system and year of publication. Major efforts have been made to reduce the incidence of pressure areas, and it is now estimated to be around 5% in recent data extracted from the NHS in the UK.[1]
- The economic burden to healthcare is immense and reported to be £1.4–2.1 billion in the UK per annum (equivalent to 4% of total National Health Service (NHS) expenditure).
- They cause significant mortality and morbidity including pain, infection, osteomyelitis, extended hospital stay, amputation, and death.
- About 95% of pressure ulcers are totally preventable with vigilance, and high standards of nursing and medical management.
- They are characterized initially by persistent skin erythema where pressure from friction forces injures blood vessels in the skin; this results in ischaemia, cell necrosis, and superficial ulceration.
- Deeper structures may be affected by shear forces occurring in the proximity to bony prominences, which give rise to more extensive subcutaneous destruction through damage to subcutaneous blood vessels.
- Any necrotic tissue in a pressure sore is at high risk of becoming infected, causing secondary inflammation of surrounding tissues and systemic toxicity.
- Factors that impair the normal tensile strength of skin increase the likelihood of skin breakdown. These factors include maceration of the skin by sweat and urine, and reduced skin thickness as seen in elderly people and in people with a SCI.

See Table 14.1 and Fig. 14.2 for clinical features and stages.

Table 14.1 Pressure ulcer grades

Stage/grade	Feature
I. Erythema	Non-blanchable erythema of intact skin
II. Blistering or shallow open ulcer	Partial-thickness skin loss involving epidermis, dermis, or both.
III. Full-thickness skin loss with visible subcutaneous tissue	Skin loss involving damage to subcutaneous tissue down to (but not through) fascia. Slough may be present
IV. Deeper tissue involvement with or without full thickness skin loss	Involves muscle, tendon, bone, or joint. Often includes undermining and tunnelling. Slough may be present

Risk factors for pressure ulcers

The risk factors for pressure ulcers are cumulative, in that the more risks an individual has, the greater the likelihood of skin breakdown. These factors include the following:

- Immobility after illness, especially:
  - motor weakness
  - muscle atrophy
  - obesity
  - coma/confusion
  - critically illness
  - those with bladder/bowel incontinence.
- Sensory loss due to:
  - SCI/brain injury
  - neuropathy/diabetes.
- Ischaemia due to:
  - sepsis
  - peripheral shutdown
  - arterial injury or microangiopathy
  - anaemia.
- Nutritional deficiency:
  - Weight loss
  - Low protein
  - Anaemia
  - Dehydration.
- Deformity producing abnormal loads:
  - Fractures
  - Contractures
  - Spasticity.
- Lifestyle/psychosocial factors:
  - Smoking/substance abuse
  - Family/carer support
  - Access to healthcare.

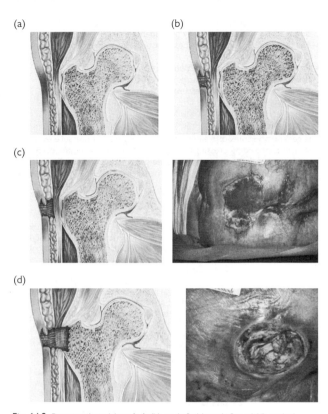

Fig. 14.2 Pressure ulcers (a) grade 1; (b) grade 2; (c) grade 3; and (d) grade 4.

Reproduced with permission from Grey J., et al. Pressure ulceration and leg ulcers in *Managing Older People in Primary Care: A practical guide*, Gosney M. and Harris T. (Eds.). Oxford, UK: Oxford University Press. © 2009 Oxford University Press. Reproduced with permission of Oxford University Press through PLSclear. http://oxfordmedicine.com/view/10.1093/med/9780199546589.001.0001/med-9780199546589-chapter-18.

Prevention

- Early risk assessment (within 6 hours of hospital admission). Multiple scales are available including the Norton, Waterlow, and Braden scales.[2–4] These measures are used in conjunction with clinical judgement to highlight risk.
- Preventive measures and education of 'at-risk' patients.
- Repositioning in chair and bed every 2–3 hours.

- Avoid lateral decubitus positions; 30° side-lying positions are preferred due to lower pressure on bony prominences.
- Management of pain, deformities, spasticity, incontinence, and contractures.
- Protection from shearing/friction forces (e.g. protecting of heels in patients with knee flexor spasms).
- Provision of customized pressure-relieving mattresses, seating, and cushions.

Management

The general principles of treatment are avoiding further pressure to the affected area, providing dressings to the wound, and elevating the body part where practical. It is important to titrate pain management against the risk of sedation and/or confusion. Other management issues are presented in Table 14.2.

Table 14.2 Management of pressure ulcers

Physical/topical measures	Relief of pressure is the most important factor (every 2 hours for those lying in bed and every 15 minutes for those sitting)
	Pressure relief mattresses
	Appropriate dressings based on ulcer status (hydrocolloid/hydrogel for minimally draining/dry yellow slough/granulating wounds; alginate-based dressing and foam for heavily draining wounds; and negative pressure dressing for cavitating ulcers)
	Use antibiotics in presence of infection and raised inflammatory markers
	Prompt debridement of necrotic tissue (using surgical instruments, irrigation, or chemical agents)
Surgery (adjunct to conservative therapy in select cases)	For grade III and IV wounds
	Formal plastic and reconstructive surgery—to provide skin and muscle flaps for weight-bearing areas (buttock, sacrum, trochanter), as a skin graft alone will often not survive the stresses and strains
	Tension free closure and pressure offloading from reconstructed area and customized seating
	Perioperative antibiotic therapy
General health	Correct dietary deficiencies, e.g. adequate protein: at least 1–1.5 g/kg/day for those with pressure ulcer(s)
	Adequate fluid intake
	Haematinics to treat anaemia
	Treatment of constipation/faecal loading
	Prevention of urinary/faecal incontinence
	Cut down on smoking
Adjuvant therapeutic modalities	Hydrotherapy (whirlpool, pulsatile lavage therapy)
	Electrical stimulation/therapeutic ultrasound/electromagnetic therapy
	Negative pressure wound therapy (vac pack)

Leg ulcers

The prevalence of leg ulcers ranges from 1 to 3 per 1000 population and can rise to 8.5% in those aged more than 65 years. The commonest causes of chronic ulcers are:
- venous ulcers (60–70%)
- mixed ulcers (15–20%)
- arterial (10%)
- systemic diseases and unusual causes (5%).

Venous ulcers are associated with chronic venous stasis (or insufficiency) and are typically seen in the lower third of leg. The dysfunction of the venous system could be due to various factors such as varicose veins, deep venous thrombosis, calf muscle complex inactivity, or heart failure. The high pressure within the veins causes leakage of plasma, proteins, fibrin, and haemosiderin into the tissues causing oedema, itching, eczema, hyperpigmentation, and induration of the skin (lipidermosclerosis). Most venous ulcers will heal with a combination of compression therapy and suitable dressings (similar principles to pressure sore dressings) and antibiotic therapy in select cases that present with systemic symptoms. A broad-spectrum antibiotic is started and then altered based on the sensitivity of the organism shown in cultures. Ulcer debridement to remove the dead and necrotic tissue will be needed in some cases to optimize healing.

Arterial ulcers are observed in the context of cardiovascular disease and peripheral arterial disease. They are also seen in end-vessel microangiopathy as in diabetes and end-stage renal disease. They are most usually seen in the toes and foot/ankle area, presenting as deep, punched-out ulcers with necrotic tissue underneath, appearing dry and with minimal surrounding oedema. The skin is often shiny, pale, or cold with reduced pulses and delayed capillary refill time.

The key principle in the management of these ulcers is to measure the ankle/brachial pressure index (ABPI) and Doppler ultrasound assessment of lower limb pulses. ABPI determines the percentage of blood flow to the feet. A reading of 1.0–1.3 indicates normal arterial blood flow and indicates high compression bandage/stockings can be used in the management (using pressures <40 mmHg for venous ulcers). A reading of 0.8–1.0 indicates mild arterial disease and compression dressings can still be used with caution and reduced pressure settings (15–20 mmHg). An ABPI of 0.5–0.8 indicates moderate arterial impairment, while less than 0.5 indicates critical limb ischaemia and compression dressings are contraindicated. Ischaemic ulcers need management of underlying arterial insufficiency including peripheral vascular angiography, angioplasty, and bypass surgery in cases of critical ischaemia.

Osteomyelitis is seen in approximately 25% of non-healing ulcers. Blood tests, X-ray, bone scan, and MRI scan help diagnose a bone infection and when diagnosed, a long course of broad-spectrum antibiotics (usually 12 weeks) is recommended. Surgical debridement will be indicated in some cases for removal of dead necrotic sequestrum. Plastic reconstruction flaps are undertaken only after infection is adequately managed. There is evidence to support hyperbaric oxygen therapy in recurrent osteomyelitis or osteomyelitis in an immunocompromised individual.

References

1. National Institute for Health and Care Excellence (NICE) (2014). *Pressure Ulcers: Prevention and Management*. Clinical Guideline [CG179]. NICE, London. ℘ http://www.nice.org.uk/guidance/cg179.
2. Norton D (1961). Preventing pressure sores of heels. *Nursing Times* 57, 695–696.
3. Waterlow J (1985). Pressure sores: a risk assessment card. *Nursing Times* 81, 49–55.
4. Braden BJ, Bergstrom N (1994). Predictive validity of the Braden Scale for pressure sore risk in a nursing home. *Research in Nursing & Health* 17, 459–470.

Further reading

Grey J, Stevens J, Harding K (2009). Pressure ulceration and leg ulcers. In: *Managing Older People in Primary Care: A Practical Guide*, pp. 211–234. Oxford University Press, Oxford.
Qaseem A, Humphrey LL, Forciea, M.A., et al. (2015). Treatment of pressure ulcers: a clinical practice guideline from the American College of Physicians. *Annals of Internal Medicine* 162, 370–379.

Useful website

℘ https://www.safetythermometer.nhs.uk/—the NHS 'Safety Thermometer' point-of-care survey instrument.

Injections in rehabilitation medicine

Introduction

Injection-based interventions are a useful addition to the rehabilitation physician's practice. These can occur in either inpatient or outpatient settings and be for musculoskeletal (e.g. joint/soft tissue injections) or neurological conditions (such as antispasticity injections and nerve blocks).

Musculoskeletal injections

Joint and soft tissue injections

- Local steroid injection is a well-proven and effective treatment for focal pain and inflammation. It is used in inflammatory arthritis, osteoarthritis, tendinopathy, tenosynovitis, bursitis, trigger points, and other 'overuse' conditions.
- Steroid injection can permit an increased ROM and facilitate rehabilitation exercises.
- Systemic absorption and side effects are minimal.
- The recommended practice is not to repeat joint steroid injections more than four times in a year.
- Contraindications are broken skin/infection at injection site, systemic illness, prosthetic joint/s, and hypersensitivity to injection agents.
- Caution is needed in patients with coagulopathies, on anticoagulants such as warfarin (avoid injections when international normalized ratio (INR) is >3).[1] For those on newer oral anticoagulants (such as apixaban or rivaroxaban) that cannot be monitored by INR levels, interruption of anticoagulants is not necessary for simple steroid/local anaesthetic injections. For other interventional procedures (such as dry needling), avoiding during peak activity (e.g. 2–4 hours after dose for rivaroxaban) is recommended.
- Injected agents are steroids and local anaesthetics, either alone or in combination. Local anaesthetic injections are commonly used for diagnostic purposes whereas combined steroid and local anaesthetic is for therapeutic use. Adding local anaesthetic helps provide transient pain relief until the steroid effect starts. It is better to warn patients that there may be a period of worse pain after the local anaesthetic wears off before the steroid takes effect on the day following injection.
- See Tables 15.1 and 15.2 for dosage and duration of action.[2] The steroid dose varies depending on the target structure, for example, the triamcinolone acetonide dose can be 40 mg for a large joint, whereas it is 5–10 mg for a hand joint.
- Dexamethasone phosphate and betamethasone phosphate are freely soluble and hence are non-particulate. Triamcinolone and methylprednisolone are particulate steroids. Triamcinolone has lower solubility than methylprednisolone, leading to a longer

Table 15.1 Dose and duration of action of commonly used steroids for injections

Steroid	Typical dose (comparative)	Duration of action (approximate)
Methylprednisolone acetate	40–80 mg	8 days
Triamcinolone acetonide	20–40 mg	14 days
Betamethasone phosphate	6–12 mg	6 days
Dexamethasone phosphate	4–8 mg	6 days

Table 15.2 Dose and duration of action of commonly used local anaesthetics for injections

Local anaesthetic	Onset of action	Duration of action (approximate)	Maximum volume of injection
1% lidocaine	1–2 min	1 h	20 mL
0.5% ropivacaine	3–15 min	6 h	60 mL
0.25% bupivacaine	30 min	8 h	60 mL
0.5% bupivacaine	30 min	8 h	30 mL

duration of action but a higher incidence of cutaneous side effects. Methylprednisolone might be preferred for injections into superficial structures for this reason.
• Patients with diabetes should be monitored for fluctuations in blood glucose. The soft tissue steroid injections are more prone to raise glucose levels than a single steroid injection. These fluctuations can persist for up to 1–3 weeks. Steroid injections are also less effective in diabetic patients when compared to non-diabetics.
• Steroid injections have been shown to suppress the hypothalamic–pituitary–adrenal axis and patients must be warned not to engage in activities with a high risk of trauma, infection, or stress for 2 weeks after the injection. This will apply to sporting activities as well.
• The most common complications of steroid injections are post-injection flare (2–10%), skin atrophy (1%), fat atrophy (1%), facial flushing (1%), and tendon rupture (1%). Less common side effects are iatrogenic infection, allergy, or life-threatening anaphylaxis.
• Injection of steroid into a tendon must be avoided as it predisposes to weakening of tendon and rupture.
• Local anaesthetics inhibit nerve excitation and provide local analgesia and nerve block. Known side effects are hypersensitivity including life-threatening anaphylaxis and cardiac and CNS toxicity if the safe limit for total dose is exceeded (Table 15.2).
• Image guidance is increasingly being used for injections. It enables the injector to plan a safe access route to target, is more accurate, less painful than surface landmark injections, and potentially has a better clinical outcome. Ultrasonography is commonly used for soft tissue injections whereas X-ray/computed tomography (CT) guidance is used for bony and joint injections, particularly spine injections.

Injection agents and procedures

Commonly injectable substances, procedures, their mechanism of action, and indications are listed in Table 15.3.

Table 15.3 Common musculoskeletal injections and procedures

Common agents	Mechanism of action	Indications
Local anaesthesia	Inhibits nerve excitation, analgesia	Bone, soft tissue, nerve pain condition
Corticosteroids	Anti-inflammatory, analgesia	Bone, soft tissue, nerve pain condition
Hyaluronic acid	Joint viscosupplementation, analgesia	Joint osteoarthritis
Autologous substances (blood, platelet-rich plasma)	Promotes tendon healing	Chronic tendinopathy
Sclerosants (polidocanol, aqueous phenol)	Sclerosis of neovascularity in tendinopathy	Chronic tendinopathy
Prolotherapy	Soft tissue inflammation by injection of hyperosmolar solution	Chronic low back pain, chronic tendinopathy
Dry needling	Promotes healing and regeneration	Chronic tendinopathy
Hydrostatic distension	Mechanical disruption of neovessels to tendon	Chronic tendinopathy
Ozone	Oxidizing agent, anti-inflammatory, promotes healing	Disc herniation
Phenol (in water/in glycerol)	Nerve block (lower concentration) and chemical neurolysis (higher concentration)	Painful neuroma, neurolysis for spasticity management, chemical sympathectomy
Alcohol	Neurolysis, analgesia	Painful neuroma, trigeminal neuralgia, neurolysis for spasticity management
Glycerol	Neurolysis, analgesia	Trigeminal neuralgia
Radiofrequency	Neurolysis, analgesia	Radiculopathies, facet pain, arthritis
Cryotherapy	Neurolysis	Painful neuroma
Cement	Structural support to bone, pain relief	Acute painful vertebral fractures

Botulinum toxin injection

- BoNT is used as a chemodenervating agent that inhibits acetylcholine release at the neuromuscular junction, in spindle cells and glandular tissue. It is used in managing spasticity seen in UMN syndrome after damage to the CNS[3,4] (🔍 see Chapter 10 for further information on spasticity). It is also used in treatment of movement disorders (such as dystonia, hemifacial spasm, and bruxism), hypersecretory disorders, eye disorders (such as strabismus), and chronic pain conditions.[3,4]

- Sialorrhoea or drooling can become a troublesome symptom in some neurological conditions such as Parkinson's disease, MND, and brain injury. Botulinum toxin injection of salivary glands can help reduce the saliva production. Parotid glands alone are injected first and in cases with no desired response, both parotid and submandibular glands are targeted. There is a risk of dysphagia in case toxin spreads beyond the salivary gland capsule.

- The three commonest commercial formulations of BoNT-A with proven efficacy in spasticity are Dysport® (manufactured by Ipsen), Botox® (manufactured by Allergan), and Xeomin® (manufactured by Merz). The three products use different biological assays and there is no internationally recognized dose comparison between the units for specific patient groups.

- The dose will vary and needs to be assessed for each individual. It is common to start with low doses and titrate upwards depending on response. Maximum doses should not exceed (a) 1000 U Dysport®/600 U Botox® in total per session or (b) 200 U Dysport®/50 U Botox® per injection site.

- Current practice recommends that injections are made as near to the motor end plates as possible; however, this area needs further research. For example, the end plates are concentrated around an inverted V-shaped zone in the middle of biceps muscle belly (Fig. 15.1).

- Multiple injections and larger volumes are preferred for larger muscles, whereas single doses of smaller volumes are more common for smaller muscles.

- The clinical effect of injection is generally seen after 4–7 days and lasts for 3–4 months in most cases.

- Injections should ideally not be repeated within 3 months due to a theoretical risk of reduced efficacy due to neutralizing antibodies following repeated BoNT injections. The incidence of antibody formation for current formulations is estimated to be less than 1%. In such cases, BoNT-B (Neurobloc® or Myobloc®) is used as there is no cross-reaction with type B toxin. Alternatively, giving a toxin holiday for 6 months might work in some patients who will start responding again to toxin A.

- Systemic side effects are rare and include flu-like symptoms, anaphylaxis, and fatigue. Occasional patients develop generalized weakness, reminiscent of botulism. This temporary complication appears more likely with larger doses. Local side effects due to spread of toxin can

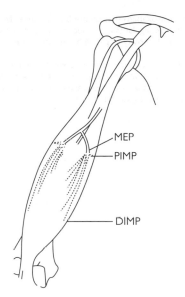

Fig. 15.1 Motor end plates of biceps brachii muscle. DIMP, distal limit of the intramuscular motor point; MEP, motor entry point; PIMP, proximal limit of the intramuscular motor point.

Reproduced with permission from Lee et al. Localization of motor entry points and terminal intramuscular nerve endings of the musculocutaneous nerve to biceps and brachialis muscles. *Surgical and Radiological Anatomy*, 32(3): 213–220. © Springer-Verlag 2009. https://doi.org/10.1007/s00276-009-0561-4.

cause weakness of adjacent muscles, dysphagia in case of neck muscle or sialorrhoea injections, or ptosis in facial injections.
- EMG guidance can be used to identify spastic muscles by hearing involuntary motor unit action potentials—the sound is greater when the needle is closer to the motor end plate. Ultrasound guidance is used to target specific muscles by allowing real-time visualization of needle advancement in to the muscle. This makes it a better option (than EMG) for targeting specific muscles but does not have the advantage of EMG for ensuring the muscle injected is spastic. There is some evidence to support superior clinical results for guided injections when compared to injections based on anatomical localization.
- Caution is needed in patients with coagulopathies, on anticoagulants such as warfarin (avoid injections when INR >3.5). Use of thinner needles (27 G) and ultrasound guidance will reduce the chances of bleeding complications. For those on newer oral anticoagulants (such

as apixaban or rivaroxaban) that cannot be monitored by INR levels, interruption of anticoagulants is not necessary. Injections could be avoided during peak activity (e.g. 2–4 hours after dose for rivaroxaban) as an extra precaution.
• BoNT should be injected only as a component of a multimodal approach to spasticity that includes prevention of aggravating factors, physical therapy, splinting/orthotics, regular review by the MDT, and measuring outcome using validated scales.

Injection techniques

A guide to the use of appropriate general techniques in listed in Box 15.1. There will be special additional techniques or precautions to take for specific procedures such as use of a centrifuge device for platelet-rich plasma injections. It is recommended that all procedures be performed in reasonably equipped settings by trained clinicians. Most of the procedures discussed in this chapter can be performed in the outpatient clinic environment, provided sterile techniques can be maintained and appropriate resuscitation equipment are available for managing adverse effects and emergencies.

There are many different ways of learning injection techniques: training on silicone models, training on cadavers, apprenticeship under an experienced injector, simulated and actual videos, and seminars. The apprentice model is regarded as the best model as the learner has the opportunity to learn from mistakes in real situations that are difficult to be simulated in other methods of learning.

Box 15.1 Musculoskeletal Injection techniques

- Relevant history, examination, and confirm diagnosis.
- Perform diagnostic ultrasound scan if indicated and for guidance.
- Exclude contraindications.
- Discuss all treatment options and shared decision-making.
- Supply appropriate information leaflet.
- Check allergies and current medication list.
- Check INR and blood glucose level if indicated.
- Obtain and record informed consent.
- Check drug name, strength, dose, dilution, and expiry.
- Use separate needles for drawing up drugs and injection.
- Use sterile non-touch technique and sterile single-use syringe and needle.
- Sterile dressing after injection.
- Dispose of sharps appropriately.
- Observe patients for 20–30 minutes post injection for immediate adverse effects. Discuss about driving risks if indicated depending on injection site.

References

1. Conway R, O'Shea FD, Cunnane G, Doran MF (2013). Safety of joint and soft tissue injections in patients on warfarin anticoagulation. *Clinical Rheumatology* 32, 1811–1814.
2. Stephens MB, Beutler AI, O'Connor FG (2008). Musculoskeletal injections: a review of the evidence. *American Family Physician* 78, 971–976.
3. Wissel J, Ward AB, Erztgaard P, et al. (2009). European consensus table on the use of botulinum toxin type A in adult spasticity. *Journal of Rehabilitation Medicine* 41, 13–25.
4. Royal College of Physicians (RCP) (2009). *Spasticity in Adults: Management using Botulinum Toxin*. RCP, London.

Further reading

Elmadbouh H. Introduction to musculoskeletal injections. In: Hutson M, Ward A (eds) *Oxford Textbook of Musculoskeletal Medicine*, 2nd edn, pp. 236–259. Oxford University Press, Oxford.
Saunders S, Longworth S (2006). *Injection Techniques in Orthopaedics and Sports Medicine with CD-ROM: A Practical Manual for Doctors and Physiotherapists*. Elsevier, Edinburgh.

Useful websites

Practical videos on joint injection techniques can be accessed online:
🔗 http://learning.bmj.com/learning/home.html.
🔗 http://www.injectiontechniquesonline.com/.

Cardiac rehabilitation

Definition

Cardiac rehabilitation (and secondary prevention) services are comprehensive, long-term programs involving medical evaluation, prescribed exercise, cardiac risk factor modification, education, and counselling. These programs are designed to limit the physiologic and psychological effects of cardiac illness, reduce the risk for sudden death or re-infarction, control cardiac symptoms, stabilize or reverse the atherosclerotic process, and enhance the psychosocial and vocational status of selected patients.[1]

While exercise training remains a cornerstone intervention, current practice guidelines consistently recommend 'comprehensive rehabilitation' programmes containing the necessary core components to optimize cardiovascular risk reduction, foster healthy behaviours (and the compliance to these behaviours), reduce disability, and promote an active lifestyle.

Epidemiology

- Incidence—common: in the UK, around 110,000 men and 65,000 women have an acute myocardial infarction (MI) every year, equivalent to one every 3 minutes. Yearly, 785,000 new and 470,000 recurrent MIs occur in the US.
- Prevalence: with improved survival and an ageing population, the number of people living with coronary heart disease (CHD) in the UK has increased to an estimated 2.3 million.
- Mortality: although mortality from CHD has fallen over recent decades, annually it still claims an estimated 1.8 million lives per annum in Europe.
- Disability: loss of physical, psychological, or social functioning following hospital discharge can lead to impaired health-related quality of life. The effectiveness and accessibility of cardiac rehabilitation and secondary preventions services after a cardiac illness have therefore never been more important.

Patient groups can benefit from cardiac rehabilitation
- Acute coronary syndrome (ACS)
- Coronary artery bypass surgery (CABG)
- Percutaneous coronary intervention (PCI)
- Chronic heart failure (CHF)
- Heart transplant and ventricular assist device
- Implantation of intra-cardiac defibrillator/cardiac resynchronization therapy.

Core components

The core components of a cardiac rehabilitation programme are illustrated in Fig. 16.1 and include:
- health behaviour change and education
- lifestyle risk factor management:
  - physical activity and exercise
  - diet
  - smoking cessation
- psychosocial health
- medical risk factor management
- cardioprotective therapies
- long-term management
- audit and evaluation.

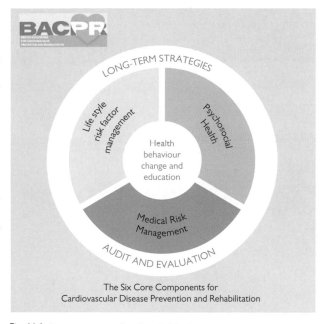

Fig. 16.1 Core components of cardiac rehabilitation.
BACPR Standards and Core Components 2017.

Delivery of the core components requires expertise from a range of different professionals. The team may include:
- physician: cardiologist, rehabilitation physician, or GP with a special interest
- nurse specialist
- physiotherapist
- dietician
- psychologist
- exercise specialist
- occupational therapist
- clerical administrator.

Assessment

All eligible patients with ACS/MI and all patients immediately post CABG or post PCI should be referred to a comprehensive rehabilitation and secondary prevention programme, either prior to hospital discharge or at the first follow-up visit. The programmes should start as soon as possible after hospital admission. Cardiac rehabilitation and secondary prevention are generally considered most beneficial when delivered soon after the cardiac event as soon as the patient is stable. To ensure effective access to rehabilitation and preventive services, referral should be considered by all healthcare practitioners with responsibility for the care of cardiac patients and within the 12 months following their acute event or cardiac surgery.

An individual tailored patient-specific plan for cardiac rehabilitation and secondary prevention should be formulated based on a patient risk assessment at discharge or as soon as possible after hospital admission and prior to initiation of the programme. This risk assessment should systematically collect and document the clinical information as shown in Table 16.1.

Exercise testing and training

Symptom-limited exercise testing prior to participation in the exercise component of a comprehensive cardiac rehabilitation programme is strongly recommended.

Exercise test parameters should include assessment of:
- symptoms of CHD
- heart rate and rhythm
- blood pressure (BP)
- ST-segment changes on electrocardiography
- exercise capacity
- perceived exertion (e.g. Borg scale of perceived exertion).

Based on this exercise test, patients can then be risk stratified to select the appropriate level of supervision and monitoring required during the exercise component of their rehabilitation programme.

Exercise training should be an individualized exercise prescription for aerobic training that is regularly reviewed by the programme team and modified if necessary.

Current recommendations for exercise prescription are as follows:
- Frequency: three to five sessions per week.
- Intensity: 50–80% of maximal exercise capacity.
- Duration: 20–60 minutes per session.
- Modality: walking, treadmill, cycling, rowing, stair climbing, arm/leg ergometry, and others using continuous or interval training as appropriate.
- Exercise-based rehabilitation programmes can also include resistance exercise.

Table 16.1 Patient risk assessment and clinical data collection

Clinical history	Screening for cardiovascular risk factors, co-morbidities and disabilities, psychological stress, vocational situation
Symptoms	Cardiovascular disease (NYHA functional class for dyspnoea and Canadian Cardiovascular Society class for symptoms of angina)
Medication	Including dose, frequency, side effects
Adherence	To medical regimen and self-monitoring (weight, BP, symptoms)
Physical examination	General health status, BMI, waist circumference, heart failure signs, cardiac and carotid murmurs, pulse, BP control, extremities for presence of arterial pulses, musculoskeletal and neurological abnormalities
ECG and cardiac imagining	Heart rate, rhythm, repolarization. Two-dimensional and Doppler echocardiography: in particular ventricular function, valvular heart disease, presence of effusion where appropriate
Blood testing	Routine biochemical assay: including full blood count, electrolytes, renal and liver function, fasting blood glucose (HbA1C if fasting blood glucose is elevated or known diabetes) and serum lipids (total cholesterol, LDL-C, HDL-C, and triglycerides)
Physical activity level by history	Domestic, occupational, and recreational needs; activities relevant to age, sex, and daily life; readiness to change behaviour; self-confidence; barriers to increased physical activity, and social support in making positive changes
Peak exercise capacity	Symptom-limited exercise testing, either on bicycle ergometer, or on treadmill. If this is not feasible (e.g. because of recent surgery), submaximal exercise evaluation and/or a walk test should be considered
Education	Clear, comprehensible information on the basic purpose of the cardiac rehabilitation programme and the role of each component (including optimal medical therapy compliance); education on the self-monitoring (weight, BP, warning symptoms and signs of instability, e.g. angina, dyspnoea) and self-management

HDL-C, high-density lipoprotein cholesterol; LDL-C, low-density lipoprotein cholesterol; NYHA, New York Heart Association.

Education

Current guidelines for education include its role in:
- positively impacting healthy behaviour
- cardiovascular risk factor modification
- improving adherence to cardioprotective medications
- providing psychosocial support, vocational guidance, and sexual functioning (➲ see Table 16.3 in 'Comprehensive risk factor management')
- improving health-related quality of life
- improving the patient's motivation and ability to comprehend a broad array of information

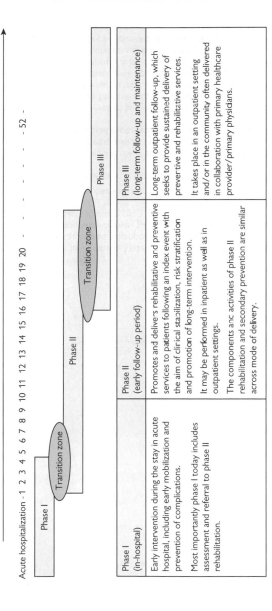

Weeks

Acute hospitalization - 1 2 3 4 5 6 7 8 9 10 11 12 13 14 15 16 17 18 19 20 - - - - - - 52 -

Phase I

Transition zone

Phase II

Transition zone

Phase III

Phase I (in-hospital)	Phase II (early follow-up period)	Phase III (long-term follow-up and maintenance)
Early intervention during the stay in acute hospital, including early mobilization and prevention of complications.	Promotes and delivers rehabilitative and preventive services to patients following an index event with the aim of clinical stabilization, risk stratification and promotion of long-term intervention.	Long-term outpatient follow-up, which seeks to provide sustained delivery of preventive and rehabilitative services.
Most importantly phase I today includes assessment and referral to phase II rehabilitation.	It may be performed in inpatient as well as in outpatient settings.	It takes place in an outpatient setting and/or in the community often delivered in collaboration with primary healthcare provider/primary physicians.
	The components and activities of phase II rehabilitation and secondary prevention are similar across mode of delivery.	

Fig. 16.2 The cardiac rehabilitation pathway following acute hospitalization.

Morrow, David, *Myocardial Infarction: A Companion to Braunwald's Heart Disease*, 2015, with permission from Elsevier.

Psychosocial support

The relationship between psychosocial and cardiac health is complex, and both direct (e.g. psychological effects on immunological function) and indirect (e.g. behaviourally mediated) mechanisms are thought to play a role. Consequently, patients may be offered a wide variety of psychological treatments to treat depression, anxiety, stress, or maladaptive behaviours, and these treatments aim to improve both psychological and cardiac health.

The concepts underpinning most of the psychosocial treatments for cardiac patients are:

- CHD and associated treatments may cause psychological distress
- psychological symptoms may cause or exacerbate cardiac disease
- unhealthy behaviours may increase when people experience psychological distress
- psychological strategies may be useful in modifying risky behaviours.

Major depressive disorder affects approximately 20% of individuals with CHD and:

- has a bidirectional relationship (i.e. CHD can cause depression)
- is an independent risk factor for CHD and its complications
- predicts worse medical outcomes including: poorer health-related quality of life, increased morbidity, and greater use of healthcare.

Comprehensive risk factor management

As summarized in Tables 16.2 and 16.3, risk factor management plays a pivotal role in comprehensive cardiac rehabilitation and secondary prevention.

Physical activity counselling

Regular physical activity is associated with a reduced risk of fatal and non-fatal coronary events in healthy individuals, those with coronary risk factors, and cardiac patients over a wide age range. A sedentary lifestyle is one of the major risk factors for cardiovascular diseases. Regular physical activity is therefore suggested by guidelines as a very important non-pharmacological component for risk factor control in primary as well as secondary prevention.

Smoking cessation

Smoking is associated with an increased risk of all types of cardiovascular and coronary artery diseases. Stopping smoking after a heart attack is considered one of the most effective preventative initiatives. Evidence points towards the risk of cardiovascular disease approaching the risk of never-smokers within 10–15 years of cessation. However, stopping smoking is a complex and difficult process because the habit is strongly addictive both pharmacologically and psychologically. The most important predictor of successful quitting is motivation, which can be increased by professional assistance. Sign posting to smoking cessation services is an important part of cardiac rehabilitation and secondary prevention.

In addition to psychosocial interventions which can encourage smoking cessation, nicotine replacement therapy, bupropion or varenicline, can be offered to assist cessation. No increase in adverse cardiac events for bupropion was found but concerns about adverse cardiac events caused by varenicline have been raised.

Nutritional counselling and weight management

Dietary behaviour has direct effects on weight, serum lipids, BP, blood sugar and insulin sensitivity, cardiac rhythm, endothelial function, and oxidative stress, all factors associated with cardiovascular health and disease. Poor diet may therefore increase the risk of coronary events and healthy eating is expected to decrease the risk.

Systematic reviews of patients with coronary artery disease or undergoing PCI have suggested an 'obesity paradox' whereby obesity appears protective against an adverse prognosis. Based on this evidence, current guidelines agree that clinicians should encourage weight maintenance/reduction through an appropriate balance of lifestyle, physical activity, structured exercise, diet, and formal behavioural programme when indicated to achieve or maintain a BMI between 18.5 and 24.9 kg/m^2.

Table 16.2 Assessment, clinical interventions, and expected outcomes for behavioural interventions following acute MI

Area of interest / Treatment goal	Evaluation/assessment	Intervention	Expected outcomes
Physical activity counselling • *Minimum 2.5 hours/ week of moderate aerobic activity, in multiple bouts each lasting ≥10 minutes* • *30 minutes a day/ 5–7 days per week* • *Complementary resistance training 2 days a week*	Assess current physical activity level and determine domestic, occupational, and recreational needs Evaluate which activities are relevant Assess readiness to change behaviour, self-confidence, and barriers	*Recommend:* gradual increases in daily lifestyle activities over time, incorporated into the daily routine, i.e. minimum 5 days a week *Emphasize:* sedentary lifestyle as a risk factor *Advise:* individualize physical activity according to patient's age, past habits, co-morbidities, preferences, and goals *Reassure:* regarding the safety of the recommended protocol *Encourage:* involvement in leisure activities which are enjoyable *Forewarn:* inform patients on the risk of relapses *If physical activity interruption has occurred, physical, social, and psychological barriers should be explored, and alternative approaches suggested*	Increased participation in physical activities Improved psychosocial well-being Prevention of disability Improved aerobic fitness and body composition
Smoking cessation *Non-smoker*	Smoking status and use of other tobacco products Amount of smoking (per day, and number of years) Determine readiness to change; if ready, choose a date for quitting	All smokers should be encouraged professionally to stop smoking all forms of tobacco permanently Follow-up: referral to special programmes, and/or pharmacotherapy (including nicotine replacement) are recommended, as is a stepwise strategy for smoking cessation. Offer behavioural advice and group or individual counselling Consider bupropion or varenicline if not contraindicated	Long-term smoking abstinence

| Nutritional counselling *Heart health diet* | Daily caloric intake and dietary content of fat, saturated fat, sodium, and other nutrients

Assess eating habits | Education: regarding dietary goals and how to attain them; Healthy food choices:
• Wide variety of foods: low-salt foods
• Mediterranean diet: fruits, vegetables, wholegrain cereals and bread, fish (especially oily), lean meat, low-fat dairy products
• Replace saturated fat with the above-listed foods and with monounsaturated and polyunsaturated fats from vegetable (oleic acid as in olive oil and rapeseed oil) and marine sources to reduce total fat to <30% of energy, of which <1/3 is saturated
• Avoid: beverages and foods with added sugars and salty food
• Integrate: behaviour-change models and compliance strategies in counselling sessions | Patient understands basic principles of dietary content

Patient adheres to prescribed diet |
| Weight control management
BMI: 18.5–24.9 kg/m^2
Waist circumference:
80 cm women/94 cm in men | Measure weight, height, and waist circumference. Calculate BMI | BMI: it is useful to consistently encourage weight control through an appropriate balance of physical activity, caloric intake, and formal behavioural programmes when indicated

Waist circumference: it is beneficial to initiate lifestyle changes and consider treatment strategies for metabolic syndrome as indicated | To reduce body weight by 5–10% in 6 months

Consider referring patient to specialist obesity clinic if goal not reached |

Table 16.3 Assessment, clinical interventions, and expected outcomes for psychosocial management and vocational advice following MI

Area of interest *Treatment goal*	Evaluation and assessment	Intervention	Expected outcomes
Psychosocial management *Absence of clinically significant depression and psychosocial problems*	Screen for psychological distress using interview and/or other standardized measurement tools Screen for substance abuse of alcohol and/or other psychotropic agents	Offer individual and/or small group education and counselling on adjustment to heart disease, stress management, and health-related lifestyle change (i.e. profession, car driving, and sexual activities), relaxation techniques Whenever possible, offer spouses and other family members, domestic partners, and/or significant others access to information sessions Teach and support self-help strategies and ways of obtaining effective social support. Provide vocational counselling in case of work-related stress Treatment of depression in collaboration with mental health specialist and primary care	Emotional well-being Absence of clinically significant psychosocial problems and acquisition of stress management skills Improved health-related quality of life
Vocational advice *Return to prior activities unless contraindications*	Before discharge, return to prior activities must be discussed with the patient, unless there is a medical contraindication The presence of any barriers to return to work following illness should be assessed	All procedures to help individuals to overcome barriers to return to work and so remain in, return to, or access employment: i.e. retraining and capacity building, reasonable adjustments and control measures, disability awareness, condition management, and medical treatment	Return to prior activities
Sexual functioning *Return to prior activities unless contraindicated*		Offer individual and/or small group education and counselling on sexual activities	Return to prior activities unless contraindicated

Cardioprotective medications and adherence

Based on current evidence, patients should be prescribed from the following classes of cardioprotective disease-modifying medications for secondary prevention following ACS:

- ACE inhibitors or angiotensin receptor blockers
- β-blockers
- Cholesterol-lowering drugs: high-dose statins
- Dual-antiplatelet therapy including aspirin and thienopyridines.

International guidelines recommend long-term treatment with these medications except for dual-antiplatelet treatment and β-blockers which are recommended for 1 year and then continuing with only long-term aspirin. If the left ventricular function is normal (ejection fraction >40%), NICE recommends considering stopping β-blocker treatment.[2]

Adherence to therapy

Despite the strong evidence for each of these therapies, the rates of prescriptions and adherence rates for cardioprotective medications is, however, suboptimal. Although nearly 90% of patients are discharged with appropriate medications after an acute MI, there is a steady decline in medication adherence over a period of 5 years. Studies have found a significant improvement in adherence to cardioprotective medications over 3 years with participation in a cardiac rehabilitation programme. To fully realize the long-term benefits of secondary prevention, good communication is needed between secondary and primary care. In the UK, GPs are incentivized to provide long-term care for people with CHD through nurse-led clinics in primary care.

Risk stratification

Table 16.4 can help as a guide for the exercise professional to determine the appropriate level of supervision and monitoring. The recommended risk stratification tool has been adapted from the American Association of Cardiovascular and Pulmonary Rehabilitation guidelines.[3] The guidelines recommend that there must be direct supervision of the exercise for at least 6–18 workouts or 30 days after the event or post-procedure. For those with moderate risk, direct supervision at least 12–24 sessions or 60 days after the event or post procedure is recommended, and high-risk patients should be monitored for at least 18–36 exercise sessions or 90 days after the event or post procedure.

The content of the exercise prescription will depend on the on the level of risk as categorized in Table 16.4. The Association of Chartered Physiotherapists in Cardiac Rehabilitation (ACPIR Standards)[4] recommends that deconditioned individuals may require a prescription that is adapted to their needs and some individuals may have to reduce their sedentary time and maintain their usual level of physical activity. Detailed guidance on the impact of risk stratification on exercise prescription is also given.[4]

The risk stratification can also be used to establish the prognosis of future major cardiovascular events and chances of survival. The risk of mortality within the first year can be estimated using the following categories: low risk is 2%, moderate risk is 10–25%, and high risk is greater than 25%.

Table 16.4 Risk stratification tool

High risk if any one or *more* of the factors are present	• Left ventricular ejection fraction <40% • Survivor of cardiac arrest or sudden death • Complex ventricular dysrhythmias at rest or with exercise • MI or cardiac surgery complicated by cardiogenic shock or CHF or post-procedure ischaemia • Abnormal haemodynamics with exercise • Significant silent ischaemia (ST depression ≥2 mm) with exercise • Angina pectoris/dizziness/light-headedness or dyspnoea at low level of exercise (<5.0 METs) • Maximal functional capacity <5.0 METs • Clinically significant depression or depressive symptoms
Low risk if *all* of the factors are present	• Left ventricular ejection fraction >50% • No resting or exercise-induced complex dysrhythmias • Uncomplicated MI, CABG, angioplasty, atherectomy, or stent (absence of CHF or post-event ischaemia) • Normal haemodynamic and ECG responses with exercise and in recovery • Normal haemodynamic and ECG responses, including absence of angina • Maximal functional capacity at least 7.0 METs • Absence of clinical depression or depressive symptoms
Moderate risk if meeting neither high-risk or low-risk standards	• Left ventricular ejection fraction = 40–50% • Angina at 60–75% of maximal functional capacity or in recovery • Mild to moderate silent ischaemia (ST depression <2 mm) with exercise or in recovery

METs, metabolic equivalents.

Benefits and risks of cardiac rehabilitation

The benefits of cardiac rehabilitation for individuals after myocardial infarction and revascularization and for those with heart failure include the following:

Reduction in mortality

Earlier meta-analysis of randomized controlled trials showed reduced overall mortality associated with cardiac rehabilitation. However, a 2016 Cochrane review of exercise-based cardiac rehabilitation for CHD reports an absolute risk reduction in cardiovascular mortality but no significant reduction in overall mortality.[5]

Reduced hospital admissions

The risk of hospital readmission is reduced in patients with heart failure receiving exercise-based cardiac rehabilitation.

Improvement in psychological well-being and quality of life

Improvements in depression, anxiety, and hostility scores in patients with CHD have been observed after cardiac rehabilitation. Patients with depression who complete their cardiac rehabilitation programmes have a reduction in depressive symptoms when compared to those who drop out or do not undergo rehabilitation. Significant improvement in health-related quality of life has been confirmed in systematic reviews of patients with CHD and heart failure who participated in rehabilitation.

Improvement in cardiovascular risk profile

Even before the use of statins for the secondary prevention of CHD, studies had demonstrated the beneficial effects of diet and exercise in improving lipid profiles. More intensive cardiac rehabilitation programmes have shown significant improvements in systolic BP, BMI, serum triglycerides, high-density lipoprotein cholesterol, total cholesterol, blood glucose, and peak oxygen uptake.

The risk of a serious cardiovascular event related to a cardiac rehabilitation intervention is very low—equivalent to 1.3 cardiac arrests per million patient-hours in a large French study. A US study reported 1 case of ventricular fibrillation per 111,996 patient-hours of exercise.

There is no evidence to suggest that exercise training programmes cause harm in terms of an increase in the risk of all-cause death in either the short or longer term in patients with stable CHF.

Maintaining long-term behaviour change

Of those patients referred to cardiac rehabilitation and prevention, few complete the programme and less than 50% maintain an exercise regimen for as long as 6 months after completion. Factors reported as predicting attendance and adherence to include illness perception, geographical location, financial and work constraints, sex, age, social support, depression, and a dislike of group-based rehabilitation sessions.

Effective interventions for improving adherence include daily self-monitoring of activity, action planning, and adherence facilitation by cardiac rehabilitation staff. Interventions that are multifaceted are likely to be more effective.

For those who have difficulty accessing centre-based cardiac rehabilitation, or those who dislike groups, home based cardiac rehabilitation programmes are sometimes available. The most widely used programme in the UK is the 'Heart Manual'—a 6-week intervention that uses written material and a relaxation CD and is delivered by a trained healthcare facilitator who makes home visits and provides telephone support. This has been shown to be just as effective as centre-based programmes.

Despite robust evidence of clinical and cost-effectiveness, uptake of cardiac rehabilitation varies worldwide and by patient group, with participation rates ranging from 20% to 50%. Poor uptake has been attributed to multiple factors, including physicians' reluctance to refer some patients, particularly women and those from ethnic minorities or lower socioeconomic classes, and lack of resources, capacity, and funding (Box 16.1).

Box 16.1 Barriers to cardiac rehabilitation

- Poor referral rates, especially in certain groups:
  - Women
  - Ethnic minorities
  - Elderly
  - Rural population
  - Lower socioeconomic class.
- Poor patient adherence: low enrolment and higher dropout rates.
- Lack of endorsement by a doctor.
- Obesity: high BMI.
- Multiple morbidity with poor functional capacity.
- Poor exercise habits.
- Cigarette smoking.
- Depression.
- Problems with transport.
- Poor social support.
- Lack of leave from work to attend centre-based sessions.

Adherence to cardiac rehabilitation programmes is influenced by factors such as psychological well-being, geographical location, access to transport, and a dislike of group-based rehabilitation sessions. The most effective way to increase uptake and optimize adherence and secondary prevention is for clinicians to endorse cardiac rehabilitation by inviting patients still in hospital after a recent diagnosis of CHD or heart failure to participate and for nurse-led prevention clinics to be linked with primary care and cardiac rehabilitation services. Novel ways of providing cardiac rehabilitation are emerging using the Internet and mobile phones. Self-management and collaboration with caregivers can also improve uptake and outcomes.

References

1. Balady GJ, Williams MA, Ades PA, et al. (2007). Core components of cardiac rehabilitation/secondary prevention programmes: 2007 update: a scientific statement from the American Heart Association Exercise, Cardiac Rehabilitation, and Prevention Committee, the Council on Clinical Cardiology; the Councils on Cardiovascular Nursing, Epidemiology and Prevention, and Nutrition, Physical Activity, and Metabolism; and the American Association of Cardiovascular and Pulmonary Rehabilitation. *Journal of Cardiopulmonary Rehabilitation and Prevention* 27, 121–129.

2. National Institute for Health and Care Excellence (NICE) (2013). *Myocardial Infarction: Cardiac Rehabilitation and Prevention of Further Cardiovascular Disease.* Clinical Guideline [CG172]. NICE, London. ⬥ http://www.nice.org.uk/guidance/cg172.

3. American Association of Cardiovascular and Pulmonary Rehabilitation (2005). *Guidelines for Cardiac Rehabilitation and Secondary Prevention Programmes*, 5th edn. Human Kinetics, Champaign, IL.

4. Association of Chartered Physiotherapists in Cardiac Rehabilitation (ACPIR). (2015). *Standards for Physical Activity and Exercise in the Cardiovascular Population*, 3rd edn. ACPIR, London.

5. Anderson L, Oldridge N, Thompson DR, et al. (2016). Exercise-based cardiac rehabilitation for coronary heart disease: Cochrane systematic review and meta-analysis. *Journal of the American College of Cardiology* 67, 1–12.

Further reading

British Association for Cardiovascular Prevention and Rehabilitation (2012). *BACPR Standards and Core Components for Cardiovascular Disease Prevention and Rehabilitation 2012*, 2nd edn. UKBACPR. ℘ www.bacpr.com/resources/46C_BACPR_Standards_and_Core_Components_2012.pdf.

Dalal HM, Doherty P, Taylor RS (2015). Cardiac rehabilitation. *BMJ* 351, h5000. ℘ http://www.bmj.com/content/351/bmj.h5000.

Leon AS, Franklin BA, Costa F, et al. (2005). Cardiac rehabilitation and secondary prevention of coronary heart disease: an American Heart Association scientific statement from the Council on Clinical Cardiology in collaboration with the American Association of Cardiovascular and Pulmonary Rehabilitation. *Circulation* 111, 369–376.

Menezes AR, Lavie CJ, Milani RV, et al. (2014). Cardiac rehabilitation in the United States. *Progress in Cardiovascular Diseases* 56, 522–529

Piepoli M, Corrà U, Adamopoulos S, et al. (2014). Secondary prevention in the clinical management of patients with cardiovascular diseases. Core components, standards and outcome measures for referral and delivery. *European Journal of Preventive Cardiology* 21, 664–681.

Smith SC Jr, Benjamin EJ, Bonow RO, et al. (2011). AHA/ACCF Secondary Prevention and Risk Reduction Therapy for Patients with Coronary and other Atherosclerotic Vascular Disease: 2011 update: a guideline from the American Heart Association and American College of Cardiology Foundation. *Circulation* 124, 2458–2473.

Tayor RS, Zwisler AO (2016). New concepts in cardiac rehabilitation and secondary prevention after myocardial infarction. In: Morrow DA (ed), *Myocardial Infarction: A Companion to Braunwald's Heart Disease*, pp. 419–433. Elsevier, St. Louis, MI.

Useful websites

Association of Chartered Physiotherapists in Cardiac Rehabilitation (ACPIR Standards): ℘ http://acpicr.com/sites/default/files/ACPICR%20Standards%202015_0.pdf.

British Heart Foundation: ℘ http://www.bhf.org.uk/heart-health/living-with-a-heart-condition/cardiac-rehabilitation.

Healthtalkonline: ℘ http://www.healthtalk.org/peoples-experiences/heart-disease/heart-attack/cardiac-rehabilitation-support; ℘ http://www.healthtalk.org/peoples-experiences/heart-disease/heart-attack/topics#ixzz3IzyXycCp.

NICE 2013 http://publications.nice.org.uk/cardiac-rehabilitation-services-cmg40/1-commissioning-cardiac-rehabilitation-services.

Respiratory issues
in rehabilitation

Introduction and epidemiology

Respiratory aspects of rehabilitation fall into two broad and overlapping categories. One is that of pulmonary rehabilitation which traditionally has focused on exercise, behaviour change and educational based intervention for those with chronic lung disease, predominantly chronic obstructive pulmonary disease (COPD). The other is rehabilitation in the context of neurogenic respiratory impairment, which is relevant to persons with both degenerative and monophasic-onset neurological conditions. These categories are overlapping as techniques from one may have relevance to the other.

COPD is a common condition with prevalence varying from 7% to 12% of the population worldwide.[1] It is more frequent in men than women and in current or previous smokers, although 36% of those with COPD have never smoked. It is associated with several co-morbidities, the commonest of which are hypertension and asthma. Sarcopenia is found in approximately 15% of people with COPD, compared with about 7% of the general population. Impairment of lung function for any reason is also common, 6.5% having restrictive and 13.7% of the general population having obstructive impairment in a US study.[2]

Pulmonary rehabilitation

Pulmonary rehabilitation was initially used for people with COPD but its efficacy has since been proven in other chronic respiratory conditions.

The American Thoracic Society and European Respiratory Society (ATS/ESR) definition of pulmonary rehabilitation from their 2013 consensus statement is:

> Pulmonary rehabilitation is a comprehensive intervention based on a thorough patient assessment followed by patient tailored therapies that include, but are not limited to, exercise training, education and behavior change, designed to improve the physical and psychological conditions of people with chronic respiratory disease and to promote long term adherence to health enhancing behaviours.[3]

Respiratory conditions for which there is randomized controlled trial evidence that pulmonary rehabilitation is effective

- COPD
- Asthma
- Interstitial lung disease
- Cystic fibrosis
- Bronchiectasis
- Lung transplantation
- Pulmonary hypertension.

There are ongoing studies in other conditions such as lung cancer. The common underlying features of these conditions suggest that a rehabilitation approach can be helpful, in that they all affect activity and participation; emotional, social, and psychological well-being; and cause deconditioning, dyspnoea, fatigue, and loss of muscle mass and strength. There are specific impairments in different respiratory conditions that may be included in a pulmonary rehabilitation programme, such as:

- warm up and use of bronchodilators to avoid exercise-induced bronchospasm in asthma
- allowance for desaturation in interstitial lung disease, following lung volume reduction surgery and pulmonary hypertension, for instance, including use of supplemental oxygen
- awareness of and adaptation for infection risk in cystic fibrosis
- airways clearance in bronchiectasis.

Indications for starting a pulmonary rehabilitation programme and selection of patients

There is evidence that an individualized pulmonary rehabilitation programme benefits patients with different severities of lung disease and function. Those with early-stage disease may benefit more from prevention, establishing good exercise and dietary habits, and from the earlier enhancement of self-efficacy; while those with later-onset disease can benefit from seeing the improvement in their activities that the programme can result in.

Pharmacological management of the chronic respiratory disease should be optimized before starting the programme.

Common indications for referral for pulmonary rehabilitation, taken from the 2013 ATS/ERS consensus statement,[3] are shown in Box 17.1. The underlying theme is that referral is appropriate when the underlying respiratory disease is adversely impacting any aspect of life.

Many patients have co-morbidities, particularly cardiovascular disease, diabetes mellitus, and obesity. While the programme will have to be individualized to take these into account, it is also likely to benefit these conditions as well. ECG, echocardiogram, and cardiopulmonary exercise testing may be considered in order to establish a safe exercise prescription. A condition that puts the patient at risk would be contraindicated (e.g. uncontrolled cardiac disease), but it would be relatively rare that a programme cannot be adapted.

Pulmonary rehabilitation programmes can start in or outside of hospital. Those starting in hospital can begin in the intensive care unit (ICU) or acute ward and assist in reducing the deconditioning that occurs during acute illness.

Box 17.1 Common indications for referral to pulmonary rehabilitation

- Dyspnoea or fatigue and chronic respiratory symptoms.
- Impaired health-related quality of life.
- Decreased functional status.
- Decreased occupational performance.
- Difficulty performing ADLs.
- Difficulty with the medical regimen.
- Psychosocial problems attendant on the underlying respiratory illness.
- Nutritional depletion.
- Increased use of medical resources.
- Gas exchange abnormalities including hypoxaemia.

Elements of a pulmonary rehabilitation programme

Exercise training

People with chronic respiratory disease experience dyspnoea at low levels of exercise and also become physically deconditioned. Both of these will respond to exercise training. The underlying principles are the same as for any person, namely:

- the training load must exceed the person's usual degree of exercise
- there should be a progressive increase in training load
- the type of training should reflect the person's goals (e.g. if the aim is to improve walking then seated exercise will have little or no benefit)
- there is a role for exercise to promote both improvements in endurance and strength.

The frequency and level of endurance and strength training follow the principles of the American College of Sports Medicine Guidelines for exercise testing and prescription (⊃ see Chapter 16), with the same recommended frequency, but with intensity, repetitions, and loads adapted to the individual's abilities.

Endurance training

The modes of exercise used are bicycle (usually a static bike) or walking. There are different advantages to each and a combination can be used:

- Cycling eliminates some weight bearing, which may be beneficial in those with osteoarthritis or low levels of fitness.
- Cycling is associated with less exercise-induced oxygen desaturation.
- Cycling is useful in training quadriceps which may assist in standing up and in knee stabilization while walking.
- Walking relates more to everyday function.
- It is easy to count steps using a variety of apps, allowing targets for walking to be easily incorporated into everyday life.
- Both can be incorporated into leisure activities to supplement the programme and assist in continuing exercise long term.

Training can be in the form of continuous exercise at the same intensity and duration or interval training. Intervals can be useful for those who cannot manage a more sustained form of exercise. There is no evidence yet of benefit of one over the other as long as the training load is similar, but they offer different forms of exercise that can be used to individualize and vary a programme. There is evidence in other conditions that high-intensity interval training produces a better metabolic response than continuous training.

Resistance training

This will result in improvements in muscle mass and strength and a reduction in the sensation of dyspnoea that will complement endurance training. Improving muscle strength has the generic advantages of strengthening muscles weak secondary to whatever pathology the person has, in reducing falls, an overall improvement in health, and a possible improvement in bone mineral density. It may also be used to strengthen specific muscle groups according to the needs of an individual patient—for instance, to assist in specific ADLs or in a role or pastime that the person has. The exercises should be prescribed according to the abilities and preferences of the individual and the resources available, and should be progressive. For example, a person needing safe and independent stair climbing would aim at lower limb strength training, especially quadriceps and gluteals, to reach that goal. Conversely, if they wished to prepare dinner for the family then upper limb exercises would be relatively more important.

International recommendations for adults are that strength training should be performed at least twice per week and involve the major muscle groups. This should be the standard to aim for, but may have to be decreased in some individuals.

Inspiratory muscle training

Inspiratory muscle training is specifically directed at inspiratory muscles. It is usually performed by breathing in against a measured resistance using a specific device. It is uncertain how much, or if, inspiratory muscle training adds to a whole-body exercise programme, but it is known to be effective alone and is potentially useful for individuals who are unable to cycle or walk.

Flexibility, posture, and core training

There is no evidence that these modes of training add to endurance and resistance training, but it is thought the resulting improvements in posture should aid respiration. They also have a role in warming up and cooling down, which are important parts of exercise programmes in order to avoid injury.

Neuromuscular electrical stimulation

This has been shown to benefit those who are unable to exercise by walking or cycling, for instance, in the ICU or persons with very low exercise tolerance who cannot get out of the house. It has been shown to preserve muscle mass and reduce the incidence of critical care neuropathy and myopathy in those in the ICU. It is contraindicated in persons with implanted electrical devices.

Nutritional interventions

People with chronic respiratory conditions tend to have a higher fat mass and lower muscle mass than healthy people of the same age, irrespective of weight (i.e. obese, normal, or underweight). Advice on optimal diets and how to implement these are thus part of any pulmonary rehabilitation programme.

Behaviour change and self-management

Behaviour change is an essential part of any rehabilitation programme and is especially emphasized in pulmonary rehabilitation. The aim is to enhance the self-efficacy of a person in managing their own condition using the principles of collaborative self-management. This allows the person to work with healthcare professionals in managing their condition. In order to do this, the person needs to acquire knowledge about their respiratory condition and how to optimize their health in the context of having the condition, alongside methods to put that knowledge into practice. Aspects of knowledge that are important are shown in Box 17.2, adapted from the 2013 ATS/ERS consensus statement.[3]

CBT and related cognitive therapies can assist the person in changing and maintaining new behaviours and habits. Collaborative self-management allows a person to use a framework of problem-solving, goal setting, decision-making, and planning to use the knowledge and skills they acquire during the pulmonary rehabilitation programme.

Maintenance of benefits from pulmonary rehabilitation

Even with the emphasis on self-management, compliance with a pulmonary rehabilitation programme decreases over time. Several strategies, such as telephone follow-up or maintenance levels of input, have been trialled to extend the benefits, but with little success. However, repeating the programme has been shown to be of benefit.

Box 17.2 Knowledge the person can acquire for self-management

- How to stop smoking.
- Pulmonary anatomy and physiology, normal and pathological.
- Communicating with health and social care providers.
- Interpretation of medical tests.
- Breathing strategies.
- Secretion clearance techniques.
- Role and rationale for pharmacological therapies, including oxygen.
- Effective use of respiratory devices.
- Benefits of exercise and physical and leisure activities.
- Energy conservation during ADLs.
- Healthy nutrition.
- Avoiding irritants.
- Early recognition and treatment of exacerbations.
- Coping strategies.

Neurogenic respiratory impairment

Neurological conditions can affect respiratory control in various ways, as shown in Fig. 17.1 and Table 17.1. Many individuals will have a combination of these different factors affecting their respiration.

Further, secondary changes can occur:
- Reduced chest wall compliance secondary to atelectasis, increased connective tissue, and ankylosis.
- Increased risk of infection due to atelectasis and retained secretions.
- Chronic respiratory infection (e.g. by *Pseudomonas* spp.).
- Difficulty in voice production due to decreased respiratory volumes and/or control.
- Increase in metabolic demand in conditions where respiratory rate is increased to compensate (e.g. MND).

These primary and secondary impairments result in four broad effects on respiratory function:
- Resting inspiration and expiration
- Respiration during exertion
- Respiration during sleep
- Coughing and control of secretions.

Other system impairments that are common in patients who are unwell and immobilized for any reason can have a further impact on the respiratory system, such as:
- poor dental hygiene leading to an increased risk of lower respiratory tract infection (LRTI)
- dysphagia, leading to aspiration and infection

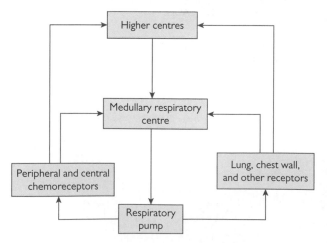

Fig. 17.1 Control of respiration.

- gastro-oesophageal reflux leading to chronic and acute aspiration
- constipation/ascites reducing diaphragmatic movement
- thromboembolic disease leading to pulmonary embolism.

Coughing is a complex process that depends on the ability to increase intrapleural pressure against a functioning glottis. It relies on intact abdominal, respiratory, and bulbar muscle function. Many neurodegenerative conditions cause impairments affecting these structures, leading to a weak and inadequate cough.

Table 17.1 Structures affected in neurological disease that are involved in respiration

Structure affected	Role on Respiration	Examples
Prefrontal cortex		Stroke, TBI
Midbrain		
Brainstem (lateral pons and ventrolateral medulla, nucleus tractus solitaries, and raphe neurons)	Overall control of respiration	Stroke, TBI, MS
Spinal cord	Provides motor control and sensory feedback of structures involved in respiration	SCI, MS, UMN component of MND
Chest wall muscle spindles and sensory nerves	Provide feedback to modulate respiratory control	SCI
Inspiratory muscles of respiration	Provide ventilatory movement necessary for respiration at rest, during exertion and coughing	Diaphragmatic paralysis in high SCI or MND
Expiratory muscles of respiration	Provide ventilatory movement for respiration during exertion and coughing	Most conditions affecting trunk musculature
Accessory muscles of respiration	Provide increased ventilatory movement during times of extra demand, such as exertion and LRTI	Muscle conditions. MND, unilaterally in stroke
Pharyngeal and laryngeal musculature	Protect and keep airway clear during swallowing and sleep	Bulbar onset MND, inclusion body myositis, myotonic dystrophy

LRTI, lower respiratory tract infection; MND, motor neuron disease; MS, multiple sclerosis; SCI, spinal cord injury; TBI, traumatic brain injury.

Symptoms of neurogenic respiratory impairment

Resting inspiration and expiration

The impact on resting inspiration and expiration tends to occur very late in neurogenic respiratory failure, unless the person also has another respiratory condition. Therefore, symptoms at rest should be considered as a red flag indicating possible respiratory failure (Box 17.3). Examples of symptoms are:

• dyspnoea in end-stage MND
• symptoms of sleep-disordered breathing
• developing a LRTI
• chest pain associated with pulmonary embolism or LRTI.

Respiration during exertion

A person with a neurological condition can experience high levels of perceived and actual exertion even during minor physical activity, due to the impact of the neurological impairment on the motor system and to deconditioning.

The metabolic demand during walking combined with a reduced VO_2 in many disabling conditions may lead to breathlessness. However, it is rare for respiratory symptoms to be the main factor limiting exertion in neurological disease, therefore other reasons for such symptoms should always be considered. If a person's neurological condition reduces their mobility, respiratory failure can be masked because they do not reach higher levels of exertion. In muscle conditions, the poor ability of muscle to respond to an increased respiratory drive, and possibly a reduction in peripheral feedback, means that increased respiratory effort is often not observed and the sensation of dyspnoea is reduced.

Coughing and control of secretions

A red flag for worsening neurogenic respiratory impairment, especially ability to cough, is the development of LRTIs. It is therefore important to ask about LRTIs, how they were treated, what length of antibiotic course was necessary, whether the person was treated at hospital or home, and whether they received any chest physiotherapy. Because neurogenic dysphagia is also common in the same patients questions about swallowing should also be asked (➔ see Chapter 9).

Box 17.3 Red flags for worsening respiratory function in patients with neurological conditions

• Use of accessory muscles (if patient can activate these).
• Falling asleep while talking.
• Falling asleep while eating.
• Severe morning headache.
• Dyspnoea.
• Lethargy, unexplained by other possible causes.
• Chest infections.

Some patients with chronic cough, especially at night, may have gastro-oesophageal reflux or a postnasal drip—both may be more frequent in neurological conditions affecting bulbar and upper GI musculature.

Respiratory secretions can be a problem for those with severe restriction of ventilation. It is important, but can be difficult on history alone, to distinguish these from sialorrhoea associated with dysphagia (➔ see Chapter 9).

Sleep-disordered breathing

Sleep-disordered breathing is the generic term for the various abnormalities of respiration occurring during sleep (Table 17.2). Many conditions lead to a combination of these impairments; for instance, in the amyotrophic lateral sclerosis form of MND sleep-disordered breathing can be due to central and obstructive apnoeas and to respiratory muscle weakness causing sleep hypoventilation.

Symptoms of sleep-disordered breathing include:

- headaches on waking (with differential of headaches secondary to neck posture during sleep or to increased intracranial pressure in those at risk)
- unrefreshing sleep
- poor appetite or nausea on waking
- sleepiness and falling asleep during the day (can measure using the Epworth Sleepiness Scale)
- peripheral oedema
- snoring
- arousals and restless sleep
- witness account of apnoeas during sleep
- nocturia.

Table 17.2 Syndromes that can be described under the term 'sleep-disordered breathing'

Syndrome	Examples of relevant conditions
Central sleep apnoea/hypopnoea	MS, multiple system atrophy, TBI
Obstructive sleep apnoea/hypopnea	Friedreich's ataxia, anyone with co-morbid obesity
Sleep hypoventilation	Muscular dystrophies, Guillain–Barré syndrome, spinal cord injury

Respiratory investigations

The aims of requesting respiratory investigations during rehabilitation are to:
- identify specific issues that may benefit from intervention
- assess the effect of therapeutic interventions
- provide information for onward referral to respiratory medicine.

The investigations described in the following sections should be readily available to the rehabilitation team. ➔ See the *Oxford Handbook of Respiratory Medicine* for more in-depth information on these and other investigations.

Overall assessment of respiratory function

Vital capacity or forced vital capacity can be used as a screening test for declining respiratory function. It is of prognostic value in some conditions, for instance, Duchenne muscular dystrophy. It can be useful to have a baseline measurement for inpatients who may experience a respiratory decline if their condition relapses (e.g. Guillain–Barré syndrome or chronic inflammatory demyelinating polyneuropathy); or for assessing worsening of respiratory function in those with progressive neurological conditions.

Measuring vital capacity when lying down can indicate diaphragmatic function is declining, with a fall of 25% from the sitting position being significant. A visual test of diaphragmatic function is to look for paradoxical abdominal movement during a full inspiration.

More detailed measurements of respiratory muscle function can be made using maximal expiratory (MEP) and inspiratory (MIP) pressures. However, these are less discriminatory if used for guiding intervention as they as will decrease early on in many neurological conditions and many patients find them difficult to perform, reducing the reliability of the tests.

Persons with impaired bulbar function will find it hard to make a mouth seal to give reliable forced vital capacity, vital capacity, MEP, or MIP measurements, even when using adapted mouthpieces. Sniff tests are useful in such instances—either just observation of sniff or measurement of sniff nasal inspiratory pressure (SNIP). SNIP values have been shown to have an association with nocturnal in conditions such as amyotrophic lateral sclerosis.

Measuring cough

Cough can be measured very easily using a peak flow device to give cough peak flow by asking the patient to cough into the device, although it is also dependent on a good mouth seal. Similar to sniff, observing cough provides useful information. It can be instructive to measure cough peak flow before and after cough augmentation techniques, which will indicate the improvement in coughing that these techniques can make. Reduction in cough peak flow can be used as an indicator of declining respiratory function during a LRTI. For those with a usual cough peak flow of greater than 160 L/min, decreasing below that value can be predictive of the need for hospital admission.[4]

Blood gases

These can be taken from arterial or capillary blood. Earlobe capillary blood gases are a more acceptable test when available. The primary aspect to consider in neurogenic respiratory failure is whether the patient is becoming hypercapnic (a partial pressure of carbon dioxide ($PaCO_2$) of >6.0 kPa), being a strong indicator for use of non-invasive ventilation (NIV) if the person has decided they want to use this intervention.

Sleep studies

Measuring respiratory function during sleep indicates how the respiratory system is performing when drive from the neurological and musculoskeletal systems is lowest, which has an impact on sleep-disordered breathing (➲ see 'Symptoms of neurogenic respiratory impairment').

Full polysomnography is a specialist test and not widely available. Overnight oximetry can be used as a screening tool for sleep-disordered breathing, to supplement history, examination, and the other investigations described. Aspects to consider are the minimum oxygen saturation, the average frequency of dips in SaO_2 of at least 4% per hour (oxygen desaturation index), and the pattern of desaturation over time and compared with pulse rate.

Interventions for neurogenic respiratory impairment

These can be divided into prevention of infection, augmentation of coughing, and assistance with ventilation. There is some overlap in these—for instance, augmenting cough will help to prevent infection.

Prevention of infection

- Vaccination against common respiratory pathogens (e.g. influenza, pneumococcus).
- Good oral hygiene, with appropriately adapted toothbrush and use of mouthwash.
- Optimizing nutrition and hydration.
- Although there is no clear evidence, it may help to avoid exposure to infectious agents (e.g. carers with an upper respiratory tract infection, avoiding admissions, or reducing length of stay in secondary care).
- If infections are repeated and other measures have failed, low-dose prophylactic antibiotics are sometimes used.

Cough augmentation

Expectoration may be helped by physical manoeuvres:

- Breath stacking using glossopharyngeal breathing or a lung volume recruitment bag. This increases inspiratory volume, increasing cough peak flow so producing a more effective cough.
- Cough assist using a cough assist device (exsufflator/insufflator).

Manually assisted cough by a physiotherapist or taught carer.

- Suctioning to remove remaining secretions. This may be a reason for use of a tracheostomy.

Secretions can be made looser, and thus easier to expectorate, using medication such as N-acetylcysteine. Often the reason for retaining or being unable to wean a tracheostomy is because of the need to suction secretions.

Even very simple strategies such as hoisting a patient out of bed or sitting out may provide some extra movement to assist in clearing secretions.

Improving respiratory muscle strength

There is some evidence that respiratory resistance exercises can improve respiratory muscle strength in various conditions, for instance, MS and amyotrophic lateral sclerosis,[5] but the effects on activities, participation, and hospitalization are uncertain

There are various forms of mechanical assistance with ventilation:

- Phrenic nerve stimulation. This is sometimes used in those with high cervical cord injuries and may have a positive impact on survival.
- NIV can be used for symptom management and there is evidence in some conditions, such as MND and Duchenne muscular dystrophy, that it also prolongs life and improves quality of life. It is less effective when there is bulbar involvement. It is important to start to discuss NIV from an early stage in progressive conditions in order for the person to make

an informed choice. It is often of major benefit to individual patients but
the issues of using the machine and mask, and sometimes an increase
in carer burden, should also be included in discussions with patients in
order for them to make an informed choice.

• Invasive ventilation. Sometimes this will have been used during the acute
  illness, for instance, in major trauma, TBI, or Guillain–Barré syndrome.
  At other times, there will have been an elective decision to use it, such
  as in some neurodegenerative conditions. When instituted during acute
  illness it is often possible to wean, but not always and such patients will
  need high levels of support.

Interventions for sialorrhoea

Although this problem is due to dysphagia it has a major effect on the respiratory system.

Pharmaceutical interventions:

• Glycopyrronium (oral or via gastrostomy).
• Atropine eye drops in mouth.
• Ipratropium bromide spray to mouth.
• Hyoscine (oral or transdermal).
• BoNT injection to salivary glands. While this tends to be used after
  other methods have failed, it has the advantage of directly targeting the
  saliva, whereas the other anticholinergic medications listed will have
  systemic effects that may include increased thickness of chest secretions.
• Salivary gland irradiation has been used as a last resort in those in whom
  the previously listed interventions have failed.

Combining interventions

It is helpful to use the previously described interventions as part of an emergency or a respiratory care plan. The exact plan will depend on the individual, but having a written plan available can help to reduce the severity of
intercurrent illness or avoid hospital admission. There are various methods
in different countries to make such a plan available to patient, carers, and
healthcare staff. This can also be combined with information about treatment that the person does not want, for instance, using an 'advance decision to refuse treatment'.

References

1. Landis SH, Muellerova H, Mannino DM, et al. (2014). Continuing to Confront COPD International Patient Survey: methods, COPD prevalence, and disease burden in 2012–2013. *International Journal of COPD* 9, 597–611.

2. Ford ES, Mannino DM, Wheaton AG, et al. (2013). Trends in the prevalence of obstructive and restrictive lung function among adults in the United States. *Chest* 143, 1395–1406.

3. Spruit MA, Singh SJ, Garvey C, et al. (2013). An official American Thoracic Society/European Respiratory Society statement: key concepts and advances in pulmonary rehabilitation. *American Journal of Respiratory and Critical Care Medicine* 188, e13–e64.

4. British Thoracic Society ℛ https://www.brit-thoracic.org.uk/guidelines-and-quality-standards/physiotherapy-guideline/.

5. Ferreira GD, Costa AC, Plentz RD, et al. (2016). Respiratory training improved ventilatory function and respiratory muscle strength in patients with multiple sclerosis and lateral amyotrophic sclerosis: systematic review and meta-analysis *Physiotherapy* 102, 221–228.

Further reading

British Thoracic Society (2014). *BTS Quality Standards for Pulmonary Rehabilitation in Adults*. ℛ https://www.brit-thoracic.org.uk/document-library/quality-standards/pulmonary-rehabilitation/bts-quality-standards-for-pulmonary-rehabilitation-in-adults/.

Chetta A, Aiello M, Tzani P, et al. (2007). Assessment and monitoring of ventilator function and cough efficacy in patients with amyotrophic lateral sclerosis. *Monaldi Archives for Chest Disease* 67, 43–52.

Netzer N (2001). Overnight pulse oximetry for sleep-disordered breathing in adults. A review. *Chest* 120, 625–633.

Panossian L, Daley J (2013). Sleep-disordered breathing. *Continuum (Minneap Minn)* 19, 86–103.

Mobility and gait

Background

Mobility is a function that allows us the freedom to move between places in everyday life. As such, mobility is often a key treatment focus in those whose functional mobility has been affected by pathology. Reduction in mobility leads to activity limitations and participation restrictions, may increase dependence on others, and adversely affects the quality of life of the person, carers, and family. Rehabilitation can aim to improve mobility by:

• reducing the underlying impairment
• restoring abilities that will improve mobility, such as strength, endurance, balance, and so on
• compensating by achieving mobility in different ways or altering the environment to aid mobility and improve access.

This chapter will concentrate on walking mobility. The different forms of wheeled mobility are covered in ➜ Chapter 22.

Anatomy and physiology of mobility

Walking involves the coordination of the musculoskeletal and nervous systems. Musculotendinous and ligamentous structures are key factors in providing stability, and determining ROM across joints. The brain, spinal cord, peripheral nerves, and muscle spindles control muscle movements. Impairment at any level of this system will therefore affect motor control and lead to disorders of gait.

An understanding of the basic anatomy of the lower limbs is required to conceptualize the dynamic process that occurs during walking. It is also useful to think about the lower limbs as segments which move in sagittal, coronal, and transverse reference planes perpendicular to each other.

The gait cycle

Gait describes the pattern of walking, occurring as a series of gait cycles. Each gait cycle is a series of age-dependent and predictable phases for those whose gait is unimpaired by pathology.

Gait has two distinct phases: the stance (during which the limb is in contact with the floor) and the swing phase (where it is being moved forwards in preparation for the next step). Each of these phases has a number of recognized subphases to allow greater definition of specific events. A widely accepted breakdown of the gait phases (Fig. 18.1) is as follows:

• *Initial contact*: the time point during which the foot contacts the floor, signifying the start of the gait cycle and of stance phase.
• *Loading response*: a short phase (first 10% of the gait cycle) during which weight is transferred onto the stance limb and the forefoot is lowered to the floor. Weight is simultaneously offloaded from the opposing limb, which is about to enter its swing phase.
• *Mid-stance*: during this phase (10–30% of the gait cycle) the walker stands on one limb (single leg stance) while the opposing limb is in its swing phase and moves from behind to in front of the stance limb. Stability of the stance limb is important during this phase.
• *Terminal stance*: this phase (30–50% of the gait cycle) ends when the opposing limb contacts the floor. Progression forwards is made and momentum is maintained prior to transfer of weight onto the opposing limb for the next step.
• *Pre-swing*: this is the final 10% of stance phase (50–62% of the gait cycle) and is the second period of double support whereby weight is transferred onto the opposing limb. It ends as the foot is lifted off the floor and enters the swing phase.
• *Swing phase* is divided into three phases to describe the foot moving off the floor (initial swing, 62–75% of gait cycle), crossing the stance limb (mid swing, 75–87% of gait cycle) and extending forwards to prepare for ground contact (terminal swing, 87–100% of gait cycle).

The main muscles activated during each phase of the gait cycle are shown in Fig. 18.1, with the muscles involved smoothly increasing and reducing the degree of contraction between each phase. The small muscles of the foot are not described here, but are important as they maintain the structure of the foot during gait.

Neural control of gait consists of an interplay between cerebral cortex, midbrain, cerebellum, brainstem, spinal central pattern generators, and peripheral feedback. The spinal central pattern generators produce an automatic symmetrical stepping pattern but, in humans, this is insufficient to produce a functional gait even walking over a smooth level surface. Supraspinal input is necessary to integrate lower limb sensory feedback (proprioception, muscle spindles, touch, etc.) and the senses (auditory, visual, and vestibular) along with input from cerebellum, basal ganglia, and cerebral cortex to initiate smooth, modulated movement.

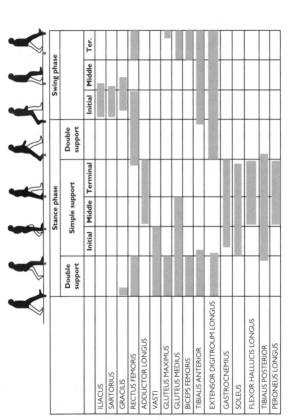

Fig. 18.1 Muscle activation in one limb during the gait cycle.

Canavese, Frederico, and Deslandes, Jacques, *Orthopaedic Management of Children with Cerebral Palsy*, Nova Science Publishers, Inc. (2015), Chapter 16, Normal Gait by Bonnefoy-Mazure, Alice, and Armand, Stephane – Figure 6, p210.

The effect of pathology on gait

Walking can be affected by pathologies of the nervous and/or musculoskeletal systems. Some pathologies give rise to typical gait patterns (Table 18.1). For example, patients with the spastic diplegic form of cerebral palsy often walk with a scissoring gait. Increased lateral trunk lean may be seen to

Table 18.1 Typical gait deviations

Gait deviation	Observation	Common reasons
Trendelenburg	Pelvis on swing side drops as patient stands on one leg	Abductor weakness in the stance side
	Lateral trunk lean to the stance side to lift the swing side	Unilateral hip pain (various causes)
Anterior trunk lean	Forwards lean of the trunk during stance	Hip extensor weakness
		Ankle equinus
Scissoring	The non-weight-bearing proximal leg adducts or swings across the other leg during swing phase	Adductor spasticity
Circumduction	Swing side leg is swung out in a circle to ensure ground clearance	Stiff knee, ankle plantarflexion, leg length discrepancy, weak hip flexors
Hip hiking	Swing side of the pelvis is hitched upwards to ensure ground clearance	As for 'Circumduction'
Steppage	Exaggerated, high stepping pattern of the hip and knee in swing	Usually compensatory to ensure ground clearance either for ankle plantarflexion (tightness or weakness) in swing, or reduced proprioception where the patient is unaware of foot positioning during swing
	Patient looks at ground when using vision to compensate for proprioceptive loss	
Vaulting	Patient rises onto their toes in stance to ensure ground clearance	Calf shortening (e.g. spasticity) or drop foot or stiff knee gait on the swing side
Genu recurvatum	Knee hyperextends during the stance phase	Calf shortening or quads weakness
Drop foot	Ankle drops into plantarflexion in swing	Tibialis anterior weakness
Ankle equinus	Ankle held in plantarflexion and equinovarus	Ankle action dystonia and/or calf contracture
Ataxic gait	Gait is broad based, movement is exaggerated and uncoordinated	Cerebellar pathologies or lower limb proprioceptive loss

compensate for weakness of hip abductors and spasticity of adductors. Patients with quadriceps weakness, such as spinal bifida or following polio, often use knee hyperextension during stance (even using their hands to stabilize their knee) to provide a secure leg on which to stand while the other leg moves forwards. They may flex the trunk forwards to facilitate the knee locking and to maintain forwards momentum. After a stroke, patients often present with a mixed pattern of weakness as well as extensor spasticity which results in a very stiff leg. They therefore use a range of compensations such as circumduction, vaulting, or hip hiking to ensure ground clearance while swinging the limb forwards to achieve progression.

Conditions affecting the basal ganglia lead to changes in the fluency of gait. In Parkinson's disease steps are small with uncontrolled acceleration (festinating), difficulties in stopping and turning, freezing, and a flexed posture. In small vessel vascular disease steps are small but with a regular rhythm (*marche à petits pas*), and in normal pressure hydrocephalus gait is wide based and shuffling. Lastly, patients with painful conditions adapt their gait pattern to minimize the loading through their painful joint, often with a shorter stance time on the painful side to further reduce the pain.

Patients presenting with spasticity may have problems with coordinating movements in the lower limbs during walking partly because uncontrolled muscle overactivity and co-contraction often cause unwanted movements, such as hip adduction, persistent knee flexion, and/or ankle equinovarus. The antagonist muscle groups (such as the ankle dorsiflexors) often cannot generate sufficient force to control this movement. Secondary compensations occur, such as hip hitching to allow the lower limb on the hemiparetic side to clear the ground.

History and examination of mobility

Asking the person, or their carers, the following questions can assist in assessing mobility and planning rehabilitation:

- Current walking ability:
  - Distance
  - Time and speed
  - Balance
  - Difficulties with specific aspects of walking (e.g. turning, getting up, and stopping)
  - Falls and trips—frequency, circumstances, precipitants, injuries, changes made to avoid them, environmental impact on falls, and ability to get up from the floor.
- Environmental factors that will affect walking ability:
  - Surface.
  - Gradient.
  - Distractions (e.g. talking, crowds).
  - Mobility aids and the circumstances these are used in. Many patients will vary their walking aid according to environment (e.g. a walking frame outdoors, a walking stick. or furniture or walls in indoors, versus a wheelchair for longer distances).
  - Footwear—how long do shoes last? Where do they wear? How do they affect walking? Does the height of the heel or style (e.g. boot) affect walking pattern and fatigue?
- Health factors associated with walking ability:
  - Fatigue
  - Upper limb and trunk impairments
  - Pain
  - Spasticity
  - Cognition
  - Co-morbidities.
- History of how walking ability has changed.
- Effect of reduced mobility on activities and participation (e.g. getting to the bathroom, in and out of shower, up and down stairs, carrying shopping, getting around in workplace, moving between classrooms at school, impact on leisure activities, and keeping up with others).
- The effect of previous interventions and rehabilitation aimed to improve gait or mobility, such as medication, surgery, physiotherapy or orthoses; for example, does the person walk better with orthoses on? Does use of baclofen help spasticity but reveal weakness? Has the person had orthopaedic surgery to improve gait? What were the effects of this?
- Their self-perceived problems with walking and how these affect goals and expectations with regard to mobility.

Examination should be holistic and guided by the history. It should include a detailed neuromusculoskeletal examination (➔ see Chapter 5).

Observation of the person's gait allows an analysis of how their gait deviates from normal and identification of some aspects of strength and spasticity that may only be apparent when walking. Ideally, gait should be viewed in both the sagittal and coronal planes. It is helpful to initially look at overall gait quality before considering movements at individual joints. The common features to observe in someone's gait are:

- symmetry
- pattern recognition of well-known gait patterns (e.g. Parkinsonian, scissoring, hemiplegic, LMN foot drop, etc.)
- velocity
- cadence
- stride and step length
- turning
- starting and stopping
- exertion, features such as of breathlessness, sweating, and fatigue.

As previously described, the clinical observation of gait is potentially time-consuming and it takes many years to develop mastery. Many hours of practice in interpreting gait is necessary to become accurate and efficient. To optimize your performance, it is worthwhile taking any opportunity to observe gait, whether it is in the waiting room, the shopping centre, or during the consultation itself. It is important to be familiar with different normal and abnormal gaits to recognize the range of normality, as well as to determine whether observed changes are primary (as a direct result of an impairment) or secondary (to compensate for an impairment).

Gait analysis

The gold standard for interpretation of gait is three-dimensional (3D) computerized gait analysis. This gives a biomechanical assessment of gait that identifies and measures specific gait-related impairments impossible or difficult to identify by observation alone. These data can be used to provide a specific treatment plan that aims to improve mobility. Occasions when gait analysis can be useful are as follows:

- When there are many impairments associated with a person's gait, so that it is difficult to identify and assess them.
- When it is hard to distinguish secondary and primary gait deviations.
- When different rehabilitation interventions are being considered, but where it is hard to judge the relative importance of the impairments involved (e.g. spasticity and weakness when considering strengthening, stretching, orthotic interventions, and BoNT injections).
- As a clinical outcome measure for the chosen intervention.
- Research, using gait parameters as baseline or outcome measures.
- When orthopaedic surgery to improve gait is being considered.

The parameters measured during gait analysis are as follows:
- Kinetics:
  - Moments and powers
  - Ground reaction forces.
- Kinematics:
  - Joint angles.
- EMG:
  - Muscle firing patterns throughout the gait cycle.

Data collection for gait analysis is achieved by the following:
- Placement of surface markers over the lower limb joints to determine measurement of angles at and between joints, and of moments around each joint. Marker system can be passive (e.g. Vicon, BTS, or Qualisys systems using camera tracked retro-reflective markers, requiring postprocessing to label each marker) or active (e.g. Codamotion system, where markers emit a unique infrared signal, allowing automatic marker tracking).
- Surface EMG, which records when specific surface muscles are active during the gait cycle.
- Force plate, measuring ground reaction force (GRF) and allowing calculation of forces, power, and moments. Combined with video, it allows video vector analysis of how the GRF aligns with the body during walking.
- Walkway, fixed cameras, and sensors systematically collecting data in a replicable way.
- Software to analyse and display collected data.

The end result is a 3D picture of how joint angles, moments, ground force, and muscle activation in different segments vary throughout the gait cycle and of velocity, cadence, step, and stride length. Energy cost can be calculated using various methods. The parameters measured can be compared with and without different walking aids and orthoses, or before and after specific interventions. Figs. 18.2 and 18.3 show examples of how the data can be presented.

The data collected require interpretation. This is ideally done by an experienced and knowledgeable MDT consisting of a clinical scientist, physiotherapist, and doctor, which results in a report and recommendations for those involved in the person's rehabilitation.

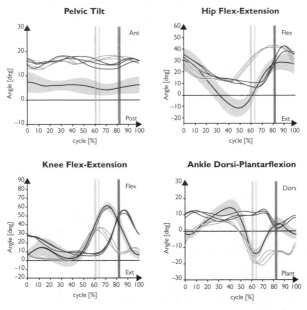

Fig. 18.2 Example data from a patient post stroke showing drop foot in swing, knee locking during stance, and poor knee flexion in swing, with hip flexion and anteriorly tilted pelvis on the right side (light purple).

With permission from Gait and Motion Laboratory, University Hospitals of Derby and Burton NHS Foundation Trust.

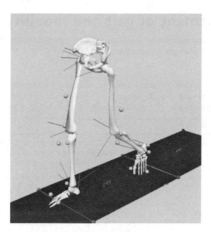

Fig. 18.3 Skeletal model from computerized motion analysis software showing joint centres and axes of rotation of each joint.

With permission from Gait and Motion Laboratory, University Hospitals of Derby and Burton NHS Foundation Trust.

Measurement of gait and mobility

There are many outcome measures used to assess mobility. Many of the common examples are provided in Table 18.2.

Table 18.2 Common scales measuring different mobility aspects. Most are accessible via the Rehab Measures website (🖰 http://www.rehabmeasures.org/default.aspx)

Scale	Comments
10-metre walk	A practical timed measure often used in clinic, requires precise instruction as to the speed and manner of walking in order to be comparable
6-minute walk test	Assesses walking over a longer time frame, so can assess early effects of fatigue; again needs precise instructions and route
Timed up and go (TUG)	As getting up and sitting down are important practical activities associated with walking the TUG can be very useful to measure and observe functional gait
Rivermead Mobility Index	A mostly self-reported scale assessing mobility in different situations of increasing difficulty, such as turning over in bed, moving from bed to chair, walking outside
Berg Balance Scale (BBS)	This assesses static balance, an important component of mobility. Low BBS scores are associated with increased falls risk
Dynamic Gait Index	Consists of observations of gait in different situations such as stepping over items, climbing stairs, and changing speed

Mobility aids

Many mobility aids are available to meet individual requirements, usually aiming to facilitate walking and improve safety. For some, the use of an aid may help offload force through a painful joint, but others may be dependent on the support of the walking aid to permit walking.

Falls occur when a person's centre of gravity moves outside of their base of support: walking aids improve safety by increasing the base of support. This occurs at the expense of transferring some force from the lower limbs to the upper limbs, meaning that users must have sufficient upper limb function for their use, and problems can occur with wrist or shoulder pain due to the additional upper limb loading.

The choice of mobility aid depends on the functional needs of the individual as it will depend on the degree of support required, hand dexterity, and functional ability of the person to propel, stop, and turn the device. Usually a physiotherapist will be involved in the prescription of a walking aid when a more complex aid than a simple walking stick is required. Many patients choose to purchase their own choice of walking aid, giving them a more flexible or aesthetically pleasing choice.

Common mobility aids include the following:
- Walking stick:
  - Improves stability and confidence.
  - Can help off-load a painful joint.
  - Provides counterbalance for some gait patterns.
  - Range of handles available to suit choice and hand function (e.g. Fischer handles) and some are height adjustable/collapsible for ease of transport.
  - Similarly, walking sticks can have a number of feet, offering increasing stability to the base of support (e.g. tripod or quad stick).
- Crutches:
  - Stability provided from more proximal joints.
  - Used where more weight needs to be taken off the lower limb (i.e. total/partial non-weight bearing) or hand function poor.
  - Gutter crutches allow the arm to be flexed at the elbow, taking weight along the forearm rather than through the wrist and hand.
- Walking frames:
  - Used where more stability is required for increased weight bearing through the frame, or where balance is poor.
  - Versions can have four fixed feet, two fixed feet and two wheels, or with four wheels, depending on requirements.
  - Some versions can have three wheels, are foldable for ease of transport, and can have hand-operated brakes to prevent the frame from rolling away when in use. Optional baskets can allow the user to carry items, and some have a back rest and seat so that the user can sit and rest when required.
- Other mobility aids:
  - Less commonly required, some aids provide additional support (e.g. incorporating pelvic, trunk, and leg support or a walking saddle). These frames may be used by patients with more severe limitations (such as those with cerebral palsy with limited mobility).

Rehabilitation of gait

Some of the interventions used in specific conditions are described in other chapters, but there are general principles that hold true for most conditions. These are described as follows:

- *Goals*. Negotiating goals that are specific and measurable while also achievable in a realistic timeframe can be difficult. Often there are differences in opinion between the person aiming to use walking to achieve a specific activity or participation-based goal in the near future and the physiotherapist aiming to achieve a quality of walking that will reduce effort and avoid longer-term musculoskeletal injury. Usually, it is possible to reach a compromise, but not always. Like any area of rehabilitation, keeping the focus on activity and participation retains a sense of perspective and reality.
- *Walking mobility* consists of standing up and sitting down as well as walking. Independence in all these processes is vital to rehabilitation of mobility. Similarly, avoiding falls and getting up from falls are also crucial components. Issues regarding falls are presented in following section (→ see 'Falls').
- *Strengthening*. Appropriate muscle strengthening has been shown to improve gait parameters in many medical conditions. Strengthening includes the lower limb muscle groups but also core and upper limb muscles. It should also have secondary effects of strengthening the entire musculotendinous complex and beneficial effects on glucose and fat metabolism.
- *Endurance*. Many activities in daily life require adequate stamina and reliability of gait throughout the day. Therefore, improving endurance optimizes mobility, as well as having beneficial effects on cardiovascular and metabolic fitness.
- *Concurrent endurance and strength training*. Beneficial effects of combining strength and endurance training have been recognized in athletes in recent years. A small number of rehabilitation-based studies have shown a similar effect in those with pathologies such as COPD and stroke, suggesting a more generalized benefit.
- *Flexibility*. Flexibility is important in maintaining musculotendinous length, reducing discomfort and in avoiding further injury. Incorporating practices that enhance flexibility are fundamental in rehabilitation programmes to improve walking mobility.
- *Balance*. Adequate balance is required in order to avoid falls, stand, reach, and carry items.
- *Psychological approach*. As with any rehabilitation intervention, the psychological approach of the person to their rehabilitation is crucial to its success. Personal learning styles can be identified which assist in knowing which approaches may benefit an individual most, such as their preferences regarding individual and group rehabilitation in order to maintain an exercise programme in the longer term; to assist the person in identifying goals and in overcoming fears concerned with falling, using walking aids, and walking in different situations.

- *Variety*. Different sports or activities can also be used as rehabilitation interventions to improve walking and will contain differing components of strengthening, endurance, flexibility, and cognition. Common examples are Pilates, yoga, swimming, tai-chi, Nordic walking, and dancing.
- *Work and education*. Mobility is an aspect of most jobs, therefore, including mobility goals in workplace rehabilitation is important. Decisions often have to be made as to whether walking or wheelchair mobility will be the main form of work mobility, with or without associated environmental modifications.

Falls

Avoiding and reducing falls is important both for safety and for the practical purpose of completing any activity associated with walking. Studies include specific diagnostic groups (such as MS, stroke, and osteoarthritis), the elderly, and specific environments (such as care homes and hospitals). Many falls guidelines exist (❯ see 'Further reading') but most include the following elements:

- Identification of those at high falls risk, including:
  - age over 65 years
  - those with conditions affecting muscle strength, balance, cognition, coordination, lower limb proprioception, vision, or level of consciousness
  - those using walking aids (indicating problems with walking)
  - those with a fear of falling, as fall-related anxiety affects attention and impairs motor control
  - previous history of falls.
- Multifactorial risk assessment:
  - Falls history to include frequency, situation, timing, and outcome of falls, trips, and stumbles.
  - Medication review.
  - Cardiovascular history and examination, looking for evidence of cardiovascular risk factors for fainting, carotid sinus hypersensitivity, arrhythmia, and conduction block.
  - Neurological history and examination, looking for evidence of weakness, poor balance, spasms, ataxia, movement disorders, and cognitive and visual impairment.
  - Urological history to assess urinary frequency, urgency, nocturia, and urinary tract infections, which may contribute to falls.
  - Assessment of fear of falling which may increase falls risk and result in reduced physical activity.
  - Factors increasing secondary complications of a fall (e.g. osteoporosis, living alone).
  - Assessment of how the person gets up from falls.
- Interventions:
  - Balance training.
  - Strength training.
  - Assessment of the environment in which the person falls.
  - Changing medications where possible to reduce those causing a reduction in balance or alertness or postural hypotension.
  - Education regarding falls and how to prevent them.

Further reading

Belda-Lois JM, Mena-del Horno S, Bermejo-Bosch I, et al. (2011). Rehabilitation of gait after stroke: a review towards a top-down approach. *Journal of Neuroengineering and Rehabilitation* 8, 66.

Ivey FM, Prior SJ, Hafer-Macko CE, et al. (2017). Strength training for skeletal muscle endurance after stroke. *Journal of Stroke and Cerebrovascular Diseases* 26, 787–794.

National Institute for Health and Care Excellence (NICE) (2013). *Falls in Older People: Assessing Risk and Prevention*. Clinical Guideline [CG161], updated 2016. NICE, London. ᕫ http://www.nice.org.uk/guidance/cg161.

Perry J, Burnfield JM (2010). *Gait Analysis: Normal and Pathological Function*. SLACK Incorporated, Thorofare, NJ.

Pons JL, Moreno JC, Torricelli D, et al. (2013). Principles of human locomotion: a review. In: *Engineering in medicine and biology society (EMBC), 2013 35th Annual International Conference of the IEEE*, pp. 6941–6944. IEEE, Piscataway, NJ.

Whittle M (2002). *Gait Analysis: An Introduction*. Butterworth Heinemann, Oxford.

Young WR, Williams AM (2015). How fear of falling can increase fall-risk in older adults: applying psychological theory to practical observations. *Gait & Posture* 41, 7–12.

Zambom-Ferraresi F, Cebollero P, Gorostiaga EM, et al. (2015). Effects of combined resistance and endurance training versus resistance training alone on strength, exercise capacity, and quality of life in patients with COPD. *Journal of Cardiopulmonary Rehabilitation and Prevention* 35, 446–453.

Useful websites

ᕫ http://www.anzfallsprevention.org/resources/—a website from the Australian Committee on Safety and Quality in Healthcare regarding falls prevention with falls guidelines for different environmental settings.

ᕫ http://www.knowledge.scot.nhs.uk/fallsandbonehealth.aspx—links to resources concerned with falls prevention and optimization of bone health.

ᕫ http://www.rehabmeasures.org/default.aspx—a website with descriptions of and links to many measures used in rehabilitation.

Family and relationships

The caregiving role of family

When an individual experiences a serious, sudden-onset illness that requires hospitalization and ongoing care, family members are often relied upon to provide a wide range of different types of assistance. This may include emotional support, physical assistance with daily activities, and practical support and advocacy to navigate complex healthcare services. In the most recently available Survey of English Housing (from 2002), the proportion of people aged 16 and over with caring responsibilities for a sick, disabled, or elderly person increased with age from 8% of 16–29-year-olds to 24% of those in the 45–64 years age group. The proportion then decreased to 16% among those aged 65 or over. People aged 45–64 are likely to have caring responsibilities for elderly parents and sometimes for a spouse or partner with age-related health problems, hence the high proportion of carers in this age group.

Family members require a range of supportive measures during the process of transition into a caregiving role. This may include information and education about the patient's health condition and possible treatments, or information about available community services. Healthcare professionals need to work with family members from early in the patient's admission through to discharge by providing information on the patient's health condition and anticipated level of future functioning. Support may also address the family member's personal needs by enhancing problem-solving skills, coping skills, or provision of counselling. Most supports are offered during or shortly after discharge from acute care or rehabilitation; however, it is often the experience of families that care needs change and in some conditions, increase over time; for example, increasing behavioural problems associated with dementia increases caregiver load, burden, and stress over time, and can lead to caregiver depression.

Family and carers are important 'environmental factors' influencing the impact of a health condition and have the potential to enhance health outcomes through the provision of a safe and supportive discharge destination (http://www.who.int/classifications/icf/en/). People without the benefit of family supports are more likely to require residential care following rehabilitation, particularly when care needs are high.

Caregiver support: 'Timing It Right'

It is clearly acknowledged that the patient's care needs will change as their abilities change and as they progress through their recovery. However, what is less clear is how the caregiving role of family also changes. When considering how healthcare professionals can more effectively support family caregivers, the 'Timing It Right' framework provides a structure to facilitate understanding of caregiver needs.[1] This framework highlights family caregivers' changing experiences and corresponding support needs across the care continuum. 'Timing It Right' highlights five different phases of caregiver support: (1) event/diagnosis, (2) stabilization, (3) preparation, (4) implementation, and (5) adaptation. The first two phases occur during acute care, the third occurs during acute care and/or inpatient rehabilitation, and the final two phases occur in the community. This approach has been developed and trialled to support families of patients with stroke; however, the principles are equally applicable to other sudden-onset conditions that require ongoing support.

Family caregiver support needs

Phase 1: event/diagnosis

The family caregiver's focus at this stage is usually in the present, with little thought for the long-term future. Their focus is on the current health event and treatment, and whether or not the event is deemed life-threatening. This stage is characterized by a high degree of uncertainty, and caregivers are often anxious and express concern for their family member's immediate survival. Family members can be best supported by providing information on diagnosis, prognosis, and current treatment. Emotional support may assist family members to manage their own emotional reaction and the uncertainty surrounding the medical event/diagnosis.

Phase 2: stabilization

Once a patient's medical condition has stabilized, caregivers generally move into a phase characterized by initial relief, followed by information seeking in order to understand the extent of impairment or disability that the patient may experience now and in the future. Information on the cause of the event and current care needs is a priority. If information is not readily available or information is mixed, confusing, or delayed, family caregivers may again experience increased anxiety and worry. Initial training from healthcare professionals to assist with the provision of physical care may commence if the family members are 'ready'. Some family caregivers may also wish to participate in the rehabilitation process during this time, others may not, preferring to provide an emotional support role rather than a role of physical assistance.

Phase 3: preparation

At this time, the patient's medical condition has stabilized and the clinical emphasis is on preparing the patient to return home. This period can be short if discharge occurs directly from an acute care environment, or can be extended if a period of inpatient rehabilitation is required. As discharge approaches, family caregivers become increasingly concerned with their abilities to provide care at home and wonder if they will be 'up to the job'.

They specifically want information and training from healthcare professionals to assist with the provision of physical care in the home (if needed) and to learn about signs of potential problems that could signal new adverse health events. Many would also like to receive appraisal and feedback about their caregiving activities to enhance their skills and build their confidence in performing these activities. Family caregivers may also seek information about community services and assistance so they can submit applications to appropriate organizations. In addition to preparing for the patient's return home, many caregivers may experience additional strain as they struggle to partially re-establish existing family and work routines.

Phase 4: implementation

The implementation phase occurs when the patient returns home and responsibility for providing care shifts from healthcare professionals to family caregivers. During this phase, caregivers are attempting to apply the skills they learnt during the acute or rehabilitation stage to helping the patient adapt to living at home. Their focus is often on developing routines and the provision of physical assistance, coordinating medical follow-up, and assisting with transport and secondary prevention (e.g. managing medication). Family caregivers often report that they did not receive enough training prior to hospital discharge and that a large amount of their learning occurred via 'trial-and-error' once home. Healthcare professionals can support family caregivers by continuing to offer training, ideally in the home environment as training received in the hospital setting may not easily adapt to the home environment. During this phase, it is important for caregivers to receive appraisal and feedback about their caregiving activities with the aim of addressing any potentially problematic activities before they cause harm to either the patient or the caregiver, and to enhance caregiver's confidence in their caregiving activities.

It is acknowledged that formal healthcare services will be variable during this phase, depending on service availability and accessibility in the area that the patient lives. When in-home support is not possible, technology may be used to access other forms of support such as telephone or Internet-based support. A telephone-based problem-solving intervention for family caregivers over the 12-month period following hospital discharge can be effective in reducing caregiver depressive symptoms, reducing physical complaints, enhancing leisure time, and enhancing caregiver competence.[2]

During this phase, family caregivers start to experience the personal consequences of providing care including the resulting emotional, physical, social, and role changes. Healthcare professionals can best support family caregivers by providing strategies to assist caregivers in managing these personal consequences (e.g. accessing respite, and utilizing other sources of support including family and friends), and facilitating access to local caregiver support groups. Support groups for caregivers are often proposed at the time of hospital discharge; however, the extent of care being provided by the caregivers at this time may make attendance at support groups or educational sessions difficult. Therefore, timing is critical to ensure that support strategies are suggested and facilitated at the right time for family caregivers.

Phase 5: adaptation

After the period of adjustment that signals the implementation phase, many caregivers report an adaptation phase. At this stage, the patient's abilities have tended to stabilize, outpatient programmes have been completed, and ongoing healthcare focuses on monitoring, often by a GP rather than specialist team. Caregivers may become increasingly confident in their abilities to support ADLs and begin to shift their emphasis towards assisting the patient to participate in valued activities and interests (i.e. community reintegration). As a result, caregivers may report the need for additional information to help the stroke survivor to resume participation in social activities, driving, sex life, employment, and travel.

At this stage, family caregivers may also begin to report difficulties dealing with competing demands and roles in their lives. Caregivers who have put other responsibilities on hold often feel the need to resume these responsibilities. Caregivers may also need guidance to help manage their competing roles. If the caregiving demands become more manageable at this stage, caregivers may have more time to participate in support groups where their needs for information and support may be met by others in a similar situation. It is also in this stage that family caregivers may also take greater notice of the restrictions that caregiving has imposed on their own abilities to socialize with family and friends, and typically report needing a break. Timely respite care is an important support strategy at this phase.

This framework, originally developed for stroke, can be generalized to other medical conditions, especially those with a sudden onset and a period of hospitalization, such as spinal cord or brain injury. This approach could also guide healthcare professionals' interactions with family caregivers when dealing with conditions more commonly experienced by older people including falls, heart conditions, or cancer.

Caregiver strain and burden

Caregiver strain and burden is commonly experienced, encompassing difficulties assuming and functioning in the caregiver role as well as associated alterations in the caregiver's emotional and physical health that can occur when the care demands exceed the caregiver's resources. As outlined in the previous section, caregivers experience different challenges throughout the rehabilitation process that can significantly impact their functioning and quality of life.

Supports that may be effective in reducing caregiver strain include the following:

• Cognitive behavioural intervention approaches that may help caregivers to identify helpful and unhelpful behaviours, and develop skills to solve problems and implement new behaviours to facilitate effective coping. Structured programmes based on cognitive behavioural approaches may include activities such as education or relaxation training, may be provided in individual or group settings, and may be delivered in person, by telephone, or by other methods.

• Psychoeducational interventions encompass a broad range of activities that combine education and other activities such as counselling and supportive interventions. Psychoeducational interventions may be delivered individually or in groups. This type of intervention generally includes providing caregivers with information about rehabilitation needs, services, and condition-specific information; training to provide care and respond to disease-related problems; and problem-solving strategies for coping. Interventions may include the use of booklets and videos, and may be interactive among healthcare professionals and patients and caregivers, self-directed via the use of CDs and other materials or delivered online.

• Emotional support interventions include activities such as general counselling related to emotional and other issues. Supportive interventions may be provided by healthcare professionals or may be structured as peer group support. Interventions can be one-on-one individualized sessions, support group sessions, or specific interventions with caregivers, families, etc.

• Mindfulness-based stress reduction (MBSR) is a consciousness discipline that is grounded in Eastern philosophy and traditions, focusing on awareness of the present moment. It aims to teach people to deal more effectively with experience through awareness of feelings, thoughts, and bodily sensations. MBSR has been studied in caregivers of patients with cancer for its effect on caregiver strain and burden

Relationships, partnerships, and friendships

Relationships of all types are vulnerable following a significant physical injury or disability. Furthermore, specific neurological injuries (such as ABI) are associated with complex sequelae that jeopardize friendships, relationships with family members, and relationships with intimate partners.[3] This is an area of rehabilitation that many healthcare professionals feel underprepared for and typically refer to clinical psychology or social work colleagues to offer advice and support to the patient, their partner, and family members.

Physical disability introduces challenges into relationships and can increase stress and reduce relationship satisfaction. The role of healthcare professionals can be to re-establish previous ways of coping and communicating or to develop new ways of coping.[4] There is also the need to support those who are not in relationships to develop new relationships and friendships if desired.

The biopsychosocial model put forward in ➲ Chapter 13 can be applied more broadly to understand the different aspects of disrupted relationships and potential strategies for improving relationships in the context of physical rehabilitation.

Biological factors: physical changes

Physical impairments such as pain, fatigue, reduced physical fitness, or reduced mobility can impact a patient's ability to access community-based activities thereby reducing opportunities to meet with others and maintain friendships. Physical injury and changes in appearance can affect self-confidence and patients that experience prejudice or negative feedback may be reluctant to go out into the community. Rehabilitation goals should include supporting patients to access social groups in the community, engage in leisure activities with friends and family members, and develop greater independence with community mobility in order to support the development and maintenance of relationships.

Intimate relationships can also be affected by physical dysfunction that restricts physical mobility, flexibility, and spontaneity. Rehabilitation goals related to enhanced physical intimacy may vary from simple activities such as transfer training to ensure partners can sit together on the couch or be together in bed, through to developing and trialling strategies to engage in sexual activities using adapted positions, techniques, or aides. Hormonal and physiological changes to sexual drive and sexual ability are further outlined in ➲ Chapter 13.

Biological factors: cognitive and communication changes

Cognitive changes associated with ABI are directly associated with memory failures such as forgetting names, agreed social plans, appointments, birthdays, previous conversations, and information about a person. These can impact friendships and relationships, leading to an ever-reducing social circle. Executive dysfunction and social cognition deficits can result in reduced empathy; social judgement failures; disinhibited, impulsive, and inappropriate behaviour; tangential conversation; and poor social problem-solving. Slowed speed of information processing is likely to mean that injured individuals cannot keep up with group conversations. These factors can significantly impact social relationships, and people with ABI may experience confusion and frustration with social situations, such that they avoid social events. Furthermore, language impairments restrict what can be expressed or asked for in words and have a profound impact on communication. Communication difficulties often reduce levels of social participation and negatively impact intimate relationships.

Rehabilitation targeting communication, cognitive, and behavioural changes can be tailored to achieve specific relationship goals such as taking turns in listening and talking, trying to understand another person's point of view, joint problem-solving, and strategies to ensure their own physical or emotional safety when meeting new people.

Psychological factors

Psychological adjustment is a gradual process and a well-documented part of rehabilitation. Understanding and accepting change following a physical disability takes time, as the patient starts to create a new sense of identity. These emotional changes may result in frustration, which will often impact interactions with others, and influence how others relate to the patient.

Re-establishing a sense of intimacy with partners is identified as a source of enormous personal support. Patients report that the ability to share problems was a comforting experience, because they felt that they had an ally in the struggle.[5]

Social and environmental factors

Social groups hold beliefs about relationships and disabilities, which they may or may not be aware of, including the misperceptions that people with disabilities are not interested in sex and that sex is not important to older people. Misinformation and prejudice about what is a healthy relationship or a healthy sex life is common, and can lead to an absence of conversations about these important issues.

Environments can facilitate or inhibit development and maintenance of relationships. Rehabilitation settings are not optimally designed to facilitate relationships. Common areas are often large with few spaces to spend family time or intimate time with partners. Most patients desire discharge home to resume cohabitation with their partner and family. Living with a partner facilitates the transition home. Patients report it is easier to slip into life again and that it makes it possible to go home on short visits earlier on in the rehabilitation period, which was highly appreciated and contributed to the recovering process.[5]

References

1. Cameron JI, Cignac MAM (2008). 'Timing It Right': a conceptual framework for addressing the support needs of family caregivers to stroke survivors from the hospital to the home. *Patient Education and Counseling* 70, 305–314.
2. Pfeiffer K, Beische D, Hautzinger M, et al. (2014). Telephone-based problem-solving intervention for family caregivers of stroke survivors: a randomized controlled trial. *Journal of Consulting and Clinical Psychology* 82, 628–643.
3. Palmer S, Herbert C (2016). Friendships and intimacy: promoting the maintenance and development of relationships in residential neurorehabilitation. *NeuroRehabilitation* 38, 291–298.
4. Bowen C, Yeates G, Palmer S (2010). *A Relational Approach to Rehabilitation: Thinking about Relationships after Brain Injury*. Karnac, London.
5. Angel S (2015). Spinal-cord-injured individual's experiences of having a partner: a phenomenological-hermeneutic study. *Journal of Neuroscience Nursing* 47, E2–E8.

Vocational rehabilitation

Work and employment

Work is important for the health and well-being of individuals, regardless of whether it is paid or unpaid employment. The ICF defines employment as 'engaging in all aspects of work, as an occupation, trade, profession or other form of employment, for payment or where payment is not provided, as an employee, full or part time, or self-employed'.[1] Employment is known to be a critical component of personal identity and personal growth, disability adjustment, social integration, and life satisfaction, in addition to economic self-sufficiency. In its broadest sense, work is 'an activity involving mental or physical effort in order to achieve a result'.

People with disabilities experience a significantly higher than average level of unemployment. In March 2013, the economically inactive rate for working age people with a disability was 44.3%. This figure is nearly four times higher than for people without a disability (11.5%). In addition to a higher level of unemployment, people with disabilities are more likely to remain unemployed long term. Over 50% of people with a disability claiming Employment Support Allowance have been out of work for more than 5 years.[2]

The reasons for low employment rates are varied and complex. The most commonly cited barriers to work among adults with disabilities are a lack of job opportunities (43%) and difficulty getting transport to and from work (29%). Considerably fewer adults with disabilities have a formal qualification (11%) in comparison to their non-disabled peers (30%), considerably reducing employment opportunities, particularly for higher-paid work. In addition, workplaces vary in their willingness to facilitate employment for people with disabilities. In a recent survey, only 34% of people who work in the private sector and 55% of those who work in the public sector think their workplace welcomes people with disabilities.[2]

The common medical conditions in 2.7 million individuals in the working age group (16–64 years) on Employment and Support Allowance in the UK in 2011 are shown in Table 20.1.

Table 20.1 Medical conditions of individuals on Employment Support Allowance

ICD medical condition	% of total
Mental and behavioural disorders	43
Musculoskeletal conditions	16
Symptoms, signs, and abnormal clinical and laboratory findings (not elsewhere classified)	12
Neurological conditions	6.5
Injury, poisoning	5.5
Circulatory conditions	4
Respiratory conditions	2

ICD, International Classification of Disease.

Vocational rehabilitation

Definition

Vocational rehabilitation (VR) is a facilitatory process, designed to assist people with health conditions to secure employment and to integrate into the community. The focus may be on accessing employment, resuming employment, or maintaining employment.

VR is required for people with congenital or early-onset disabilities who require assistance to first enter the employment market (accessing employment) and also for people who become incapacitated during their working life (resuming employment). It is also critical to ensure maintenance of employment, as research has shown that long periods off work reduce the likelihood of resuming work. For example, after 6 months of back pain, there is an approximately 50% chance of returning to work, which falls to 25% at 1 year and 10% at 2 years. Few individuals return to any form of work after an absence of 1–2 years, irrespective of further treatment.

VR is complex, and for successful outcomes, health professionals need to consider the relationships between personal and environmental factors, availability of services, and the legislative framework, and how these interrelationships influence a worker's occupational ability or disability. The VR process for people with MS is outlined in Fig. 20.1, highlighting the complex influences on work outcomes. While this schematic relates to adults with MS, this process applies to people with other conditions impacting on work.

Although it makes sense for VR to take place in the community (as that is more closely related to the work environment), it is important to begin addressing this aspect of rehabilitation in the inpatient setting. This can start the process of patients considering their prognosis in the context of return to work, assist in them maintaining a constructive relationship with their employers, add meaning to inpatient goals, and include referral to VR services following discharge.

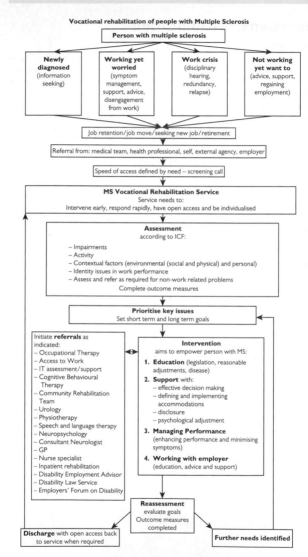

Fig. 20.1 Schematic view of vocational rehabilitation.

Reproduced with permission from British Society of Rehabilitation Medicine (BRSM). *Vocational Assessment and Rehabilitation for People with Long-Term Neurological Conditions: Recommendations for Best Practice*, p.34. London, UK: British Society of Rehabilitation Medicine. Copyright © 2010 British Society of Rehabilitation Medicine. https://www.bsrm.org.uk/downloads/vr4ltncv45fl-websecure.pdf.

Modifiable and non-modifiable factors

Factors associated with positive employment outcomes can be thought of as modifiable and non-modifiable.[3] This categorization provides a clear process for health professionals involved in VR to direct resources and rehabilitation towards factors that can be changed, rather than work-related factors that cannot be changed.

Table 20.2 provides an example of such categorization factors associated with resuming employment following a SCI. Independence in community-based transport (public transport or private transport) is strongly associated with positive employment outcomes and is an area that should be targeted by rehabilitation health professionals. Workplace-related environmental factors, both the physical environment and the psychosocial environment or 'workplace culture', strongly influence return to work outcomes, and can be a positive facilitatory factor or a barrier to re-engaging in work.

Table 20.2 Example modifiable and non-modifiable factors associated with resuming employment by ICF domain

ICF domain	Modifiable	Non-modifiable
Health condition		Aetiology
		Pre-injury chronic conditions
		Time since injury
		Severity of injury
		Time period of injury
Body structures and function	Motor status	Associated injuries
	Secondary health conditions	
Activity and participation	Use transportation independently	Pre-injury employment
	Able to drive	
	Able to live alone	
	Functional independence	
	Wheelchair skills	
	Mobility	
	Community integration	
	Post-injury employment [GOAL]	
Environmental: *Facilitators*	Area environmental factors	
	Assistive technology	
	Social support	
	Vocational Rehabilitation	
Barriers	Accessibility	
	Disability discrimination	
	Financial disincentives	
	Insurance	
Personal	Personal attitude	Age
	Post-injury education	Age at injury
		Sex
		Race
		Pre-injury education

Workplace and worker assessment

The ultimate goal of VR is to achieve 'fit' between the capacities of an individual and the demands of a job and workplace. Therefore, workplace and worker assessment are the first critical steps to understanding what the employee's capacities are and what the job and workplace demands are. A job analysis will ideally involve the employee, employer (or representative), and an experienced VR provider (health professional). A job analysis should gain a thorough understanding of:

• current work status of the person commencing/resuming work
• current rehabilitation/treatment regimen
• previous work-relevant injuries/illnesses and whether there are specific ongoing work guides applicable to these injuries/illnesses
• co-morbidities which may impact ability to perform duties
• functional tolerances—postural, strength, and movement
• details of duties performed at the time of onset of symptoms
• details of usual duties (if different from previous point)
• work processes, work flow, and frequency and duration of tasks
• work practices used by the worker to perform usual duties
• hours of work, usual work days, usual work roster, overtime (regular or intermittent), shift patterns, seasonal work, and provisions for rest breaks
• usual job rotations
• machines, tools, equipment, and work aids used
• licensing/training for specified duties or operation of machinery
• relevant environmental factors
• relationships with team leaders/supervisors and co-workers
• other roles/jobs performed (e.g. secondary employment, parenting, or significant caring responsibilities)
• list of duties the worker considers he/she can currently perform
• list of duties the worker considers he/she is currently unable to perform or has issues with and why.

The various health conditions, both physical and psychological, that can affect work raise a challenge for universal assessment of work readiness. To tackle this issue, a collaborative project involving the ICF Research Branch, WHO, International Labour Organization (ILO), World Confederation for Physical Therapy (WCPT), World Federation of Occupational Therapists (WFOT), and the International Society of Physical and Rehabilitation Medicine (ISPRM), developed an ICF-based Core Set to describe the functioning and health of individuals who participate in multidisciplinary VR. This core set forms the basis of a generic work assessment tool, the Work Rehabilitation Questionnaire (WORQ), designed to evaluate the person factors, social factors, and environmental factors that may limit engagement in productive work.[4] WORQ can be accessed at ℬ http://www.myworq.com/.

Vocational rehabilitation interventions

Research on interventions that aim to improve work participation is widely available, frequently focusing on specific diagnostic group, such as workers with low back pain, arthritis, or neurological conditions. These interventions often contain common strategies or elements, such as workplace assessment, changes in the work environment or organization, job accommodations, strengthening programmes, vocational counselling, guidance, education, and self-management strategies. These common interventions appear applicable irrespective of the person's underlying diagnosis. This multicomponent approach is likely to be more effective than interventions consisting of a single component. Ideally, specialist VR services will include a range of healthcare professionals including occupational therapists, physiotherapists, psychologists, physicians, social workers, and nurses. This multidisciplinary approach reflects the complexity of the problems.

For example, a recent report identified that people with MS sought VR services that highlighted the importance of managing task performance. They highlighted three separate but complementary processes including the need to:
- improve performance (e.g. through physiotherapy to improve mobility)
- compensate for changing performance (e.g. taking a taxi to work) and/or
- modify performance (e.g. by reducing the demands of the task).

Strategies should *not* solely focus on reducing impairment but on performance of an activity, and may require referral to occupational therapy, physiotherapy, speech and language therapy, neuropsychology, and specialist rehabilitation and neurological services, both medical and nursing. These services can minimize the impact of symptoms that impact work such as cognitive difficulties, visual decline, fatigue, heat sensitivity, and poor mobility. An essential component in work performance is increasing self-belief, developing good self-management skills, and self-efficacy. These are best addressed by a MDT.

Employment can be maximized if people with disabilities or specific medical conditions have access to appropriate assessment, job redeployment, and workplace accommodations including the use of assistive devices. One clear way of reducing the demands of working and diminishing associated fatigue is to reduce travel time and complexity. Advances in technology means that working from home is a viable option for many people with significant disabilities or chronic conditions.

Suitable duties

As part of the VR process, three types of suitable duties are typically considered when returning the worker to the workplace:
- Pre-injury duties—reduced hours of the pre-injury duties that the worker has the capacity to perform.
- Modified duties—components of some of the pre-injury duties that have been included or removed to match the worker's current capacity.
- Alternative duties—duties that are different from the pre-injury duties but allow the worker to stay at work or return to work.

Workplace accommodations and identification of suitable duties are most likely to occur when health professionals work closely with the employee and employer. Both employees and employers require education and access to support for times of potential conflict to prevent breakdown of employer/employee relationship. Accommodating unpredictable absences from work can pose significant problems for employers. Anecdotally, many employers express concern that work may aggravate the worker's condition and education on how to manage the condition in the work place is critical.

VR in the US has shifted from work hardening programmes, based away from the work site, to the delivery of services on site. This has the advantage of maintaining the employee in a worker role, even if on modified duties. This is better for employers, health services, and society. For the individual, this approach may avoid low self-esteem and loss of confidence in (or even actual decline of) ability. In the UK, 'fit' notes have replaced 'sick' notes, with the aim of returning a person to the workplace when fit to carry out some work-related activity, often with modifications to working pattern or environment, rather than waiting for them to become fully fit.

References

1. World Health Organization (2001). *The International Classification of Functioning, Disability, and Health (ICF)*. World Health Organization, Geneva.
2. Disability in the UK (2016). *Facts and Figures*. Papworth Trust. ℘ http://www.papworthtrust.org.uk.
3. Trenaman L, Miller WC, Querée M, et al. (2015). Modifiable and non-modifiable factors associated with employment outcomes following spinal cord injury: a systematic review. *Journal of Spinal Cord Medicine* 38, 422–431.
4. Finger M, Escorpizo R, Bostan C, et al. (2014). Work Rehabilitation Questionnaire (WORQ): development and preliminary psychometric evidence of an ICF-based questionnaire for vocational rehabilitation. *Journal of Occupational Rehabilitation* 24, 498–510.
5. Department for Work and Pensions (2013). Fit note (last updated 2018). ℘ https://www.gov.uk/government/collections/fit-note.

Further reading

British Society of Rehabilitation Medicine (BSRM) (2003). *Vocational Rehabilitation: The Way Forward*, 2nd edn. Report of a working party. BSRM, London.
British Society of Rehabilitation Medicine (BSRM) (2010). *Vocational Assessment and Rehabilitation for people with Long-Term Neurological Conditions: Recommendations for Practice*. BSRM, London.

Websites

Health and Safety Executive, UK—guidance: ℘ http://www.hse.gov.uk/guidance/index.htm.
The Council for Work & Health: ℘ http://www.councilforworkandhealth.org.uk/.

Orthotics

Definition and classification

An orthosis is an externally applied device used to modify, support, or enhance the functional characteristics of a body segment. Other terminology used to describe orthoses includes splints, braces, and supports. The practice of orthotics can include selecting, prescribing, designing, fabricating, fitting, applying, and evaluating orthoses to achieve specific rehabilitation goals. Orthoses can be custom-made, for example, by an occupational therapist, orthotist, physiotherapist, or rehabilitation engineer; or can be ordered 'off the shelf' as a prefabricated device. Orthoses can be fabricated from a variety of materials depending on the need for external support. Material selection is closely aligned with the purpose of orthotic fabrication, for example, to 'block' range of movement, to provide 'traction' for contracture management, or to 'assist' active movement. Casts made from plaster or fibreglass are used to immobilize fractures or provide stretch in the presence of contractures. A wide range of thermoplastic materials can be moulded to support the joint at a specific angle to facilitate function or maintain alignment. Softer materials such as neoprene provide less support to enable movement rather than immobilizing joints (primarily in the upper limb (UL)).

Types of upper limb orthoses

UL orthoses including splints, casts, and garments can be classified into three primary categories—static, dynamic, and hybrid:
- *Static orthoses* have no movable parts or joints incorporated into the design, and are primarily used to provide joint support, stabilization, protection, or immobilization. Static orthoses may be used in fracture management, inflammatory conditions such as arthritis, or peripheral nerve injuries where the body segment needs to be stabilized and protected.
- *Dynamic orthoses* have moving parts that promote, control, or restore movement. Dynamic orthoses can increase motion through traction or provided external assistance for weak musculature. Each orthosis is designed to provide 'pull', through the use of elastic bands, springs, or mechanical devices, to create force in a particular direction, applied at a specific joint to result in increased motion of the joint or muscle. Dynamic splints are often used in rehabilitation following tendon repair.
- *Hybrid orthoses* incorporate features of static and dynamic orthoses in one device. These orthoses cross multiple joints with the intention of restricting or limiting movement at some joints while allowing or facilitating movement at other joints. This hybrid activity is achieved through the elastic property of the materials used in fabricating these splints (e.g. Lycra®, neoprene, or foam).

Upper limb orthotic goals

The primary purpose of UL orthotic prescription, and the associated rehabilitation programme, is to regain or preserve UL function, in particular, prehension of the hand (Box 21.1). In this respect, the UL is significantly different to the lower limb (LL), which primarily serves to maintain body weight. Conversely, it is the role of the shoulder, elbow, forearm, and wrist to position the hand purposefully in space to enable gross and fine motor skilled movement.

Box 21.1 Upper limb orthotic goals

- Immobilize or protect weak, painful, or healing musculoskeletal structures by limiting load or motion.
- Prevent or correct developing deformities, including scarring and contractures.
- Enable movement or function, through substitution of weak or absent muscles or providing an attachment for other assistive devices.

Immobilization

The first goal is probably the most common indication for prescription of an UL prosthesis. Immobilization may provide joint protection, rest, or enable wound healing. Orthoses prescribed for joint protection, to reduce joint damage, or to help manage pain will also have a prescribed wearing regimen. For example, an orthosis for joint protection in the presence of arthritis will be worn at all times, in order to achieve the intended goal of controlling load across damaged joints and slowing disease progression. In contrast, an orthosis for joint protection following trauma might only be worn when symptoms of pain are present.

Immobilization for rest provides a supported 'resting' position (Fig. 21.1) that ideally creates balance between muscle and ligament tension to minimize complications associated with inflammation, pain, or contracture. The resting position is 10–20° wrist extension, neutral pronation/supination of the forearm, 20–45° metacarpophalangeal (MCP) flexion, and allowing between 10° and 30° interphalangeal (IP) flexion.[1] The thumb should be

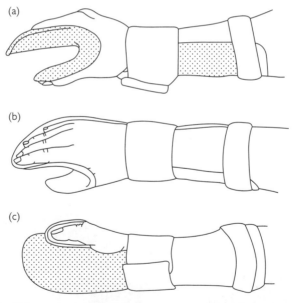

Fig. 21.1 Wrist–hand orthosis—static resting hand splint: (a) lateral view; (b) dorsal view; (c) volar view.

Reproduced with permission from McKee P. *Orthotics in Rehabilitation: Splinting the Hand and Body.* Philadelphia, USA: F. A. Davis Company. Copyright © Pat McKee, Illustrations by Sarina Wheeler.

immobilized opposite the fingers in palmar abduction and extension. The webspace should be maximized for both gross grasp and fine motor pinch.

Immobilization may also be undertaken to enable healing of soft tissues in a specific position, such as following skin graft surgery. The hand position will be primarily determined by the damaged structures and any surgery undertaken. In the case of surgical repair, the orthosis is designed to control loading across damaged limb segments and to promote healing. This requires careful balancing between immobilization for healing and guarding against loss of movement. Potential complications which are part of the normal healing process should be regularly monitored and orthotic adjustments should accommodate these processes, for example, through monitoring and adjusting an orthosis in the presence of oedema.

Immobilization may also be indicated in the presence of pain, particularly when pain limits engagement in function and is alleviated by external support. Musculoskeletal pain may arise from overstretching a muscle, ligament, or tendon; or may occur following abnormal movement in a joint or muscle. Joint pain may be caused by inflammation, and be present throughout the range of movement, only at the extremes of range, at all times, or only during activity. For example, a shoulder orthosis such as the Omo Neurexa™ (Ottobock) corrects alignment of the humeral head with the joint socket to alleviate pain, and correctly position and stabilize the shoulder (℅ https://www.ottobock.com.au/orthotics/products-from-a-to-z/omo-neurexa/).

Prevent or correct deformities

Immobilization of a body part, for example, following significant injury to promote healing as outlined in the previous section (➜ see 'Immobilization'), may result in a reduction of the normal ROM due to contraction of the joint capsule and shortening of tendons and muscles that cross the joint. In these cases, progressive stretching is required through the application of a series of orthoses, either static or dynamic, that are modified on a regular basis.

Clinical situations of UMN injury (CNS injury) or LMN disease or injury (brachial plexus injury, peripheral nerve injury, Guillain–Barré syndrome) require correct positioning to prevent deformity or contracture of the UL. In these cases, the neurological injury predisposes to musculoskeletal changes in the segment leading to deformity or contracture. While there is a strong professional opinion supporting the ability of orthoses to correct deformity and prevent contracture in these cases, the research evidence base is less convincing.

A range of orthoses may be used to prevent the formation of contractures including static, dynamic, and hybrid splints. Static splints or casts may be used to position joints to maintain stretch on soft tissues (Fig. 21.2). For example, in adults with brain injury, serial elbow casting may be used to increase the range of elbow extension in patients with developing flexor contractures. How aggressively an orthotic programme is pursued will be determined by the degree and duration of deformity.

Dynamic orthoses can also be applied to prevent post-surgical deformities. For example, a dynamic flexion splint following flexor tendon repair provides controlled motion, protecting the healing tendon from excessive tension, while allowing limited glide to prevent adherence of the tendon and development of a contracture. Hybrid splints made from Lycra® or similar positioning garments can provide low-load stretch while allowing some movement. These are used in adult burns and neurological rehabilitation, and more extensively in paediatric rehabilitation.

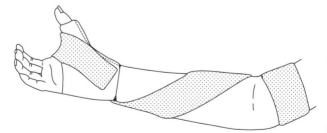

Fig. 21.2 Prefabricated TAP (tone and positioning) splint—reduces muscle tone by abducting the thumb and supinating the forearm.

Reproduced with permission from McKee P. *Orthotics in Rehabilitation: Splinting the Hand and Body.* Philadelphia, USA: F. A. Davis Company. Copyright © Pat McKee, Illustrations by Sarina Wheeler.

Enable movement or function

Orthotics can also be prescribed to facilitate or enable movement. Some orthotics are designed for very specific functional tasks, for example, a handwriting splint or an orthosis to enable steering wheel control while driving a car. A common goal for UL orthotic prescription is to support weak muscles or compensate for loss of movement. This can be achieved through application of static, dynamic, or hybrid orthoses for adults with various medical conditions including cervical level SCIs, brachial plexus injuries, or peripheral nerve injuries.

The types of UL movements that a therapist aims to facilitate through orthotic prescription include reach, grasp, release, carry/transportation, and in-hand manipulation. A 'wrist cock-up splint' is a commonly fabricated splint designed to provide proximal stability (wrist) in order to facilitate greater use of a more distal aspect of the UL (fingers). The wrist cock-up splint holds the wrist in a neutral to slightly extended position (preventing wrist flexion), and in doing so, provides forced opportunities for active finger extension during motor retraining activities, or more generally during activities of daily living. By blocking wrist flexion, passive finger extension is prevented, demanding active finger extension to open the hand for prehension and also for object release. Orthoses to enable movement in the presence of post-surgical weakness often have a dynamic component, for example, radial nerve injuries often require a dynamic wrist–hand–finger orthosis to assist with wrist and finger extension. This extensor force is achieved through use of rubber bands or spring wire (Fig. 21.3).

UL orthoses with integrated electrical stimulation

Commercially available orthotic devices are available with surface-base electrodes built into the design to provide stimulation for weak muscles, particularly focusing on finger and thumb activation. This form of functional electrical stimulation uses the platform of the orthosis to position the forearm and wrist in an ideal position for function, allowing activation of finger and thumb flexion or extension as required. Good proximal control at the shoulder and elbow increase the functional benefit of this style of orthotic device.

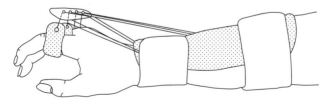

Fig. 21.3 Forearm-based orthosis for radial nerve injury with MCP-assisted extension.

Lower limb orthotics

LL orthoses are primarily prescribed to assist with walking in individuals with gait disturbances caused by musculoskeletal or neuromuscular disorders. Walking is one of the most commonly cited rehabilitation goals across many diagnostic groups. Orthotic devices may enhance walking by reducing pain, preventing or correcting deformities that may limit ambulation or by immobilizing specific LL joints. Many neoprene orthoses for the LL appear to work by increasing proprioceptive feedback rather than providing structural support. Thus goals for LL orthotic prescription reflect the goals previously cited for UL prosthetic prescription.

LL orthoses are typically fabricated from metal, plastics (including thermoplastics), or lightweight carbon graphite, depending on the length of time the device will be required for, the load applied to the orthosis, and other forces applied across the device. Various strapping materials are used including leather or Velcro® to ensure correct fit to the LL body segment. Thermoplastic moulded orthotics are the most commonly used in current practice, as the orthosis can be customized to provide better conformation and fit, are generally lighter, fit better inside footwear, and are aesthetically more acceptable to patients than metal and leather style braces.

Correct biomechanical alignment is critical to maximize ambulatory ability. Close correlation between the centres of rotation of both orthotic and the anatomical joint is required to avoid pain, joint swelling, and skin breakdown. Biomechanical malalignment can adversely affect functional ambulation. Ongoing monitoring through inpatient and outpatient rehabilitation programmes provides an opportunity to complete any required adjustments to enhance function and achievement of ambulatory goals.

Gait analysis

Clinicians routinely use informal visual analysis of gait to evaluate the dynamic alignment of an orthosis. Gait deviations and compensations can be observed during ambulation, with our without gait aids. While visual analysis does not provide quantitative information, clinical observation and patient feedback remain the primary sources of information on orthotic fit and alignment. Formal gait analysis provides greater objectivity but requires more equipment and time for analysis. This is true whether using highly sophisticated instrumented gait analysis in a gait laboratory, measuring kinematics (temporal and spatial measures, motion and force analysis) or using less sophisticated approaches such as video recording to enable slow motion and instant replay. ➲ See Chapter 18 for further information on gait analysis.

Foot orthoses

Customized foot orthoses are an effective tool in managing most abnormal biomechanics of the foot and associated foot pain. Foot pain is a common complaint and may be due to joint disease or to nerve injury from unsupported weight-bearing structures. Foot orthoses can be corrective or accommodative devices. When used to correct malalignment, the bones of the foot must be flexible enough to allow the foot position to achieve improved alignment using more rigid materials such as thermoplastics, acrylic laminates, or carbon graphite composites. In contrast, accommodative devices are made from soft, open or closed cell foam alone or in combination with a semi-rigid material to provide cushioning or support to feet with existing deformities. The goal of these orthoses is to prevent further deformity while improving function using the following design features:

- *Medial longitudinal supports*—used for simple flat feet and for lateral plantar nerve compression.
- *Arch supports*—prevention of subtalar valgus subluxation, as found in rheumatoid arthritis and osteoarthritis.
- *Metatarsal domes*—transfer weight away from the metatarsal heads to the metatarsal shafts to relieve the pain from metatarsophalangeal joint disease and subluxation.
- *Heel insoles*—for traumatic heel and leg pain and plantar fasciitis.

Modified shoes

Modifications to commercial footwear or fabrication of fully customized footwear is an aspect of LL orthotic practice that can successfully treat many simple problems that affect ambulation, by accommodating existing foot deformities, reducing pressure on painful areas of the foot, improving safety, or limiting movement in painful joints.

- *Wedges or flares*—are extensions attached either medially or laterally to the sole of the shoe to provide mediolateral stability. The flare may be added at the heel only or extend the length of the shoe. Flares are not intended to correct deformities but rather to control motion of the foot. In contrast, wedges are designed to accommodate rigid deformities or to correct flexible deformities of the hind foot.
- *Shoe raises or elevations*—these components are used to compensate for acquired or congenital leg length discrepancies. In general, decreasing leg length discrepancies to less than 2 cm between the limbs is adequate to improve gait efficiency and reduce pelvic tilt. When added to the contralateral shoe of a patient with neurological impairment in limb clearance, shoe raises can also facilitate swing phase of the affected LL. Elevations can be applied at the heel only or along the entire shoe length, internally or externally on the shoe sole.
- *Rocker soles*—the main purpose of a rocker sole is to allow the foot to move from heel strike to toe-off without metatarsal bending. This reduces pressure on the metatarsal heads and can assist gait by increasing forward propulsion.

Ankle–foot orthoses

A well-fitting ankle–foot orthosis (AFO) (Fig. 21.4) can influence LL posture in the direct area of the ankle and foot, but also more proximally; which may in fact be the indirect effect that is being sought. Thus, AFOs may be used to reduce swing phase problems and to influence stance phase impairments resulting from three main conditions that reduce locomotor function:

- Conditions that result in weakness of the muscles controlling the ankle–foot complex.
- UMN lesions that result in hypertonicity or muscle spasticity.
- Conditions that result in pain or instability through loss of structural integrity of the LL and/or foot–ankle complex.

Equinovarus deformity is the most commonly observed pathological LL posture associated with CNS injuries. This can result in an unstable base

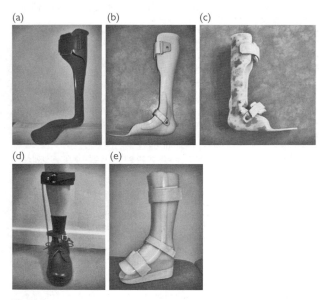

(a) (b) (c)

(d) (e)

Fig. 21.4 Various ankle–foot orthoses (AFOs). (a) The posterior leaf spring orthosis has a narrow sprung segment at the ankle level. (b) A rigid AFO. (c) An AFO may incorporate hinges. (d) A conventional AFO/caliper—here an inner iron with a T strap to correct varus deformity. (e) A Charcot restraint orthosis walker (CROW) is bivalve, total contact with liner.

Reproduced with permission from Mitchell J. and Cooke P.H. Orthoses of the foot and leg in *Oxford Textbook of Trauma and Orthopaedics* (2 ed.), Bulstrode C. et al. Oxford, UK: Oxford University Press. © 2011 Oxford University Press. Reproduced with permission of Oxford University Press through PLSclear. http://oxfordmedicine.com/view/10.1093/med/9780199550647.001.0001/med-9780199550647-chapter-009004.

of support during stance phase and heel contact may be limited or missing. Limited ankle dorsiflexion prevents forward progression of the tibia over the stationary foot during stance phase, causing knee hyperextension, lack of propulsion, and interference with terminal stance. Significant plantarflexion is observed during swing phase, producing difficulty with foot clearance and increasing risk of falls. Use of an AFO to control the ankle position during swing and stance phase is recommended.

A thermoplastic AFO is indicated for patients who lack ankle muscle power but have normal hip extension strength, full knee extension range of movement, and nil or minimal flexor spasticity. The footplate and ankle component (non-articulated) positions the foot and ankle in slight dorsiflexion, which produces a knee extension force during stance phase. Adaptations to the AFO may be required if ankle inversion is also present, requiring an inversion strap or pad. Additionally, if ankle clonus is triggered during stance phase, a dorsiflexion stop, set just before the clonus appears, may prevent the stretch response from triggering clonus

An AFO (Fig. 21.4) uses a mechanical lever arm to control the ankle and when appropriately designed, can also influence movement at the knee joint. Orthotics utilize a three-point pressure system (Fig. 21.5). In an AFO, the large primary force ($F_{Primary}$) is applied in a posteroinferior direction over the anterior surface of the ankle joint. The two correcting or counterforces are applied in the anterior direction ($CF_{Posterior}$) and in an upward direction

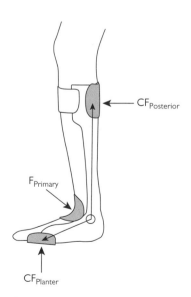

Fig. 21.5 Three-point pressure system.

($CF_{Plantar}$). Greater distance to these counter forces produces a longer lever arm, therefore requiring smaller forces to counterbalance the primary force. The two correcting forces should sum to equal the primary force, ensuring that the sum of forces is zero in a well-balanced orthosis.

LL orthoses with integrated electrical stimulation

Successful use of AFOs with integrated neuromuscular electrical stimulation has been recently reported. Several designs are commercially available, and are being increasingly used in clinical situations. These fall into two main groups; those that detect stance phase through a force transducer in the shoe (e.g. NESS L300™), or those using a tilt sensor (e.g. WalkAide®). These devices electrically stimulate the peroneal nerve via an external electrode to produce dorsiflexion, meaning that they are less or ineffective for people with LMN lesions. Implantable electrodes are currently being trialled.

Knee–ankle–foot orthoses

Knee–ankle–foot orthoses (KAFOs) are used when there is weakness in both ankle and knee muscles. Uncontrolled knee flexion during early stance phase is associated with LL instability. This is evident during early stages of neurological recovery when flaccidity and muscle weakness negatively affect LL strength and control. When the patient is unable to control excessive knee flexion, an external orthosis such as a KAFO may be required to achieve stance stability and the goal of ambulation. Plastic moulded KAFOs integrate standard ankle and knee components, but the uprights and bands are made of lightweight thermoplastic that closely fits the patient's LL.

Various orthotic knee joints and locking mechanisms are available (Fig. 21.6). A single axis or free joint (Fig. 21.6a) allows full flexion and extension while providing mediolateral and rotational stability to the knee joint. A drop lock (Fig. 21.6b) holds the knee in extension in standing, providing stability in all planes. It must be unlocked for knee flexion to occur when returning to sitting position. An offset knee joint (Fig. 21.6c) is positioned behind the anatomical knee axis, providing enhanced biomechanical stability. This form of knee joint is available with and without a locking mechanism. An adjustable knee joint (Fig. 21.6d) offers an adjustable knee joint that can accommodate for changing range of motion or for fixed contracture at the knee.

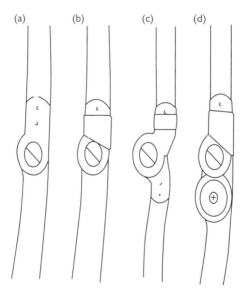

Fig. 21.6 Various orthotic knee joints and locking mechanisms.

The most common form of locking mechanism is a drop lock, which descends over the distal part of the joint to lock the knee joint in extension. For patient who cannot use a drop lock due to reduced UL strength or reduced balance, an alternative is the pawl and bail-locking mechanism, which allows the medial and lateral locks to be disengaged at the same time by applying pressure on the bail from a rigid surface such as the edge of a chair. This mechanism is often used for patients with paraplegia who must maintain bilateral UL via crutches for stability.

Knee orthoses

Sporting injuries requiring surgery or knee rehabilitation can also lead to knee instability and a knee orthosis (KO) may be indicated. Various KO designs are available, in part driven by the expanding field of sports medicine (Table 21.1). Most KOs consist of calf and thigh cuffs, joined by uprights on either side of the knee with an adjustable range knee joint in the centre. Traditional KOs with short lever arms are not effective under high load or strain. KO designs with longer lever arms and components that allow a degree of rotation have been developed for higher-level activity and athletes.

Table 21.1 Orthoses for knee conditions

Mild collateral ligament injuries	A neoprene KO may allow quadriceps and hamstring exercises while maintaining a degree of safety
More severe collateral ligament injuries	A hinged KO may be useful for deformities of <20°
	Orthoses are rarely useful for deformities of >20°
Cruciate ligament injuries	More complex stabilization from brace to prevent anteroposterior movement.
Disrupted knees	Straight leg polythene jackets

Hip–knee–ankle–foot orthoses

These devices are designed to hold both LLs in a stable extended position for upright standing. People wearing a hip–knee–ankle–foot orthosis (HKAFO) traditionally use either a hop-to gait with a walker or a swing-through gait with a pair of crutches for ambulation. As the HKAFO encompasses the hips, pelvis, and sometimes the trunk, they tend to be much more cumbersome to use, more challenging to don and doff, more expensive to fabricate, and require more maintenance than AFOs and KAFOs. HKAFOs only partially restore functional mobility, often with high energy cost.

HKAFOs designed to be used with a reciprocal gait, use a lateral weight shift from one limb to the other as the basis for orthotic-assisted reciprocal gait. Several different models exist including the hip guidance orthosis (HGO), the ORLAU Parawalker, the reciprocating gait orthosis (RGO), and the Advance Reciprocating Gait Orthosis (ARGO). The underlying goal for all of these orthoses is to achieve mobility with a lower energy cost than expended in a typical swing through gait pattern.

Recent advances in orthotics

Until recently, people with foot, ankle, or knee orthoses have not been able to enjoy walking in wet areas. Carbon fibre technology combined with plastic injection moulding has resulted in high strength joint structures made of water-resistant material which allows users to walk in wet areas such as a pool or the beach. An example is the Aqualine™ Waterproof Orthosis System available from Ottobock (https://www.ottobock.com.au/orthotics/products-from-a-to-z/aqualine/).

Spinal orthoses

Orthoses are also used to correct spinal deformities or to prevent progression of deformity. Spinal orthoses can control gross movement of the trunk in different planes, such as flexion or extension of the spine. Custom-made orthoses are used for patients born with scoliosis to slow the rate of progression of deformity (full details of these orthoses are beyond the scope of this chapter). Lumbosacral corsets are the most commonly prescribed orthoses for lower back pain. Cervical orthoses for neck pain are also used, for example, for patients with rheumatoid arthritis of the cervical spine.

Reference

1. Wilton JC, Dival TA (1997). *Hand Splinting: Principles of Design and Fabrication.* W.B. Saunders, London.

Further reading

Edelstein JE, Bruckner J (2002). *Orthotics: A Comprehensive Clinical Approach.* Slack Inc, Thorofare, NJ.
Lusardi MM, Jorge M, Nielsen CC (2013). *Orthotics and Prosthetics in Rehabilitation.* Elsevier, St Louis, MI.
McKee P, Morgan L (1998). *Orthotics in Rehabilitation: Splinting the Hand and Body.* F.A. Davis Company, Philadelphia, PA.

Wheelchairs and seating

Introduction

Freedom of movement is an essential component of independence and mobility is closely associated with quality of life. People who have difficulty with independent walking often require a wheelchair to assist with mobility. The ICF model can be used to guide the provision of wheelchairs and seating through consideration of the individual personal factors and preferences, environmental limitations, the person's desired activities and participation in life roles, as well as the person's health condition or impairments of body structure and function. Various health conditions can cause mobility impairments ranging from requiring occasional wheelchair through to full-time use by a person who is unable to sit unsupported (Table 22.1). Therefore, wheelchair prescription and provision needs to fit the intended purpose as well as the underlying medical impairment. Neurological and musculoskeletal conditions are the most common conditions associated with wheelchair use. In addition, frail older people and people with chronic conditions (e.g. COPD) may also require a wheelchair for mobility, as well as people with cognitive impairments such as pervasive developmental disorders, intellectual impairments, and some forms of dementia such as Alzheimer's disease. It is important that all rehabilitation team members have the opportunity to be involved in decisions regarding wheelchair prescription.

Table 22.1 Medical conditions associated with impaired mobility and wheelchair use

Neurological	Musculoskeletal
Cerebral palsy	Acute pain
Spina bifida	Chronic pain
Muscular dystrophy	Joint inflammation
Stroke	Contractures
Brain injury	
SCI	
MS	
Parkinson's disease	
Huntington's disease	
Guillain–Barré syndrome	

Wheelchair prescription: a team approach

The complexity of wheelchair and seating prescription requires a team approach involving the patient and caregivers, usually occupational and physical therapists, a rehabilitation engineer (if specialist adaptations are required), a rehabilitation physician, in some cases a speech and language therapist, and the equipment supplier.

A thorough assessment should include collecting information on the patient's medical condition, potential changes to the condition (particularly for degenerative conditions), current mobility status, previous use of wheelchairs or other mobility devices, factors that may have a secondary impact on mobility such as cognitive or visual perceptual abilities, fatigue, sensation (for pressure management), and medications.

A physical examination should include lower and upper body strength and ROM, coordination, muscle tone, and proprioception. Specific joint restrictions should be noted, for example, due to arthritis. During the assessment, consideration should be given to the most effective form of wheelchair control (e.g. manual push), or in cases of insufficient UL strength and control, switch controlled, chin or head control, breath controlled, and so on.

Stability in sitting should also be assessed by evaluating unsupported sitting on a plinth. The presence of kyphosis, scoliosis, or other deformities should be noted and categorized as fixed or flexible. Evaluating pelvic position is critical: identify anterior or posterior tilt, pelvic obliquity or rotation. Hip and knee ROM should be assessed and accommodated if reduced due to fixed contractures. Poor stability usually indicates the need for specialized seating and positioning (➜ see 'Specialized seating and positioning'). Pressure mapping systems can also be used to measure the skin interface pressure between the seated surface and the skin of the wheelchair user.

In addition to assessing factors associated with the person's medical condition, the wheelchair purpose and mobility goals should be established:
- Will the chair be used indoors or outdoors, or both?
- What floor surfaces exist in the person's home? Access and egress?
- What is the typical outdoor terrain over which the chair will be used?
- What activities will the person engage in while using their wheelchair?
- Will it be self-propelled or attendant-propelled?
- Will it be transported in a vehicle?
- Will the wheelchair user access public transport?

Formal assessments such as the Wheelchair Outcome Measure (WhOM) can be useful to ensure a client-centred approach to goal setting.

Manual wheelchairs

Self-propelled wheelchairs

Manual wheelchair users with the upper-body capacity to propel a wheelchair tend to use a self-propelling wheelchair or independent manual mobility system. These wheelchairs are either fixed frame or have a folding frame. In order to propel, these chairs have large rear wheels and small front wheels, called castors (Fig. 22.1 shows the basic manual wheelchair components). Fixed-frame wheelchairs are generally sturdier and easier to push, while folding chairs are often heavier making them harder to push, but are more transportable (usually folded in the rear/boot of a car).

Lightweight or ultralight wheelchairs (Fig. 22.2a) are preferred for self-propulsion as this may reduce longer-term joint stress, particularly shoulder injuries. Correct set-up of wheelchairs to reduce secondary shoulder injuries is critical for patients who will self-propel. For this reason, a healthcare professional should prescribe and configure manual self-propelled wheelchairs, and hire wheelchairs which are not individually fitted should be avoided for longer-term use.

High-performance sports wheelchairs are typically used by people who are very proficient at using their wheelchair. These chairs are typically rigid framed and often slightly less stable in order to gain greater manoeuvrability and speed. High-performance wheelchairs enable people with disabilities to engage in leisure and sports. Many wheelchair sports have organizations to provide support and opportunities to engage with other sportspeople including wheelchair basketball, fencing, rugby, sailing, and tennis.

Camber refers to the angle of rear wheel tilt. Most wheelchairs generally have 8° camber. This is to bring the wheels inward and closer to the

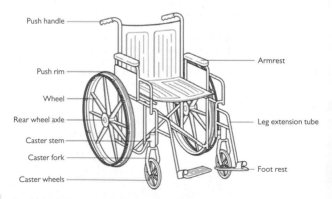

Fig. 22.1 Basic manual wheelchair components.
https://clinicalgate.com/wheelchairs-and-seating-systems/.

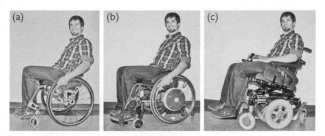

Fig. 22.2 Wheelchairs with different levels of support to the user: (a) lightweight rigid frame manual wheelchair; (b) manual wheelchair equipped with power-assisted wheels; (c) a mid-wheel drive power wheelchair with joystick control.

body making it easier to push using arms. It also increases the lateral stability of the wheelchair. High-performance sports wheelchairs have an increased camber when compared to standard manual wheelchairs.

Adjusting the axle position affects the seat position relative to the wheels, seat angle, and wheel alignment. These adjustments influence propulsion biomechanics and are utilized to suit the function and preferences of the individual.

Power-assisted wheelchairs (Fig. 22b) have force/moment sensing push rims that provide additional torque to the rear axle as the user propels the wheelchair. This adaptation is designed to enable individuals to complete mobility tasks faster and more efficiently. Power-assist is particularly useful when navigating up steep inclines. Additionally, effort (measured via oxygen consumption and heart rate) and pain can be significantly reduced when using power-assist, making it a good compromise between a manual wheelchair and a power wheelchair.

Attendant-propelled wheelchairs

These wheelchairs are used by people who cannot independently push or propel. Attendant-propelled wheelchairs for adults tend to have small wheels at the front and rear; and for children these resemble a buggy or pushchair. When prescribing an attendant-propelled wheelchair, it is important to consider the needs of both users: the rider and the attendant. For the comfort of the attendant, the weight should be minimized and push handles adjusted to the height of the attendant. If the rider is going to be sitting for extended periods of time, a tilt-in-space option will increase comfort and reduce the incidence of pressure areas. Appropriate head support is needed for wheelchairs with a tilt-in-space option (Fig. 22.3).

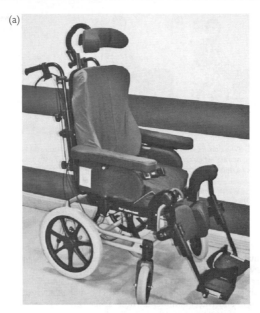

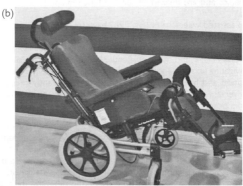

Fig. 22.3 (a) Wheelchair in standard position; (b) tilt-in-space wheelchair in 'tilt position' (note the angle between wheelchair back and seat remains at 90°).

Reproduced with permission from Talbot K. et al. Disability management in *Motor Neuron Disease: A Practical Manual.* © 2009 Oxford University Press. Reproduced with permission of Oxford University Press through PLSclear. http://oxfordmedicine.com/view/10.1093/med/9780199547364.001.1/med-9780199547364-chapter-11.

Wheelchairs for specific client groups

- *Amputee wheelchairs* are designed with the rear axle set behind the user. This is required to balance the posterior shift in the patient's centre of gravity caused by the absence of a leg or legs.
- *One-arm drive wheelchairs* are used by patients with a hemiparesis and have two push rims on one side that control separate wheels. These can often be difficult to control. An alternative for people with hemiplegia is a lever drive wheelchair; however, these are also difficult to manoeuvre.
- *Bariatric wheelchairs* are being prescribed to accommodate patients with obesity. Regular wheelchairs can usually support a body weight up to 135 kg. Bariatric wheelchairs can accommodate people with a body mass up to 450 kg.

Powered wheelchairs

Powered (or electric) wheelchairs can provide independent mobility to people who fatigue quickly or have insufficient upper-body strength to propel a manual wheelchair. Historically, health professionals have been concerned that prescribing a powered wheelchair will result in the person losing muscle power and/or gaining weight due to reduced exercise. Recent research has highlighted that people do not usually increase their weight but do increase their activity, improve their independence, and increase quality of life.

Powered wheelchairs are usually driven using a joystick as shown in Fig. 22.1c. Joystick ends can also be modified for easier grip, such as adding a ball shape or T-bar. Joystick alternatives are available for people who have limited UL function. These include foot controls, head or chin controls, scanning interfaces, and breathing controls (also referred to as sip-and-puff). Breath-controlled switches are used by people with high-level quadriplegia, controlling the wheelchair drive via a straw mounted near their mouth. These systems are becoming less popular with newer technology such as head array sensors and micro-proportional joysticks. Switch-activated sensors can be set up using a single switch or a switch array. Single-switch systems are typically slower to use (as a scan is required each time the switch is used, i.e. forward, backward, left, and right) but less motor control is required for a single switch. In contrast, a switch array provides faster wheelchair drive control but requires greater motor control to use.

Cognitive factors also require assessment when prescribing a power wheelchair to ensure adequate speed of processing, good problem-solving, and safety awareness. Visual perceptual skills should also be evaluated.

Stand-up wheelchairs

There are many health benefits to standing upright. Stand-up wheelchairs enable the patient to stand for periods of time, which is associated with decreased bladder infections, reduced osteoporosis, and decreased spasticity. There are also potential psychological benefits from a stand-up wheelchair, enabling communication at eye-level with the communication partner. This may be particularly beneficial in workplace and social settings (Fig. 22.4).

There are also many environmental restrictions to being seated at all times. Wheelchairs users can overcome some of these restrictions through the use of a stand-up wheelchair. Access to wall-mounted cupboards and storage areas in the home and workplace, access to shelving when shopping, engaging in leisure activities, and so on. Biomechanical considerations of centre of gravity are critical for stand-up wheelchair users.

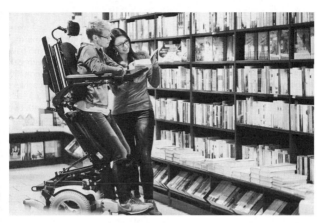

Fig. 22.4 Standing wheelchairs can enable fuller participation in social activities.
http://ortopinos.com/producto/silla-ruedas-electrica bipedestacion-quickie-jive-up/.

Scooters

In general, scooters are a good option for individuals to retain some mobility, when specialized seating is not required. Therefore, people who have limited ability to ambulate long distances, for example, people with cardiopulmonary disease, may find scooters a suitable option for community mobility. In contrast, people with neuromuscular disorders may not achieve the required seating support in a scooter.

Scooters can be three-wheeled (one central wheel at the front with two rear drive wheels) or four-wheeled. Scooter seats are similar to a typical car seat, proving comfort but fewer seating options or adaptability. Steering is achieved using handlebars, similar to a bicycle, which is intuitively easier for most people than the joystick of a power wheelchair; however, greater UL strength is required to steer. Scooters are less manoeuvrable than power wheelchairs, and a trial in the patient's home environment is recommended before purchase. In general, three-wheeled scooters have more manoeuvrability, while four-wheeled scooters offer greater stability. Improved batteries now enable greater community access and the increased use of scooters in public spaces has reduced social stigma.

Specialized seating and positioning

Specialized seating is the component of a seating and wheelchair system which is specifically prescribed to meet one or more of the following aims:
• Improve postural control.
• Improve sitting stability and balance.
• Reduce the effort required to maintain posture.
• Maintain tissue integrity.
• Allow distribution of load to provide maximal pressure relief.
• Prevent or delay the onset or worsening of deformities.
• Enhance comfort and length of sitting time.
• Decrease cardiorespiratory burden through postural support.
• Optimizes function.

By achieving the above-listed aims, important functional goals can be achieved such as to:
• enable good positioning for swallowing and feeding
• encourage bladder drainage and bowel function
• enable good positioning for eye contact and communication
• increase sitting time to engage in ADLs, particularly community access, employment, and studying
• reduce carer burden.

Armrests
Armrests provide support and comfort, as well as providing a surface from which to push when performing sit-to-stand transfers from the wheelchair. There are a variety of arm rests available depending on the goals of wheelchair use, including desk arms, full-length arms, and swing-away arm rests.

Footplates and leg rests
• Footplates provide a safe and secure place upon which to rest the patient's feet. They may also assist with positioning, particularly if heel loops or positioning straps are used. Footplates can be swing-away to assist with standing transfers, removable to assist with transporting the wheelchair in a vehicle, or can be fixed. Fixed footplates are more frequently used with ultralight or sports wheelchairs to reduce the overall mass of the wheelchair.
• Leg rests provide support along the posterior of the calf. These are usually prescribed for users of tilt or recline wheelchairs, and for users who need to elevate their feet to prevent distal swelling.

Head support
A moulded head support is critical for wheelchairs that have recline or tilt-in-space functions. Head supports may also serve as a mounting area for switches to activate the wheelchair or other environmental controls.

Cushions

The most basic cushion is composed of foam and can be used for infrequent or short-duration sitting (<4 hours per day). Cushions providing more pressure relief are made from gel, fluid, air, or a combination of materials. These cushions aim to distribute pressure over a large area of the sitting surface (buttocks and thighs) to reduce the effect of high pressure over susceptible areas such as the sacrum or ischial tuberosities. In addition to pressure relief, a good cushion should also provide postural stability, reduce shearing forces, and it may need to insulate from heat or conduct heat depending on the person's condition.

It is often difficult to achieve all of the desired seating outcomes with one cushion, so compromise may be needed. For example, air-filled cushions provide high levels of pressure relief, but some manual wheelchair users find the surface too unstable for propulsion-related activities.

Back support

The standard sling-back of a wheelchair offers little support and encourages a kyphotic sitting posture. A back-support that fixes to the upright poles of the backrest can provide stability for people with reduced trunk control. Lateral supports can be added if needed. Typically, people with greater support needs, such as those using attendant-propelled manual wheelchairs or power wheelchairs will also require trunk support. Contoured back rests and lateral supports can be fitted to accommodate a fixed deformity or to modify a flexible deformity, depending on the aims of the seating system and the goals of the patient.

Recline and tilt-in-space

Recline and tilt-in-space functions aim to relieve pressure, improve posture (particularly by controlling the hip to trunk angle), provide comfort, and also to assist with personal care tasks performed by carers:
- Recline helps to stretch hip flexors and also assists carers with access to catheters, enables toilet access, and positioning of slings for hoist transfers.
- Tilt-in-space keeps the hip and knee angles constant while shifting weight off the ischial tuberosities. Patients who are unable to independently weight shift to relieve pressure should have a tilt-in-space wheelchair.

Technology
- Infrared controllers allow power wheelchair users to operate infrared enabled devices with their wheelchair control (e.g. DVD player, television).
- Computer mouse emulators allow the driver controls to access a wireless computer mouse.
- Integrated devices (e.g. iPortal™) allow the driving controls of a power wheelchair to access all features on an iPhone™, iPad™, or Android™ device.

Further reading

Useful website

The Wheelchair Outcome Measure (WhOM): 🔗 https://millerresearch.osot.ubc.ca/tools/mobility-outcome-tools-2/the-wheelchair-outcome-measure-whom/.

Technical aids and assistive technology

Background

Technology now has a ubiquitous presence in the everyday lives of most people. Contemporary smartphones can be used to access the Internet, take photographs, record audio and video, play music, conduct banking, track daily walking distances, monitor sleep activity, control home appliances, and perform numerous other functions—including still making an occasional telephone call. This convergence of functions means that several stand-alone pieces of equipment are no longer required. Convenience and portability increases and new possibilities are created for the end user.

This single device now has the *potential* to perform a vast number of different functions and be used in a range of activities for purposes such as work, leisure, learning, and communication. Purchasing the latest smartphone, however, does not immediately mean that the end user will want to, need to, or be able to use all of the available functions. Device selection, configuration, and use are often highly individualized and depend on the device user, their past experiences, skills, interests, and requirements.

Conceptually, there are parallels with this everyday technology and the selection and use of assistive devices. Assistive technology has the *potential* to support people to engage in a number of life areas and activities, the *potential* to increase participation, and the *potential* to improve quality of life. This potential is often only realized following a highly individualized process to identify the most suitable assistive solutions.

Scope

The purpose of this chapter is to explain key terminology and considerations in the provision of assistive technology. Generic principles and selection processes will be explored to support decision-making and provide a foundation for assistive technology practice. Developments in everyday technologies will also be highlighted to illustrate their increased potential to be used by a wider range of people.

Assistive technology products can be broadly categorized as being 'low tech' or 'high tech' (also known as digital assistive technology). Low-tech assistive technology typically includes equipment that does not require a power source such as paper-based communication aids, walking sticks, and dressing aids. Digital assistive technology includes devices that have electronic components and require power to operate such as computers, voice output augmentative and alternative communication devices, and powered wheelchairs. This handbook includes chapters presenting information about assistive devices such as wheelchairs, seating, and equipment for pressure relief (➜ see Chapter 22), orthotics (➜ see Chapter 21), and prosthetics (➜ see Chapter 41).

Within this chapter, examples of digital assistive technology will be provided to illustrate key features and considerations in the assistive technology process. Assistive technology principles, however, can be applied to both low- and high-tech assistive products.

Definitions

Assistive product (device)

Assistive products can also be referred to as 'assistive devices' or 'aids and equipment'. The International Organization for Standardization Standard 9999[1] serves to classify assistive products and defines them as:

- any product (including devices, equipment, instruments and software), especially produced or generally available, used by or for persons with disability:
  - for participation
  - to protect, support, train, measure or substitute for body functions/ structures and activities, or
  - to prevent impairments, activity limitations or participation restrictions.

Assistive technology

Assistive technology (AT) is an umbrella term referring to 'the application of organized knowledge and skills related to assistive products, including systems and services'.[2]

Assistive technology service

An AT service refers to 'any service that directly assists an individual with a disability in the selection, acquisition, or use of an assistive technology device'.[3] AT services can include:

- evaluation of individual AT needs
- provision of AT devices
- selection, design, customization, maintenance, and repair of AT devices
- training and/or technical assistance for people involved in the use, recommendation, and support of assistive devices.

Assistive solution

An assistive solution is the individualized, tailored combination of assistive devices and services to support a person's autonomy and participation in life activities. This concept reflects that the solution to an individual need can require the use of more than an assistive device. A combination of generally available products, assistive devices, environmental modifications, and personal assistance could be involved in an individual assistive solution.[4] The configuration of this combination may change according to a person's different contexts (e.g. at home, work, or school), and is likely to be different from one person to another. It is therefore not possible or viable to select assistive products based solely on medical diagnosis or without considering individual circumstances and preferences.

Priority assistive products

In 2016, the WHO released the 'Priority Assistive Products List (APL)'. The APL was developed in response to the WHO 2011 *World Report on Disability* which identified that access to assistive products was a widespread unmet need.[5] More than 1 billion people globally require at least one assistive product, yet only one in ten of these people has access to them.[6]

The APL identifies 50 assistive products (Table 23.1) determined to represent prevalent need, have the greatest potential impact on a person's life and considered essential to maintain or improve activity performance and participation.[2] The final list was established using multiphase, inclusive methodology involving stakeholders across all areas of AT. After four phases of the study, more than 10,000 people with diverse linguistic and socioeconomic backgrounds from over 160 countries had contributed to the development of the list.

The APL is intended to provide WHO Member States with information to guide the development of national policy, resource allocation, product development, and access to assistive products and associated services. The products on the APL should be available at a price the community can afford and include six broad domains: mobility, vision, hearing, communication, cognition, and environment. The final APL includes both high- and low-tech assistive products and is presented in alphabetical (not priority) order.

Table 23.1 World Health Organization 'Priority Assistive Products List'. NB: list is presented in alphabetical order, not in order of priority

Alarm signallers with light/sound/vibration	Personal digital assistant (PDA)
Audioplayers with DAISY capability (Digital Accessible Information SYstem)	Personal emergency alarm systems
Braille displays (note takers)	Pill organizers
Braille writing equipment/braillers	Pressure relief cushions
Canes/sticks	Pressure relief mattresses
Chairs for shower/bath/toilet	Prostheses, lower limb
Closed captioning displays	Ramps, portable
Club foot braces	Recorders
Communication boards/books/cards	Rollators
Communication software	Screen readers
Crutches, axillary/elbow	Simplified mobile phones
Deafblind communicators	Spectacles; low vision, short distance, long distance, filters and protection
Fall detectors	Standing frames, adjustable
Gesture to voice technology	Therapeutic footwear; diabetic, neuropathic, orthopaedic
Global positioning system (GPS) locators	Time management products
Handrails/grab bars	Travel aids, portable
Hearing aids (digital) and batteries	Tricycles
Hearing loops/FM systems	Video communication devices
Incontinence products, absorbent	Walking frames/walkers
Keyboard and mouse emulation software	Watches, talking/touching
Magnifiers, digital hand-held	Wheelchairs, manual for active use
Magnifiers, optical	Wheelchairs, manual assistant—controlled
Orthoses, lower limb	Wheelchairs, manual with postural support
Orthoses, spinal	Wheelchairs, electrically powered
Orthoses, upper limb	White canes

The importance of assistive technology

The impact of impairment and the subsequent experience of disability is influenced by environmental facilitators and barriers. Barriers to participation can include:

- the physical environment
- societal attitudes
- access to information
- availability of services and support
- access to assistive devices
- legislation and policies.

The United Nations Convention on the Rights of Persons with Disabilities (CRPD) commits Member States to eliminating these barriers in order to promote inclusion and equal opportunities for all people.[7] ATs and assistive devices are identified in several CRPD Articles as important strategies to support this process.

AT can be utilized by people to reduce or eliminate the experience of disability. Users of AT include people of all ages with a health or age-related condition and/or a sensory, physical, or cognitive impairment. Assistive products can compensate for these impairments and support users to participate in life roles and activities of choice. When provided appropriately, AT can increase autonomy, productivity, social participation, and health-related quality of life.

Assistive technology processes

A number of models have been developed to outline the process of AT provision and service delivery.[8–11] These include:

- Matching Person and Technology (MPT) model
- Human Activity Assistive Technology (HAAT) model
- Comprehensive Assistive Technology (CAT) modelling framework
- Framework for Modelling the Selection of Assistive Technology Devices
- Assistive Technology Evaluation and Selection (ATES) tool
- Integrated Multi-Intervention Paradigm for Assessment and Application of Concurrent Treatments (IMPACT2) Model
- Assistive Technology Service Method (ATSM)
- Student Environment Task Tools (SETT) Framework
- Assistive Technology Assessment (ATA) process model (Fig. 23.1).[12]

A multicentre study conducted in Europe by Friederich and colleagues[13] identified that AT selection is also often informed by occupational therapy models such as the Model of Human Occupation (MOHO), and the Canadian Model of Occupational Performance and Engagement (CMOP-E). The majority of these models have similarities including:

- supporting a holistic view
- using a person-centred approach
- engaging in a task-led, team approach to device selection
- acknowledging the complex relationships between the person, their environments, and their activities and participation.

The AT selection process can have a causal relationship with user satisfaction, cost effectiveness, and AT use or disuse.[13] The application of a model or best-practice framework aims to guide service delivery and optimize outcomes for AT users.

The assistive technology team

An effective assistive solution usually requires a team approach. This should always include the perspectives of the potential device user and their immediate circle of support (e.g. family, friends, and paid and unpaid support staff). Some people may not be able to fully articulate their perspective due to age, cognitive, or communication issues. In this instance, user input may instead be provided by a family member or relevant support person.

Professionals may also be involved at different points of the AT process, often with backgrounds in areas such as:

- occupational therapy
- physical therapy
- prosthetics and orthotics
- psychology
- rehabilitation engineering
- rehabilitation medicine
- speech pathology
- teaching/education.

Entry-level training in AT is variable. To practise responsibly, a general understanding of key AT principles is required. Expertise in specific assistive products or practice areas is often developed through engaging in

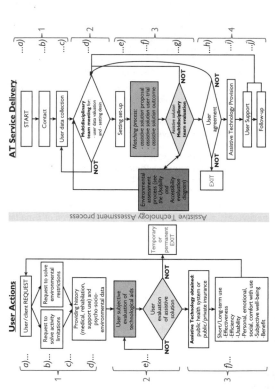

Fig. 23.1 Flowchart of the ATA process ideal model.

both formal and informal continuing professional development activities, mentoring, and through experience.

Information-savvy AT users may have the lived experience, skills, and resources to research and identify their own assistive products and solutions. Informed and expert users may require limited or no input from others to do this. Seeking input and feedback from other members of the AT team, however, can still be a valuable part of the selection process. Working as a team can lead to a dynamic information exchange, mutual benefit through the discovery and sharing of information, and stimulate discussion that may identify factors otherwise not considered. It is essential that all members of the team acknowledge any limitations in their own skills and seek additional resources, information, and support in order to provide the most effective, ethical, and sustainable AT services.

Steps in assistive technology service delivery

The steps shown in Box 23.1 were initially identified in a European study from the early 1990s involving over 21 organizations in 12 countries and remained relevant when reviewed 20 years later.[4] They are internationally recognized and considered to comprehensively describe all of the possible steps involved in AT service delivery. The organization of these steps may vary in practice and each step may not be present in all AT service systems (Box 23.1).

Evaluation of assistive solutions and articulating outcomes from technology use are an important component of service delivery and follow-up. This can be accomplished using generic rehabilitation outcome measures (➲ see Chapter 6), or through the use of AT-specific tools such as:
- the Individually Prioritised Problem Assessment (IPPA)
- the Psychosocial Impact of Assistive Devices Scale (PIADS) or
- The Quebec User Evaluation of Satisfaction with Assistive Technology (QUEST).

Box 23.1 Steps in assistive technology service delivery

- *Initiative/referral*: first contact with the service delivery system.
- *Assessment*: evaluation of needs and preferences.
- *Selection of the assistive solution*: defining the individual AT programme.
- *Selection of the equipment/trial*: choosing the specific equipment within the AT programme.
- *Authorization*: obtaining funding.
- *Implementation*: delivering the equipment to the user, fitting, and training.
- *Management and follow-up*: maintenance and periodic review.

The ATA process model builds on the steps in service provision and articulates corresponding user actions.

Reproduced with permission from Andrich, R. et al. Service delivery systems for assistive technology in Europe: An AAATE/EASTIN position paper. *Technology & Disability*, 25(3): 127–146. Copyright © 2013, IOS Press. The publication is available at IOS Press through http://dx.doi.org/10.3233/TAD-130381.

Devising assistive solutions

The multiple variables and complex factors involved in AT selection and use has resulted in a body of AT research literature primarily generated through personal opinion, surveys, single case studies and uncontrolled studies with small sample sizes.[9,14] Although there are acknowledged limitations in the available evidence, the most effective assistive solutions utilize the acknowledged steps in service delivery and incorporate the following principles:

Solution-focused

Determine what the person needs to achieve and/or what they aspire to do. Focus on devising a solution that addresses an identified problem, impairment, or activity limitation. This approach aims to determine suitable options and potential strategies to address the problem and, ultimately, may or may not involve assistive products.

Person centred

It is essential to include the AT user and their relevant circles of support in the AT process. Components of this include:
• acknowledge lived experience
• identify the person's priorities, goals, aspirations, attitudes, and interests
• establish the person's history of technology use
• consider both current and future skills, abilities, and environments of use.

Introducing an assistive product without user involvement in product selection and/or introducing a device without identifying a clear purpose are identified as main contributing factors in AT device non-use. Device non-use or abandonment wastes resources and represents a lost opportunity for a person to experience the potential of an effective assistive solution. Poor solutions can also result in negative health outcomes and possible injury.

Informed choices

Identifying a suitable solution requires access to impartial information about assistive products and other options in order to make informed decisions. This applies to all members of the AT team and can be challenging with the rapid development of technologies and the volume of information available online. It is important to understand device features, possibilities, and limitations and match these to the person's individual situation, desired activities, and abilities. Where possible, trial of the assistive product/solution should occur in context to evaluate suitability and ensure that expectations can be met.

Access to products and funding

Assistive products on the WHO APL are intended to guide policy and health initiatives to ensure key assistive devices are available to people at a price the community can afford. This is intended to be a starting point from which Member States can develop policies most relevant to address local need and circumstances. In this process, it is essential to also acknowledge that although a device may be affordable for a person to purchase, funded through policy, or other health or insurance systems, the provision of the product alone may be inadequate to realize the potential of the AT solution.

Access to support

Timely support is a key factor in enabling a person to gain the most potential benefit from an assistive solution. The support a person requires will range from discrete, episodic input, to the provision of frequent, ongoing support as an integral part of the assistive solution.

Discrete support may include:
- provision of information about assistive devices, their features, and ability to address identified issues
- assistance to identify the required components of an assistive solution
- identification of potential assistive products
- evaluation of options and trial
- justification to obtain funding (consider funding for both products and ongoing support)
- initial device set-up and personalization/customization
- training (the AT user and/or their circle of support)
- trouble-shooting technical issues
- periodic maintenance and repair
- review and evaluation of the solution.

Ongoing support could involve:
- set-up and positioning of both the person and device/s for use
- assistance to use the device
- developing and extending skills in assistive device use
- exploring new opportunities afforded by the use of a device
- routine device maintenance (e.g. cleaning, charging, updates, and trouble-shooting)
- advocacy for inclusion and opportunities for device use across different social and physical environments
- dynamic and frequent evaluation and review, particularly if a person's abilities are changing due to development, new skill acquisition, or a decline in abilities.

Funding for the support and implementation of AT is less tangible and more difficult to quantify than funding for the provision of assistive devices. In the AT process, there is the need to work with the team to establish a holistic view of the proposed assistive solution and to acknowledge, identify, and articulate the levels of discrete and ongoing support the solution is likely to require. An assistive product may not be viable if a person does not have access to the support required and this should be considered in funding allocation and policy development. Compromise in device selection or contexts of use may be necessary if the required environmental supports are not congruent with the support available.

Consideration of contexts

Assistive devices cannot sit in isolation out of a person's physical and social environments. The environment can afford opportunities and also present barriers to the implementation of an assistive solution. For example, a person may have access to a power wheelchair, carefully selected to match their individual preferences and requirements and introduced with the intention to support their mobility at home, in the community and to enable participation in their employment. To realize the potential of the assistive device, the solution needs to consider factors beyond the provision of the device itself, such as:

- whether ongoing support will be required (and available) for charging the wheelchair and/or to transfer in and out of the wheelchair
- ensuring an accessible home environment, including adequate circulation space and the ability to leave and enter the home
- an accessible built environment to mobilize in the community and workplace
- ability to access and use community transport, or provision of a modified vehicle to self-drive or be driven in
- the need for any accommodations or personal assistance in the workplace (e.g. for computer access, to set-up/position materials, etc.)
- prevalent social attitudes: what extent do they support equality and participation for all people, will advocacy be required to achieve any of the above-listed factors?

In isolation, the power wheelchair is unlikely to fulfil the intended aspirations and achieve the potential benefits of device provision. If a device is introduced in the absence of adequate information and without considering the assistive solution as a whole, there is an increased likelihood that the person will not be able to maximize the potential of the device. An assistive solution therefore needs to consider and balance these principles. With progress towards a more inclusive society, there is now increasing potential to utilize and incorporate everyday technology into an assistive solution.

Everyday technology

Most everyday technologies (e.g. desktop computers and mobile devices such as tablets and smartphones) incorporate a number of personalization features to support their access and use. This is in response to the introduction of accessibility regulations, increased public awareness, and consumer demand for improvements.[4] There is also an increased and more meaningful application of 'Universal Design' principles (Table 23.2).[15]

The rapid development of everyday technology has presented opportunities for developers to respond to these requirements and consumer demands. For example, when the Apple iPad™ was first introduced in 2010, the device could only be accessed if a person was able to reach and directly touch the screen. This limited the application and use of the device. Subsequent updates to the operating system have resulted in numerous integrated features to support access (🖰 see https://support.apple.com/accessibility for further information) and compensate for impairments in areas such as vision, hearing, physical and motor skills, literacy, and learning. Parallel to this has been the development of specific Apps and accessories (e.g. Apps for voice output communication, refreshable braille displays, and switch interfaces), which enable a wider range of people to utilize the technology once the interface has been set up, configured, and personalized to suit their requirements.

Table 23.2 Principles of Universal Design

PRINCIPLE ONE: Equitable Use

The design is useful and marketable to people with diverse abilities

PRINCIPLE TWO: Flexibility in Use

The design accommodates a wide range of individual preferences and abilities

PRINCIPLE THREE: Simple and Intuitive Use

Use of the design is easy to understand, regardless of the user's experience, knowledge, language skills, or current concentration level

PRINCIPLE FOUR: Perceptible Information

The design communicates necessary information effectively to the user, regardless of ambient conditions or the user's sensory abilities

PRINCIPLE FIVE: Tolerance for Error

The design minimizes hazards and the adverse consequences of accidental or unintended actions

PRINCIPLE SIX: Low Physical Effort

The design can be used efficiently and comfortably and with a minimum of fatigue

PRINCIPLE SEVEN: Size and Space for Approach and Use

Appropriate size and space is provided for approach, reach, manipulation, and use regardless of user's body size, posture, or mobility

Effective personalization requires an understanding of what can be possible, a knowledge of how to do this, as well as an appreciation of potential limitations. People who previously may have required the use of purpose-built or 'specialized' equipment are now afforded opportunities to successfully interface with everyday or 'mainstream' technology. Being able to use everyday technology is more inclusive and may mean that people are motivated to engage in the effort required to learn and use the technology. Widespread familiarity, confidence, and skills with everyday technology can increase access to support compared to what may be required or available with the use of specialized equipment.

Ways to access technology

There are increasing features in device operating systems and the ability to use peripheral components to enable the use of everyday technology. Once an access method is determined, there is the potential to use devices for voice output, computer control, and to control other equipment such as a television, lights, air conditioning, blinds, and doors. Without effective and reliable access, there are limited opportunities for technology use which restricts or eliminates the possibility of using technology for communication, leisure, social participation, and employment. Some options for access include:

Direct touch

Using a body part, usually fingers. May require specific positioning of the person and/or device to be effective, for example, for those with limited dexterity or upper limb range of motion.

Modified direct touch

Use of operating system software personalization options to compensate for limitations in accuracy or control, for example, altering key repeat rate, touch screen sensitivity; use of a stylus or physical pointer (Fig. 23.2); larger or smaller keyboard size; colour contrast; and size of keyboard labels. Fig. 23.2 shows how a tablet and smartphone can be accessed using a mouth stylus. An integral part of this solution is that the devices are mounted to the user's power wheelchair and positioned at a distance and angle to enable the user to make selections using the mouth pointer.

Mouse control

Includes mouse options of various sizes and ergonomic shapes, trackball, joystick, gyroscopic, and head-controlled devices. Head-control options use a camera to track the movements of a reflective sticker. The sticker is usually attached to the user's forehead, nose, or eye glasses, but could be attached to a finger or elsewhere within the camera's line of sight.

The use of a mouse necessitates the need to also consider a person's ability to accurately position the screen pointer. This may be supported by personalization to change the speed of cursor movement, the colour and size of the cursor, or the location and size of the targets on the screen. The ability to select items also needs to be considered. This may be achieved by clicking the mouse button, selection by hovering (dwelling) on a target for a predetermined time (which may require additional software), or the use of peripheral components to select using a switch activated with any body part or reliable movement.

Voice

It is possible to enter text and interact with some everyday devices using voice control. For some people, this may present a novel, convenient, and efficient way to use speech to use their device, for example, to set reminders, alarms, and calendar events, ask for directions, make telephone calls, and send text messages. For others, the use of voice control may represent the difference between being able to use a device or not.

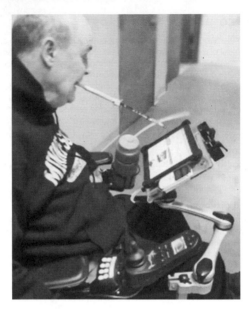

Fig. 23.2 Modified direct touch.
©BlueSky Designs.

For successful voice control, there is the need to consider factors such as ambient noise, the volume of the user's voice, their breath control, articulation, and potentially their accent. A voice-activated intelligent personal assistant (e.g. 'Ok Google' on Android™ devices or 'Siri' on Apple macOS™ and iOS™), is a hands-free way to interact with a mobile device or computer that is incorporated as a standard feature of the operating system. The potential to use this feature can only typically be realized if:

- the system recognizes the user's voice/speech
- the user knows and can execute the commands
- there is a connection to the Internet.

Eye control
Also known as eye gaze or eye tracking. These systems send out infrared light that reflects off the retina. A camera picks up the reflection and software processes eye movements and translates this into movement on the screen. Similar to mouse control, there is the need to consider the person's ability to accurately position the screen pointer and select items. Selection is possible with dwell, an external switch, or purposeful blink. An on-screen keyboard is required for text entry and specialized software may provide increased potential for personalization and improve ease of access. Ambient

light can interfere with the effectiveness of the camera and eye control systems are typically unable to be used outdoors. This is essential to consider in the development of an assistive solution using this access method.

Switch access

This necessitates use of a repeatable, reliable movement from any body part to activate a switch which then executes an action. The outcome of the action depends on the interface and system components being used. This can range from cause-and-effect control of adapted toys, to the ability to perform complex computer tasks, compose messages for voice output communication, and for environmental control.

There are numerous switches available in a range of sizes, with varying levels of activation force and differing activation methods. It is essential to consider the physical, visual, and cognitive task demands of switch access and provide opportunities to develop skills in this access method. Positioning of system components can be crucial as the person needs to be able to reliably activate the switch when required but not activate it accidentally to make erroneous selections.

Brain–computer interfaces

The potential to use brain activity as an input method was first conceived in the 1970s. Brain–computer interface (BCI) systems include invasive options that require the implantation of electrodes directly into the brain, and non-invasive options that use external electrodes. Several studies have demonstrated that it is possible to use a BCI to control devices for spelling or voice output, environmental control, and to access the Internet. Extensive support is typically required for training, set-up, and use of these systems.

Summary and conclusion

The ageing population and the increasing number of people living with chronic illness and disability affords opportunities to exploit the capabilities of technology and enable people to perform tasks they would otherwise be unable to do. Assistive solutions are individualized, tailored combinations of assistive devices and services and have the potential to enable people to engage in their chosen life roles.

This potential can only be achieved if assistive solutions are developed using a task-focused, person-led process. The solution needs to consider the interplay between the person: their preferences, skills, resources, and environments; the assistive products: features, availability, cost, and complexity; and the support: the provision and availability of timely support to implement and sustain the assistive solution. The most effective assistive solutions consider and balance all of these factors and can fulfil their potential to support well-being, participation, and inclusion in the community.

References

1. International Organization for Standardization (2016). *ISO 9999: Assistive products for persons with disability: Classification and terminology.* International Organisation for Standardization, Geneva.
2. World Health Organization (2016). *Assistive Technology* [Fact sheet]. ℘ http://www.who.int/mediacentre/factsheets/assistive-technology/en/.
3. United States Government (2004). *Assistive Technology Act of 2004.* ℘ https://www.govtrack.us/congress/bills/108/hr4278/text.
4. Andrich R, Mathiassen NE, Hoogerwerf EJ, et al. (2013). Service delivery systems for assistive technology in Europe: an AAATE/EASTIN position paper. *Technology & Disability* 25, 127–146.
5. World Health Organization (2011). *World Report on Disability.* WHO Press, Geneva. ℘ http://www.who.int/disabilities/world_report/2011/en/.
6. World Health Organization (2016). *Priority Assistive Products List.* ℘ http://apps.who.int/iris/bitstream/10665/207694/1/WHO_EMP_PHI_2016.01_eng.pdf?ua=1.
7. United Nations (2007). *Convention on the Rights of Persons with Disabilities Resolution 61/106.* United Nations, New York. ℘ http://www.un.org/disabilities/convention/conventionfull.shtml.
8. Lenker JA, Paquet VL (2003). A review of conceptual models for assistive technology outcomes research and practice. *Assistive Technology* 15, 1–15.
9. Bernd T, Van Der Pijl D, De Witte L (2009). Existing models and instruments for the selection of assistive technology in rehabilitation practice. *Scandinavian Journal of Occupational Therapy* 16, 146–158.
10. Desideri L, Roentgen U, Hoogerwerf EJ, et al. (2013). Recommending assistive technology (AT) for children with multiple disabilities: a systematic review and qualitative synthesis of models and instruments for AT professionals. *Technology & Disability* 25, 3–13.
11. Baxter S, Enderby P, Evans P, et al. (2012). Barriers and facilitators to the use of high-technology augmentative and alternative communication devices: a systematic review and qualitative synthesis. *International Journal of Language & Communication Disorders* 47, 115–129.
12. Federici S, Scherer MJ, Borsci S (2014). An ideal model of an assistive technology assessment and delivery process. *Technology & Disability* 26, 27–38.
13. Friederich A, Bernd T, de Witte L (2010). Methods for the selection of assistive technology in neurological rehabilitation practice. *Scandinavian Journal of Occupational Therapy* 17, 308–318.
14. Anttila H, Samuelsson K, Salminen AL, et al. (2012). Quality of evidence of assistive technology interventions for people with disability: an overview of systematic reviews. *Technology & Disability* 24, 9–48.
15. The Center for Universal Design (1997). *The Principles of Universal Design, Version 2.0.* North Carolina State University, Raleigh, NC. ℘ https://www.ncsu.edu/ncsu/design/cud/about_ud/udprinciples.htm.

Further reading

Assistive product information databases

AbleData: ℘ http://www.abledata.com/.
European Assistive Technology Information Network: ℘ http://www.eastin.eu/.
Independent Living Centres Australia: ℘ http://ilcaustralia.org.au/.

Assistive Technology professional associations

Association for the Advancement of Assistive Technology in Europe (AAATE): ℘ http://aaate.net/.
Australian Rehabilitation and Assistive Technology Association (ARATA): ℘ www.arata.org.au.
British Assistive Technology Association (BATA): ℘ http://www.bataonline.org/.
Global Cooperation on Assistive Technology (GATE): ℘ http://www.who.int/disabilities/technology/gate/en/.
Rehabilitation Engineering and Assistive Technology Society of North America (RESNA): ℘ http://www.resna.org/.
Rehabilitation Engineering and Assistive Technology Society of Japan (RESJA): ℘ http://www.resja.or.jp/eng/.

Personal factors in rehabilitation

Introduction

Consider yourself as an individual. Even in times of ill health you are more than just a biological machine. You have values, attitudes, and beliefs that all go towards shaping your world view. Your past is important in what you plan or hope to be doing in the future, with whom, and when. The same holds true for your patients. Following an acute or chronic disabling illness, these same personal factors form the essence of your patients' lives, and can directly impact on their rehabilitation.

A patient's perception of their journey through rehabilitation is based on their personal aspirations and expectations as filtered through the value and belief systems within which they live. From these internal constructs, the uniqueness of an individual's lived experience emerges and explains how two individuals with the same health condition or health state may respond to their situation very differently.

Contextual factors within the ICF model

The introduction of the 2001 ICF by the WHO recognized a shift in management of health conditions towards an integrated biopsychosocial model, in which individual health outcomes were acknowledged as interactions between *health conditions* and *contextual factors*. Among contextual factors are external *environmental factors* (e.g. social attitudes, physical characteristics of the built environment, legal and social structures, as well as climate, terrain, and so forth), and internal *personal factors*, which include individual characteristics that are not part of the health condition but may influence behaviour and health (ℬ http://www.who.int/classifications/icf/en/). The WHO describes personal factors as internal factors, which 'may include gender, age, coping styles, social background, education, profession, past and current experience, overall behaviour pattern, character and other factors that influence how disability is experienced by the individual'. These factors can play a positive or negative role through the patient's personal experience of the health disease or condition.

Although personal factors are recognized in the ICF model, they are not currently categorized or coded. Development of a classification system is ongoing.[1] In the rehabilitation process, personal factors can play a role in all stages of assessment, goal setting, or matching interventions to the person's characteristics. This chapter does not provide a detailed narrative on all personal factors, but focuses on the personal factors that have the ability to facilitate or inhibit the rehabilitation process. The personal factors described in the following sections are categorized using the structure suggested by Grotkamp et al.[2] acknowledging that the first categories (general characteristics and personality factors) are considered stable, while the later presented categories (attitudes, behaviours, and life situation) are potentially modifiable and may be changed during or following the course of rehabilitation.[3]

General personal characteristics

These are the inherent general characteristics of an individual that are typically unchangeable such as age, sex, and genetic factors that may have an effect on a person's health and can modify the process or outcome of rehabilitation.

For example, brain injury rehabilitation research has demonstrated age-related and gender-related differences in rehabilitation outcomes. Older age is typically associated with lower discharge functional independence scores on the Functional Independence Measure (FIM) and poorer FIM gain or FIM efficacy.[4] Similar findings have been reported in stroke research. Presence of co-morbidities and a lower baseline level of functioning prior to rehabilitation admission are usually cited as factors that contribute to reduced outcomes in older patients. However, this should be tempered by an awareness that older patients can still achieve independence or near-independent levels of functioning if provided with intensive, multidisciplinary rehabilitation.

In contrast to these findings, age differences appeared less significant in a longitudinal study (12 years) of nearly 800 patients in cardiac rehabilitation. Younger patients (<65 years) with fewer co-morbidities improved more than their age-matched peers with a higher co-morbidity index. In contrast, older patients improved to similar degrees irrespective of their stratified co-morbidity index. The authors concluded that age should not discourage referral to cardiac rehabilitation.[5]

Personality factors

In contrast to the general characteristics mentioned earlier in this chapter, personality factors are potentially modifiable. These attributes influence a person's nature in terms of their individual responses to a situation, and distinguish one person from another.[2] If these personality factors become pathological, they are not classified among the contextual factors in the ICF but among the ICF mental aspects of body functions.

Personality factors can facilitate or inhibit the rehabilitation process and may include personality traits such as relative extraversion/introversion; emotional lability/stability; openness or willingness to change; self-efficacy and self-confidence; and relative optimism/pessimism. People with extroverted personality traits tend to be gregarious, sociable, and have the emotional ability to express themselves. This personality trait has long been associated with positive rehabilitation outcomes. In contrast, social inhibition and negative affect are traits consistent with Type D personality, expressed as apprehension, irritability, high levels of insecurity in social situations, and excessive control. A recent meta-analysis highlights the predictive relationship between Type D personality traits and major adverse cardiac events such as cardiac death, and poorer health-related quality of life.[6]

When considering personality factors, the most frequently discussed and researched personal factor related to rehabilitation outcomes is self-efficacy. The construct of self-efficacy is suggested by Grotkamp et al.[2] to be an aspect of self-confidence, described as self-assuredness, self-efficacy, and the ability to assert oneself. Self-efficacy focuses on people's beliefs in their own capabilities to exercise control over their functioning and over events that affect their lives, and is therefore closely aligned with other constructs such as internal locus of control, optimism, mastery, and determination.[7] It appears that the importance of self-efficacy centres on the *perceived* rather than *actual* ability to perform or exhibit a particular behaviour coupled with a belief that the behaviour will achieve the desired results, in this context, the desired health or rehabilitation outcomes.

Multiple studies, across several health conditions, support an association between improved self-efficacy and rehabilitation outcomes. Choosing selectively from this literature, two recent systematic reviews of self-efficacy interventions in stroke rehabilitation highlight the importance association between self-efficacy and various rehabilitation outcomes. These reviews confirm the positive association between self-efficacy and improved mobility, ADLs, quality of life, and perceived health status, with a negative association between self-efficacy and incidence of depression.[8,9]

Attitudes, skills, and behaviour patterns

The attitudes, basic skills, and behaviour patterns a person uses during the process of rehabilitation can significantly influence their motivation when it comes to intervention and changes in behaviour. Positive attitudes, skills, and behaviours are essential in coping with the effects of disease and health conditions. Supportive or facilitatory skills can include the ability to develop coping strategies in dealing with the effects of a health condition, whereas some behaviour patterns, such as eating and physical activity habits, can exacerbate existing problems.

Attitudes towards health, disease, and disability are potentially modifiable personal factors, and can be thought of as a factor that *influences* health and rehabilitation outcomes and as a potential *target* of intervention.[10] Coping style and motivation can directly influence a person's attitude towards their disability and their response to intervention, which in turn can affect recovery. Previous healthcare experiences can influence an individual's expectations of the current intervention, as well as influencing their attitudes more generally towards healthcare professionals and healthcare in general.

The experience of a traumatic event (e.g. TBI or SCI) can lead to unanticipated positive change, and has been recently termed *post-traumatic growth*. Patients may experience a changed perception of themselves, as someone who is stronger than they expected or who can draw on internal resources that we previously untapped. The consequences of coping with significant trauma can also change the nature of relationships with other people, creating a greater sense of connectedness, empathy, compassion, and closeness to others, as patients realize (often for the first time) that they exist as part of a larger whole. A changed sense of what is important in life is also commonly cited as a positive experience following significant trauma.

Skills and behaviours commonly targeted as part of, or the primary focus of, rehabilitation programmes include coping strategies and development of resilience. *Resilience* has been described as a person's capacity to maintain stable psychological function following exposure to a significant event such as illness or injury. Resilience has alternatively been conceptualized as a personality trait that remains relatively stable over time, as well as a modifiable trait compromised of behaviours, thoughts, and actions that can be learnt.[11]

The relationship between resilience and rehabilitation outcomes has been demonstrated across various medical conditions. For example, a recent large longitudinal study of community-dwelling adults with MS, muscular dystrophy, post-polio syndrome, or SCI confirms the positive relationship between resilience, social and physical rehabilitation outcomes, and the negative relationship with depressive symptoms. More importantly, there was a *predictive* relationship over 3 years between high resilience and fewer depressive symptoms and increased social functioning.[12]

This evidence of a predictive relationship suggests that enhancing resilience and self-efficacy at the time of rehabilitation or immediately following rehabilitation may have the potential to reduce longer-term negative consequences of trauma or chronic medical conditions. Guccione[13] highlights some of the key principles and strategies for developing or enhancing an individual's resilience (Table 24.1).

Table 24.1 Key principles and strategies for developing or enhancing resilience

Principle	Strategy
Openly communicate the clinician's reasoning that underpins the rehabilitation care plan.	• Share results of initial examination • Include the patient directly in goal setting
Establish a realistic understanding of the patient's potential for change.	• Identify 'benchmarks' of positive prognosis, particularly the first clinical indicator of change
Encourage a patient's sense of resuming control by setting achievable goals and focusing on patient's accomplishments	• Provide explicit feedback on goal attainment and goal progress • Facilitate patient choice and preference in the rehabilitation plan whenever possible • Implement rehabilitation plan incrementally in achievable 'small bites'
Allow opportunity to engage with others who have a shared experience of similar challenges	• Recommend patient and family support groups • Provide 'vicarious learning' through group experiences as appropriate to the patient
Frame the experience as an opportunity for growth and part of a positive trajectory of adaptation	• Build upon the patient's personal history of success in meeting challenges when possible • Focus attention on what has been gained on the journey to 'who I am today' and 'where am I going tomorrow' not what was lost through illness or trauma 'yesterday'

Adapted with permission from Guccione A.A. Resilience and Self-efficacy As Mediators of Quality of Life in Geriatric Rehabilitation. *Topics in Geriatric Rehabilitation*, 30(3):164–9. Copyright © 2014, Wolters Kluwer Health | Lippincott Williams. doi: 10.1097/TGR.0000000000000022.

References

1. Mller R, Geyh S (2015). Lessons learned from different approaches towards classifying personal factors. *Disability & Rehabilitation* 37, 430–438.
2. Grotkamp S, Cibis W, Nüchtern E, et al. (2012). Personal factors in the International Classification of Functioning, Disability and Health: prospective evidence. *Australian Journal of Rehabilitation Counselling* 18, 1–24.
3. Howe TJ (2008). The ICF contextual factors related to speech-language pathology. *International Journal of Speech-Language Pathology* 10, 27–37.
4. Meiner Z, Yuvchev I, Sajin A, et al. (2015). Rehabilitation outcomes of patients with stroke: effect of age on functional outcome and discharge destination. *Topics in Geriatric Rehabilitation* 31, 138–144.
5. Listerman J, Bittner V, Sanderson BK, et al. (2011). Cardiac rehabilitation outcomes: impact of comorbidities and age. *Journal of Cardiopulmonary Rehabilitation and Prevention* 31, 342–348.
6. O'Dell KR, Masters KS, Spielmans GI, et al. (2011). Does type-D personality predict outcomes among patients with cardiovascular disease? A meta-analytic review. *Journal of Psychosomatic Research* 71, 199–206.
7. Stewart DE, Yuen T (2011). A systematic review of resilience in the physically ill. *Psychosomatics* 52, 199–209.
8. Jones F, Riazi A (2011). Self-efficacy and self-management after stroke: a systematic review. *Disability and Rehabilitation* 33, 797–810.
9. Korpershoek C, van Der Bijl J, Hafsteinsdóttir TB (2011). Self-efficacy and its influence on recovery of patients with stroke: a systematic review. *Journal of Advanced Nursing* 67, 1876–1894.
10. Geyh S, Peter C, Müller R, et al. (2011). The personal factors of the International Classification of Functioning, Disability and Health in the literature a systematic review and content analysis. *Disability and Rehabilitation* 33, 1089–1102.
11. Rainey EE, Petrey L, Reynolds M, et al. (2014). Psychological factors predicting outcome after traumatic injury: the role of resilience. *American Journal of Surgery* 208, 517–523.
12. Silverman AM, Molton IR, Alschuler KN, et al. (2015). Resilience predicts functional outcomes in people aging with disability: a longitudinal investigation. *Archives of Physical Medicine and Rehabilitation* 96, 1262–1268.
13. Guccione AA (2014). Resilience and self-efficacy as mediators of quality of life in geriatric rehabilitation. *Topics in Geriatric Rehabilitation* 30, 164–169.

Rehabilitation in critical illness

Background

Critical illness, defined in this chapter as any life-threatening illness, can be the consequence of severe traumatic injury, acute debilitating medical disease, or in the post-surgical period. People experiencing a critical illness are often being managed in an ICU setting where the main goals of the acute medical/surgical teams are to treat the disease and to minimize mortality. However, decisions and management that are undertaken in this phase of a person's hospitalization can have a significant impact on the course of events that are to follow.

This chapter focuses on those situations where the effects of the critical illness can produce additional morbidity with the potential to affect later rehabilitation. In the context of critical illness, much of this additional morbidity takes the form of readily predictable complications resulting from the disease process or the consequences of its early management. Their predictability means that some of this extra morbidity is potentially avoidable, whereas others may be mitigated through active surveillance and management, thereby lessening their impact on the person's later recovery and rehabilitation. This process of minimizing the impact of a disease or complication that is already present is a concept known as secondary prevention. Primary prevention, where an intervention is established to prevent disease before it occurs, is rarely the domain of rehabilitation.

In this sense, rehabilitation principles should be an essential and integrated part of management in the ICU setting. Even though it is occurring in ICU, the goals of rehabilitation are unchanged—to maximize the potential for the person to maximize their short- and long-term functional capacity and quality of life. To achieve this, planning remains goal directed and utilizes a team approach, with the members of the team varying according to the circumstances, for example, differing between coronary care and a neurocritical care unit. In addition, liaison with the acute treating team is of paramount importance, to determine how rehabilitation can be undertaken where there are post-intervention restrictions, such as barrier precautions, weight-bearing status, post-craniectomy precautions, and so on. There is evidence that such an approach reduces hospital length of stay (LOS), reduces overall costs, and can be associated with better functional outcomes. Despite the availability of research evidence, the take-up rate for critical illness rehabilitation has been slow, with significant funding constraints remaining in place.

The remainder of this chapter will cover general principles of secondary prevention before examining a number of specific conditions that commonly affect survivors of critical illness.

Models of early rehabilitation intervention

The provision of such care can be thought of as the hyperacute rehabilitation model, referring to the very early stage of rehabilitation for people who are in or have been stepped down from critical care or high dependency units. Research has examined rehabilitation onset as early as day 2 post admission, but this is clearly determined by the individual's capacity for safe participation. For medically unstable patients, access to immediate medical and/or surgical advice for management of complications is vitally important. The perceived risk of medical and/or surgical instability (real or otherwise) leads to situations where a person who may benefit from hyperacute rehabilitation is 'warehoused' in a clinical environment where this is not possible.

Other patients may fluctuate between medical instability and fitness for rehabilitation causing similar clinical dilemmas. This may result in patients being transferred to non-rehabilitation beds, sometimes in a different hospital, under a different acute team, and continuity of care can be lost. This scenario is also adversely affected by the common experience of having inpatient rehabilitation beds located in subacute hospitals.

This sets up a range of competing agendas. Delayed transfer to post-acute rehabilitation is a significant problem for the acute care pathway, extending patient LOS. This may be because of long waiting lists for rehabilitation services, or the presence of genuine medical issue/s preventing transfer to rehabilitation. When the patient does eventually arrive in the rehabilitation ward, a lack of earlier therapy often means they are deconditioned and require a longer stay in rehabilitation, producing a feedback loop that further drags out waiting lists.

Three main models of provision of hyperacute specialist rehabilitation within the acute care pathway have been promoted to make up for this structural deficiency:

1. A dedicated hyperacute rehabilitation unit, led by a rehabilitation medicine physician, and with a dedicated multidisciplinary nursing and therapy rehabilitation team located in, or very close to, the acute care unit. This enables transfer of patients into a rehabilitation setting while still accessing an acute environment. Hyperacute units have the drawback of requiring space within the acute care setting.
2. Dedicated rehabilitation beds within the acute ward, with rehabilitation patients being under the care of a rehabilitation medicine physician, sharing nurses and therapists with acute specialities.
3. Establish an 'inreach' rehabilitation team whose members consult in ICU and provide therapy or advice for inpatients. This is easier to achieve when the acute rehabilitation service is co-located with the acute hospital.

These models allow proximity to relevant medical/surgical expertise while providing streamlined and timely rehabilitation. Clearly, establishing a hyperacute ward requires a substantial caseload and patient throughput. It will not be practical or beneficial for all acute services.

The most common examples of such services are neurological (stroke, brain injury, or SCI) or for survivors of polytrauma. However, the success of any of these services is determined by hospital priorities, ICU culture, and staff willingness to engage with rehabilitation.

Role of rehabilitation medicine in the early acute setting

The core activities of a rehabilitation medicine physician are not dissimilar between conventional rehabilitation and that in the context of acute care. They include the following:

- Patient evaluation and management of conditions causing newly acquired and/or complex disability from a rehabilitation perspective (e.g. neurological, musculoskeletal, etc.).
- Liaison between acute surgical/medical teams and therapy teams inside or outside of the primary facility.
- Assisting in secondary prevention of rehabilitation-related complications such as pain, soft tissue shortening, behavioural management, and so on.
- Assessment and mitigation of the effect of pre-existing issues (e.g. physical, psychological, or mental health) that could further impact disability and participation.
- Evaluation of probable functional outcomes and potential to gain from rehabilitation.
- Defining rehabilitation needs and anticipating physical, psychological, and social complications, based on knowledge of a condition's natural history.
- Communicating with families to provide education, prognosis, and time frame for recovery, along with appropriate psychological support.
- Coordination of patients to appropriate rehabilitation services, whether subacute rehabilitation after acute hospital discharge or later referral into community-based rehabilitation.

Secondary prevention in critical illness

People with life-threatening illnesses are presented with a list of challenges that range from difficulty in maintaining basic homeostasis, through to being unable to make informed decisions for themselves. A non-exhaustive list of possible problems is presented in Table 25.1. The management of inter-current chronic illness that could be exacerbated while critically ill, such as diabetes mellitus or asthma, are not covered in this chapter. Information regarding rehabilitation management of these issues appears in other chapters of this handbook.

Delirium is a common problem in ICU, occurring in 30–80% of people in various studies. Fluctuating cognitive impairment represents a barrier to rehabilitation, as does moderate to deep sedation. People with delusional memories resulting from their time in ICU have increased rates of anxiety and depression, and psychological assistance may be particularly useful for affected people. Physical therapy may be less sophisticated than that done in post-acute specialist centres, consisting of ROM exercises, splinting, stretching, and progressive exercise programme (i.e. strengthening moving towards aerobic exercise, followed by increasing endurance). Functional activities are often easier to implement and can include rolling, sitting, bed mobility, transfers, standing, walking, and participating in self-care. These forms of therapy can be successfully undertaken by patients with endotracheal tubes and intravenous lines; however, it takes more coordination and care. Such early therapy has been shown to improve strength and functional capacity at the time of discharge from ICU. Intensive therapy more than doubles the likelihood of being able to walk on discharge from ICU. However, any physical rehabilitation is better than none, and participation is likely to be beneficial, even if it can only occur sporadically due to medical instability.

Table 25.1 Common classes and examples of complications in critical illness

Category		Examples
Physiological	Homeostasis	Electrolyte abnormalities
		SIADH
		Hypoxia
	Pain management	Unrecognized sources of nociception
		CRPS
	Bowel/bladder	Constipation/diarrhoea
		Urinary retention/incontinence
	GI tract/nutrition	Catabolism
		Gastric ulceration
		Unsafe/absent swallow
		GI tract malabsorption/ileus
	Immunosuppression	Increased infection risk
Immobility	Skin integrity	Pressure areas
	Respiration	Hypostatic pneumonia
		Mucous plugging
	Venous	Deep venous thrombosis
	Soft tissue changes	Muscle shortening/atrophy
		Deconditioning
		Pressure neuropathy/myopathy
Medical care	Unrecognized trauma	Occult fractures
		Rotator cuff injury
		Heterotopic ossification
	Iatrogenic infection	Catheter
		IV lines
		Postsurgical Wound/abscess
	Autonomic	Paroxysmal sympathetic hyperactivity
	Allergy	Drug
		Latex
Cognitive function	Delirium/agitation	Acute brain injury
		Drug or alcohol withdrawal
		Psychoactive medications
	Anxiety/fear	Poor-quality sleep
		Behavioural disturbance
		PTSD

CRPS, complex regional pain syndrome; GI, gastrointestinal; IV, intravenous; PTSD, post-traumatic stress disorder; SIADH, syndrome of inappropriate antidiuretic hormone secretion.

Family involvement in the intensive care unit

People in ICU with a critical illness are rarely able to make informed decisions regarding their care over their entire ICU admission. For this reason, family members are often called on to make significant decisions for their relatives. This will include decisions across the entire spectrum, from consent for minor procedures through to ending life support. For this reason, it is vital for families to be kept well informed, and to have the prognosis explained both in terms of survival and potential for long-term health and disability. Communication needs to be provided in a clear and transparent way while being sensitive to the stress that the family may be under. As discussed in the following sections in this chapter, a large minority of relatives may develop post-traumatic stress disorder (PTSD) from living through the ICU experience. Opportunistic and supportive counselling from all team members is preferred, targeting the person's response to fear and anxiety. Such an approach may not always be possible and may be of limited value even when undertaken well.

Formal meetings away from the bedside have both advantages and disadvantages for worried relatives.

Specific disease processes in critical illness

Multiple organ dysfunction syndrome

Multiple organ dysfunction syndrome (MODS) is a relatively common disorder in people with critical illness and is a common cause of death in ICU. MODS is best thought of as a continuum characterized by progressive physiological dysfunction in two or more organs or organ systems. Any or all of six main organ systems can be involved: lung, renal, neurological, GI/hepatic, cardiac, and endocrine. For example, a patient may survive the immediate insult only to develop respiratory failure, followed a few days later by liver failure, a week later developing GI bleeding, followed by renal failure. Therapy is limited to supportive care, with the main goals being to maintain adequate tissue oxygenation and safeguarding haemodynamics. Investigations can show increased C-reactive protein (CRP) levels, hyperbilirubinaemia, and cholestasis. Oliguria can develop despite a normal intravascular volume, later with rising creatinine levels and electrolyte derangements potentially requiring dialysis.

MODS can be induced by a variety of acute insults, including sepsis, severe trauma, and systemic inflammatory response syndrome (SIRS).

While the specific pathophysiology is uncertain, it is a maladaptive host response with acute inflammation occurring at a local and systemic level. Most recently, a role for complement and mitochondrial DNA have been put forward as causes of the inflammatory cascade. While MODS is potentially reversible, reported mortality rates are 30–100%, with the chance of survival poorer as more organ systems are involved, the type of systems involved, increasing age, previous chronic diseases, delayed or inadequate resuscitation, and persistent infection.

SIRS is an uncontrolled and generalized inflammatory response that suggests an increased likelihood of MODS. It has four features, and a diagnosis requires at least two to be present:

- Temperature higher than 38.0°C or less than 36.0°C.
- Heart rate greater than 90 beats/minute.
- Respiratory rate greater than 20 breaths/minute or arterial carbon dioxide tension below 32 mmHg
- White blood cell (WBC) count greater than 12,000/µL, less than 4000/µL, or including more than 10% bands.

Like MODS, it is associated with a variety of clinical insults, including sepsis, polytrauma, tissue injury, pancreatitis, ischaemia, haemorrhagic shock, and immune-mediated organ injury. SIRS is a non-specific presentation of these insults and is associated with hypoperfusion and hypermetabolism.

The pathophysiological changes that underlie MODS (poorly understood though they are) provide a common mechanism for a number of commonly recognized complications of critical illness including critical illness neuropathy/myopathy, and acute respiratory distress syndrome (ARDS), among others.

Critical illness neuropathy/myopathy

These conditions consist of an axonal peripheral neuropathy, a myopathy, or a combination of these that arises in the context of people admitted to intensive care. These conditions can occur singly or in combination with other system dysfunction as part of MODS. As before, causative factors are uncertain, but proposed causes include impairment of microcirculation, prolonged catabolism, inflammatory cytokines, impaired calcium/sodium channel function, and/or mitochondrial dysfunction (Table 25.2). Various studies show between one-quarter and one-half of individuals on intensive care for more than 7 days have documented evidence of peripheral neuropathy or myopathy. A range of factors are associated with increased risk, although it is not clear whether these factors are causative or more general indicators of greater morbidity. They include:

• hyperglycaemia
• overall severity of precipitating illness
• sepsis
• persistent inflammation
• longer intensive care stay
• prolonged catabolic state

Table 25.2 Clinical, electrophysiological, and histological features of intensive care unit-acquired weakness

Investigation	CIP	CIM	CINM
Physical examination	Distal muscle weakness	Proximal muscle weakness	Proximal and distal muscle weakness
	Distal sensory deficit	Normal sensory testing	Distal sensory deficit
	Normal or depressed deep tendon reflexes	Normal or depressed deep tendon reflexes	Depressed deep tendon reflexes
Electrophysiology studies	Decreased CMAP and decreased SNAP	Decreased CMAP and normal SNAP	Decreased CMAP and SNAP
	Normal MUAP	Decreased MUAP	Decreased MUAP
	Normal or near-normal conduction velocity	EMG shows short-duration, low-amplitude activity	EMG shows short-duration, low-amplitude activity
Histology	Axonal degeneration of distal motor and sensory nerves	Thick filament (myosin) loss, type II fibre (fast twitch) atrophy, necrosis	Axonal degeneration and evidence of loss in myosin, type II fibre atrophy, and necrosis

CIM, critical illness myopathy; CINM, critical illness neuromyopathy; CIP, critical illness polyneuropathy; CMAP, compound muscle action potential; EMG, electromyography; MUAP, muscle unit action potential; SNAP, sensory nerve action potential.

- immobility
- possible association with female sex (variably reported up to a 4:1 increased risk)
- possible association with use of glucocorticoids.

There is evidence that the prognosis for a critical care myopathy is better than that for a neuropathy. Strategies to reduce the risk and severity are:
- early mobilization—this can include mobilization while still on mechanical ventilation (e.g. by use of a cycle ergometer)
- maintaining good glycaemic control, but with caution not to cause hypoglycaemia
- minimization and early withdrawal of sedation
- resting orthoses and passive movements can be used to maintain position and range in the limbs.

Weakness with an adverse impact on physical function and rehabilitation occurs in up to 100% of patients in ICU for 4 weeks. There is a lack of a strong evidence base of the efficacy of rehabilitation, however, the goal of hyperacute rehabilitation is to maintain strength and function as much as practicable.

Acute respiratory distress syndrome

ARDS is another part of the spectrum of conditions within the umbrella term of MODS. As would therefore be expected, ARDS is a frequent complication following conditions such as pneumonia, sepsis, multisystem trauma, burns, pancreatitis, and systemic inflammation. It can complicate pneumonia but can also be a standalone problem. Respiratory difficulties stem from impaired gas exchange associated with an influx of inflammatory cells. This results in fibrosis and hyaline membrane formation. Chest X-rays show bilateral chest infiltrates.

The prognosis for survival of ARDS is better for those with fewer coexisting chronic diseases prior to hospitalization. Younger people recover at a faster rate than older. On moving to the general wards, ARDS survivors and their families often report anxiety issues, due in part to decreased levels of monitoring. Neuropsychological studies have found decreased concentration and memory loss in survivors, although this may be a consequence of neurological effects of MODS rather than an ARDS-specific problem. Long-term ARDS survivors continue to show poorer exercise tolerance and quality of life for at least 5 years post event. Participation in paid employment is reduced in ARDS survivors. The return to work rate improves over time, with non-participation closely linked to intercurrent depression rather than the diagnosis of ARDS itself. Rehabilitation has been to shown to produce better outcomes, both in terms of physical recovery and decreased psychological distress. Early intervention improves physical function both early (8 weeks) and at 6 months post discharge from ICU. This can be as simple as supplying a self-help manual to people when they are leaving ICU.

Respiratory function/pneumonia

Respiratory complications are extremely common in ICU with a multitude of risk factors being recognized (Table 25.3). It is common for patients to have bacterial colonization (rather than infection) and considerable effort is taken to minimize the risk of this becoming active infection. The risk of chest infection in ICU is high due to numerous devices being present, mechanical ventilation, pooling of potentially infected fluids above the cuff, and so on.

Interventions to control the risk of pneumonia include infection control (i.e. gloves, hand washing, etc.), avoiding large gastric volumes, regular suctioning, instituting postural change, semi-recumbent position, careful monitoring, and the use of specific antibiotics for sepsis of an organism with known sensitivities.

With regard to hyperacute rehabilitation interventions, an early decrease of sedatives can improve airway control. Some have argued for the use of ACE inhibitors as they increase cough reflex sensitivity.

Maintaining adequate pain relief may improve breathing depth, as will incentive spirometry. Data supporting the benefits of chest physiotherapy are equivocal, but the procedure involves minimal risk and may be useful. An integrated, team approach to tracheostomy weaning has practical benefit to earlier discharge.

A single randomized controlled trial showing early pulmonary rehabilitation (i.e. within 24 hours of admission to ICU) was beneficial in COPD patients requiring mechanical ventilation. Other studies have shown that mobilizing patients with mechanical ventilation is practical and improves later outcome.

Malnourishment/catabolism

Malnourishment leads to poorer outcomes, longer hospital LOS, increased mortality, immunosuppression, and increased infection risk. Nutrition is particularly important for patients with longer ICU LOS. In fact, better feeding in ICU is associated with decreased LOS.

Providing less than 25% of nutritional requirements increases the overall risk of infection and death. Providing 33–65% of nutritional needs is associated with reduced mortality, whereas overfeeding increases risk and should be avoided.

Table 25.3 Various risk factors for respiratory complications

Patient related	Treatment related
Older age	Mechanical ventilation
Decreased level of consciousness	Decreased diaphragmatic excursion
Decreased cough reflex	Enteral feeding, e.g. NG/PEG tubes
Abnormal swallow	Poor oral hygiene
Immunosuppression	Sedation
Pre-existent chronic lung disease	Thoracoabdominal surgery
CNS disease, e.g. cerebrovascular accident	Nursed supine
Burns	Immobility
Trauma	

In critical illness, rates of protein breakdown are increased, and the pattern of active protein synthesis alters compared to healthy states. This makes protein intake particularly important, as inadequate protein intake, coupled with immobility, promotes muscle atrophy. The current recommended daily intake (RDI) for protein is 0.8 grams per kilogram of body weight per day (g/kg/day) in health. Higher protein targets are often adopted in ICU, with limited data suggesting that intakes of 1.2 g/kg/day are achievable and improve strength compared with normal RDIs. Studies up to 1.5 g/kg/day have also been reported to show improvement.

Enteral nutrition is the preferred route of administration when the small bowel is functional. This may be an issue in patients with abdominal trauma or post-surgical ileus. The inflammatory changes that lie behind MODS can result in a situation where the GI tract is not working normally. However, there is currently no mechanism to test whether this is the case or not. Similarly, patients with high sympathetic drive (e.g. those with paroxysmal sympathetic hyperactivity after TBI) can have impaired GI tract blood flow with consequences for absorption of nutrients. Where these situations occur, parenteral nutrition can be delivered via intravenous (IV) access.

The means of enteral feeding can be via NG tube, PEG, or jejunostomy (sometimes referred to as a PEJ). NG tubes are less invasive and are preferred when the duration of feeding is considered to be short term. All tubes increase the risk of aspiration, which is greatest for NG tubes. This risk can be mitigated by using a head-up tilt of 45°, and considering whether continuous versus intermittent bolus feeds are more suitable for the individual patient.

Enteral feeding is cheaper than parenteral feeding, however, some research suggests that calorie delivery is less reliable than parenteral feeding. The main limitations of enteral feeding in this regard are interruptions due to digestive intolerance or due to other procedures (surgery/diagnostic, etc.) that require an empty stomach. These factors potentially restrict the percentage of predicted caloric intake that can be delivered.

Refeeding syndrome can occur when feeding is reintroduced in a person who has been starved, sometimes with as little as 48 hours of no food intake. Complications include electrolyte abnormalities (low potassium, phosphate, and magnesium), sodium retention, and fluid retention (with potential for cardiac failure). Severe cases of refeeding syndrome are associated with respiratory failure and/or death. There is debate as to the rate of refeeding, with some suggesting a slow reintroduction of enteral feeding then increasing, while other research has shown decreased mortality with faster reintroduction.

Deconditioning

Deconditioning is a multifactorial problem, being influenced by many of the same factors already discussed. They include:
- pre-illness muscle mass and fitness levels
- age
- number and severity of medical comorbidities
- nutritional status
- immobility
- length of time in ICU
- critical illness myopathy.

Older people are vulnerable to loss of muscle mass, with such losses predicting poorer physical functional capacity, loss of independence, falls, and mortality. The extent of reduced strength, fatigue, poor endurance, and associated functional limitations are the result of both any acute loss of muscle fibre alongside atrophy from previous lifestyle limitations.

Small amounts of daily protein and active exercise/movement is usually sufficient to avoid the worst effects of deconditioning. Healthy people on complete bed rest lose 3–4% strength per day and it is estimated that it takes three to four times as long to regain strength as it did to lose it. Depending on the person's pre-illness fitness, a week of bed rest can drop them below the threshold where they lack the strength for simple bed mobility. For two people experiencing the equivalent critical illness, the person with the higher exercise reserve is likely to regain sufficient muscle strength for basic self-care and mobility much faster.

Similarly, the shorter their period of immobility and catabolism, the faster they are likely to improve. The rate of improvement will be affected by the adequacy of nutrition and it is often necessary to encourage people with poor appetite to eat even if it is only 'to feed the machine' rather than for their sense of enjoyment.

The goal of rehabilitation is to maintain as much muscle mass as possible, to increase strength and thereby improve function. Even such a simple intervention as early mobilization has been shown to enhance recovery and improve functional outcomes for patients in acute and intensive care settings. This has been mostly been shown as an early benefit, although some limited data supports benefit months down the track in some research.

Deep venous thrombosis

Deep venous thrombosis (DVT) is a relatively common and predictable complication seen in critically ill patients. Most DVTs form in the lower limbs, but clotting can occur in any vein in the body. Risk factors for DVT can be divided into those intrinsic to the patient (e.g. genetic thrombophilias, obesity, smoking, cancer, age >60, pregnancy, oral contraceptive pill, hormone replacement therapy, and previous DVT) and those that are situational to the ICU setting (e.g. hypercoagulability/impaired fibrinolysis, immobility with consequent reduction in blood flow, and compromise of blood vessels, such as trauma).

The dominant risk of DVT is pulmonary embolism (PE) which is associated with increased morbidity and mortality. PE is more likely to happen where there is involvement of the proximal vessels, with proximal lower limb DVT defined as where a clot is found in the popliteal, femoral, or iliac veins. Distal DVTs are those found solely below the knee, involving peroneal, posterior, anterior tibial, and/or muscular veins. This division of proximal and distal DVTs usefully stratifies PE risk, with the overall risk of PE greater in proximal DVTs at 50% compared to 20% for distal.

Serial Doppler ultrasound is the investigation of choice; however, it can be difficult in extremely large or oedematous legs, where there is trauma, a plaster cast, or painful superficial thrombophlebitis. In these situations, D-dimer levels (a fibrin degradation product) can be assayed on venous blood. A normal D-dimer level excludes a DVT diagnosis; however, mild increases in D-dimer levels are seen in a range of non-DVT diagnoses (e.g. advancing age, recent surgery, trauma, immobility, and cancer). The low specificity of D-dimer results means that it is usually considered a second-line investigation.

The preferred management of DVT is prophylaxis to avoid the condition through the use of compression stockings, mechanical compression garments, and early mobilization. Heparin (unfractionated or low molecular weight) prophylaxis protocols are standardized in most centres. Where a DVT is identified, treatment is initially low-molecular-weight heparin and commencement of warfarin (with a goal of INR 2–3) or newer anti-coagulants such as rivaroxaban (which does not require INR monitoring). Treatment will usually be considered for a 3-month period, balancing the increased risk of bleeding against that of recurrent DVT/PE. On rare occasions, surgical intervention with thrombectomy or insertion of an inferior vena cava (IVC) filter will be considered. Prophylactic use of IVC filters is advocated in some high-risk polytrauma cases.

Pressure areas

Pressure areas (pressure sores) are caused by persistent, unrelieved pressure on the skin. In normal situations, people avoid injury to the skin through constant, subconscious fidgeting movements which minimize the duration of pressure on pressure points. However, a person with a critical illness may be unable to monitor pressure sensation or to reposition themselves, thereby running a higher risk of developing skin breakdown. The most common locations for pressure areas are overlying bony prominences such as the back of the head and ears, the shoulders, the elbows, the sacrum and ischial tuberosities, the hips, the inner knees, and the heels. Issues regarding pressure areas are discussed in more detail in ➜ Chapter 14.

PTSD following critical illness

People who survive a critical illness are at increased risk of developing PTSD. PTSD is a maladaptive response to a significantly stressful or traumatic event, irrespective of whether the event occurs to the individual or is observed to occur to someone else. It is a form of anxiety disorder where the person experiences chronic symptoms such as flashbacks, nightmares, and intrusive thoughts about aspects of the event that are associated with heightened arousal and anxiety. PTSD occurs across a spectrum, with incomplete or partial forms being recognized, and can coexist with depressive symptomatology.

As would therefore be expected, experiencing or observing the stressful events associated with an ICU stay mean that PTSD is a common complication. Estimates of the frequency of PTSD range from 5% to 60%, with between-study variability thought to be due to methodological issues such as use of PTSD screening tools rather than formal clinical diagnosis, time to assessment, loss to follow-up, and so on.

The relative risk factors for developing PTSD are not clearly linked to the reason for ICU admission (i.e. the underlying diagnosis), the presence of delirium, severity of illness, or LOS. The development of PTSD appears more linked to those with existing psychological problems, female sex, prolonged use of sedation, and reports of frightening ICU memories (real or delusional). There is inconsistent evidence to suggest that the risk of PTSD peaks in those aged 40 to 60, with lower risk expressed in those older or younger than this group.

Witnessing a person's battle to survive, and the medical interventions necessary in the ICU setting, can also exert significant stress on family members or loved ones. Sometimes, a family member's heightened emotional response may be evident from early in the ICU stay, but other people may seem emotionally strong throughout the process only to develop anxiety symptoms when their relative is out of danger. High levels of psychological distress in relatives have been found to correlate with high stress levels in patients. There is also a body of literature recognizing the impact of ICU on nursing staff. In this group, PTSD risk is reduced in nurses with active coping skills, cognitive flexibility, a sense of optimism, and positive role models. Increased PTSD rates are seen in those without these traits, those with poorer stress coping mechanisms, intrusive and pessimistic thoughts, poorer social networks, and/or the lack of a positive role model. It is likely that a similar set of personality traits would place patients and family members at risk of developing PTSD.

PTSD is associated with reduced quality of life in the long term, but it cannot be diagnosed in ICU as the chronicity of the disorder will not be reached (i.e. >3 months' duration). However, patients who may be at the highest risk of developing PTSD could be identified in ICU and monitored over rehabilitation time frames. Further, interventions have been trialled in ICU aimed at decreasing the incidence of later PTSD. A number of approaches have been proposed: minimizing aversive experiences, relieving fear and anxiety through caring behaviour, psychological intervention, and the use of ICU diaries to document and discuss patients' experiences in ICU. How effective these strategies are has yet to be fully determined. The role of pharmacological interventions within the ICU to minimize the development of PTSD has yet to be defined.

Further reading

Adler J, Malone D (2012). Early mobilization in the intensive care unit: a systematic review. *Cardiopulmonary Physical Therapy Journal* 23, 5–13.

British Society of Rehabilitation Medicine (2014). Rehabilitation for patients in the acute care pathway following severe disabling illness or injury: BSRM core standards for specialist rehabilitation. http://www.bsrm.org.uk/downloads/specialist-rehabilitation-prescription-for-acute-care-28-11-2014-ja--(ap1-redrawn).pdf.

Lee CM, Fan E (2012). ICU acquired weakness: what is preventing its rehabilitation in critically ill patients? *BMC Medicine* 10, 115.

Condition-specific approaches

Traumatic brain injury

Background and epidemiology

Traumatic brain injury (TBI) is a subset of acquired brain injuries (ABIs), a larger grouping that includes acute-onset diseases such as stroke as well as degenerative conditions such as the dementing illnesses. TBI is often considered separately to other ABIs due to differences in its presentation and how treatment is approached. TBI occurs over an extremely broad range of severities, from concussion through to profound and life-threatening damage. As the injury becomes more severe, the affected individual has an increasing risk of experiencing lifelong and complex physical, behavioural, emotional, cognitive, and social problems.

By definition, TBI occurs where there is an alteration in brain function resulting from the application of external force. TBI is extremely common, with incidence figures for hospital attendance from 200 to 400/100,000 of the population per annum, varying by country. This is an underestimate of the true incidence, however, as many people with mild injuries do not present for medical assessment. It is estimated that mild TBI comprises 85% of all injuries, with moderate TBI forming around 10%. Around 5% of all people presenting to hospital with a head injury have a severe TBI, with an estimated 30% mortality rate. Definitions for these categories are presented in Table 26.1 (➔ see 'Measuring injury severity following traumatic brain injury').

Table 26.1 Classification of head injury

Classification	Definition		
	GCS score	Coma	PTA
Concussion	14, 15	Seconds	Seconds–minutes
Mild head injury	13–15	<30 min	< 1 h
Moderate head injury	8–12	15 min—6 h	PTA <24 h
Severe head injury	<7	>6 h	>24 h

GCS, Glasgow Coma Scale, PTA, post-traumatic amnesia.

Mechanisms of injury

The mechanisms behind brain injuries can be further subclassified into three categories, each of which have the potential to affect the prognosis for survival and later recovery. These issues can be thought of as the mode of injury, the pattern of injury, and the pathophysiological response to injury. These will be considered in turn.

Mode of injury

The most common causes of TBI include motor vehicle crashes, falls, assaults, and sporting injuries, although the incidence details vary dramatically across countries. These forms of civilian TBI present with some differences to military TBI, where other patterns of concomitant injuries and the type of brain injury can be seen. Mode of injury is important in helping to determine prognosis, in that the greater the amount of energy expended on the brain, for example, in a high-speed motor vehicle crash, the greater the likelihood of severe injury.

Patterns of injury

Injury patterns can be broadly grouped in a number of ways. The classical division was into closed and open injuries, determined by the integrity of the dura mater; however, it is now recognized that blast injuries represent a third pattern:

- Closed injury, associated with rapid acceleration/deceleration. The effects of closed injury can be thought of as either focal (e.g. contusions, haemorrhages, and sub- or extradural bleeds) or diffuse (diffuse axonal injury (DAI)) (Fig. 26.1).[1,2]
- Open or penetrating injury, where the dura has been breached, runs a higher risk of post-traumatic epilepsy and infection. Bullet wounds are particularly problematic, with the extent of damage dependent on the velocity of the projectile (with higher velocity leading to much greater tissue loss) and its path through the brain.
- Blast injury, the overpressure wave associated with explosions causes injury to many body structures. Blast injuries affecting the brain often meets the criteria for mild severity but are underestimated as a cause of long-term disability, especially where they occur repeatedly over short time frames.

Pathophysiological response to injury

The brain's initial response to injury is a chain of events which are usually divided into primary and secondary phases.

Primary injuries occur as a direct result of the trauma and can include structural damage to brain tissue, blood vessels, DAI, contusions, and disruption of the blood–brain barrier.

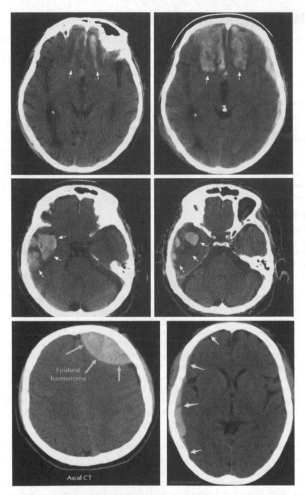

Fig. 26.1 Upper row: frontal lobe contusions (arrows). Middle row: temporal lobe burst haematoma (arrows). Lower row: extradural (left) and subdural (right).

Source: 1. reproduced with permission from Wijdicks E.F.M. Traumatic Brain Injury in *The Practice of Emergency and Critical Care Neurology* (2 ed.). Oxford, UK: Oxford University Publisher. © 2016 Oxford University Press. http://oxfordmedicine.com/view/10.1093/med/9780190259556.001.0001/med-9780190259556-chapter-41. Source 2: Reproduced with permission from Andrews P.J.D. and Rhodes J.K.J. Assessment of traumatic brain injury in *Oxford Textbook of Critical Care* (2 ed.), Webb A. et al. Oxford, UK: Oxford University Press. © 2016 Oxford University Press. Reproduced with permission of Oxford University Press through PLSclear. http://oxfordmedicine.com/view/10.1093/med/9780199600830.001.0001/med-9780199600830-chapter-342#.

Secondary injury includes other factors that influence outcome that are not due to the initial trauma. They can include issues that happen in the minutes or hours post injury (e.g. hypoxic or hypotensive brain injury), through to metabolic disruptions (e.g. metabolic acidosis) and predictable but uncontrolled cascades that increase neuronal loss over time such as free radical formation, excitotoxicity, apoptosis of healthy neurons, and so on. To date, attempts to modulate these cascades in human studies have been unsuccessful. Some forms of secondary injury can occur quite late after the trauma, for example, delayed intracerebral bleeding, infection (e.g. meningitis, abscess), and hydrocephalus.

Measuring injury severity following traumatic brain injury

For prognostic purposes, assessment of injury severity provides a rough guide to the need for and extent of investigations required following an acute event. The most common clinical scale used in this context is the Glasgow Coma Scale (GCS) which was developed to guide surgical investigations. Other indicators of outcome include duration of coma and of post-traumatic amnesia (PTA). Formal definition of these categories is given in Table 26.1 followed by a description of the GCS and PTA.

The GCS[3] is an almost universally applied system for scoring change in level of consciousness. The GCS was developed to predict the need for neurosurgical intervention by assessing three broad areas of cerebral function (Table 26.2). This gives a range of scores from 3–15, with lower scores indicating poorer cerebral function There is a loose correlation between

Table 26.2 The Glasgow Coma Scale

Item	Response	Score	Details
Eye opening	None	1	No response to pain
	To pain	2	Eyes open while pain being applied
	To speech	3	Non-specific response, not necessarily to command
	Spontaneous	4	Eyes open, not necessarily aware
Motor response	None	1	No response to pain; limbs remain flaccid
	Extension	2	'Decerebrate'; shoulder adducted, elbow extended, forearm pronated and wrist flexed
	Abnormal flexion	3	'Decorticate'; shoulder adducted, elbow/wrist flexed
	Withdrawal	4	Arm withdraws from pain, shoulder abducts
	Localizes pain	5	Arm attempts to remove the source of pain
	Obeys commands	6	Follows simple commands
Verbal response	None	1	No verbal response
	Incomprehensible	2	Moans/groans; no words
	Inappropriate	3	Intelligible, no sustained sentences
	Confused	4	Responds with conversation, but confused
	Oriented	5	Aware of time, place, person

Note: common painful stimuli used in evaluating the GCS score include supra-orbital ridge pressure, sternum rub, or pressure to the base of the fingernail.

Reproduced with permission from Teasdale G. and Jennett B. Assessment of coma and impaired consciousness. A practical scale. *Lancet*, 304(7872):81–4. Copyright © 1974 Published by Elsevier Ltd. https://doi.org/10.1016/S0140-6736(74)91639-0.

the GCS score and eventual outcome, particularly if the best GCS score in the first 24 hours is considered. However, the GCS is not as accurate a predictor of functional outcome compared to PTA duration, and there is a risk of over-interpreting the GCS in this regard.

Post-traumatic amnesia

PTA is the confusional state often seen to follow TBI, where the person is disoriented and has difficulties with laying down new memory. The duration of PTA is defined as the period of time from injury until resumption of day-to-day memory. It is worth noting that cessation of PTA is not an on/off process, and many people will display 'islands of memory' for aspects of day-to-day activity while still evidencing memory difficulties in other areas. For example, emotionally strong or aversive memories are often formed more easily in this period than semantic memory.

There are a number of tools used to evaluate PTA duration, all of which give different estimates. In the US, the Galveston Orientation and Amnesia Test (GOAT) is widely used. This gives the shortest estimates of PTA and has received criticism for being too strongly focused on biographical rather than anterograde memory. The Westmead PTA scale (WPTAS)[4] is commonly used in Australasia and the UK. It has versions covering the full range of TBI, with the WPTAS being appropriate for people with more severe injuries and the Abbreviated Westmead PTA Scale (which incorporates the GCS) for minor injuries. Despite differences in the available tools, consistent PTA measurement is recommended, particularly as PTA duration is a better prognostic indicator than GCS score in terms of rehabilitation outcomes.

Injury severity and prognosis

There is no accurate way of determining functional prognosis for survivors of TBI in the early days post injury. However, grouped data suggest that certain generalizations are possible, in that worse prognosis is correlated with:

- lower GCS score
- more prolonged PTA
- greater extent and deeper DAI (producing greater deafferentation between cortical areas)
- deeper and larger focal lesions
- more extensive lesion load
- coincident hypoxic or hypotensive injury
- recurrent brain injuries, particularly over short time frames.

However, there are too many exceptions to these general rules to make them appropriate for predicting eventual functional capacity for any given individual. As such, it is inappropriate to suggest a definitive prognosis within the first few weeks of injury. Even within the mildest TBI category there is considerable variability in functional outcome, varying between a return to normal function and lifelong disability.

Consequences of traumatic brain injury

TBI can have negative effects on every aspect of life. It is therefore important to consider the impact of an injury across the entire reach of human experience, from basic medical impairments through to how they combine to impact the person's participation in their previous life roles. These potential impacts can be thought of under the headings of medical issues, neurological impairment, cognitive impairment, personality and behavioural change, and lifestyle (Table 26.3). An overview of more specific TBI-related conditions will be discussed in ➲ 'Traumatic brain injury-related conditions'. A subgroup of patients will go on to have prolonged disorders of consciousness (PDOC) which are discussed separately in ➲ Chapter 32.

Table 26.3 A simple categorization of post-TBI difficulties

Grouping	Clinical examples	➲ See Chapter
Medical issues	Spasticity	10
	Post-traumatic epilepsy	
	Incontinence (most usually a disinhibited bladder)	12
	Hydrocephalus	
	Heterotopic ossification	
	Neuroendocrine/pituitary dysfunction—e.g. amenorrhoea	11
	Pain	
	Infection	
	Venous thromboembolism	
Neurological impairment	Motor impairment—coordination, balance, walking, upper limb and hand function	18
	Altered smell (anosmia, parosmia, etc.) and taste	
	Visual disturbance—blindness, diplopia, non-specific blurred vision, neglect	
	Impaired touch, proprioception, two-point discrimination, neglect	
	Dysphasias (receptive/expressive), impaired word finding	8
	Dysphagia	9
	Autonomic dysfunction, e.g. PSH	

Table 26.3 (Contd.)

Grouping	Clinical examples	➲ See Chapter
Cognitive impairment	Executive problems—impaired planning, organization, problem-solving, multitasking	7, 22
	Reduced speed of information processing and flexibility	
	Memory impairment, difficulty with new learning	
	Reduced attention and concentration	
	Impaired judgement and safety awareness	
Behavioural and personality change	Altered emotional control, self-centredness, egocentricity	7, 19, 22
	Impaired social and coping skills, reduced self-esteem	
	Poor frustration tolerance, impaired anger management	
	Reduced insight, disinhibition, impulsivity	
	Apathy, amotivational states, reduced initiation of actions	
	Psychiatric disorders—anxiety, depression, PTSD, first-episode psychosis	
Lifestyle/participation restriction	Restricted ADL independence, e.g. self-care, cooking, finances	
	Reduced productivity—under/unemployment	14
	Limitations in academic achievement	
	Lack of transportation alternatives	
	Inadequate recreational opportunities	
	Interpersonal relationship and marital difficulties	19
	Loss of pre-injury roles, loss of independence	
	Subjective reduction in sexual satisfaction, libido	13
	Sleep disturbance—insomnia, excessive sleepiness, fatigue, Circadian rhythm abnormalities	

Traumatic brain injury-related conditions

As outlined in Table 26.3, many of the needs of people surviving TBI are no different to the issues seen in other areas of rehabilitation (and addressed in detail in other chapters of this handbook). The most significant difference in the rehabilitation of post-TBI survivors is the extent of these issues, in that almost all areas of a person's existence can be affected by an injury.[5] However, there are a few issues that are relatively specific to TBI, and these will be discussed in the following sections. Discussion of issues concerning PDOC are presented in ➔ Chapter 32.

Post-traumatic epilepsy

Post-traumatic epilepsy is uncommon (<2–3%) in the absence of known risk factors such as:
• depressed skull fracture
• intracranial haemorrhage
• open head injuries or intracranial infection
• significant gliosis associated with focal brain damage
• seizure activity occurring more than 24 hours post injury.

Anticonvulsant therapy is usually initiated along standard guidelines, with the choice of medication linked to the risk of adverse effects (e.g. clouded cognition with phenytoin) and beneficial effects on other symptoms (e.g. carbamazepine for episodic/explosive dyscontrol syndrome).

Paroxysmal sympathetic hyperactivity

Paroxysmal sympathetic hyperactivity (PSH) is a condition that has been reported after most forms of acute brain injury; however, 80% of cases in world literature have resulted from TBI. The condition is character-ized by simultaneous, paroxysmal sympathetic (elevated heart rate, blood pressure, respiratory rate, temperature, sweating) and motor (posturing) overactivity. Untreated, the condition is a significant source of additional morbidity, leading to marked catabolism, increased neuronal death, neuro-pathic pain, and contractures from dystonia and spasticity. It is associated with more severe injuries and can be misdiagnosed as sepsis of unknown origin or narcotic withdrawal (both of which can coexist). The cardinal feature is 'triggering', where relatively benign stimuli (e.g. light touch, con-stipation, and tracheal suctioning) produce an exaggerated and transient increase in sympathetic drive. Treatment is usually based around minim-izing sources of potential nociception, pretreating patients with sedation or narcotics before painful procedures, and gabapentinoids or non-selective β-blockers such as propranolol (see Meyfroidt et al.[6]).

Heterotopic ossification

Ectopic bone formation in the soft tissues occurs in around 10% of severe TBI, most commonly around the hip and thigh, followed by the elbow. The presence of PSH dramatically increases the relative risk (RR) of heterotopic ossification (RR 59.6; 95% confidence interval 8.4–422)[7] and both diagnoses should be considered in patients with hot or painful joints. Early signs include a localized inflammatory response, swelling, pain, and decreased ROM. Heterotopic ossification can permanently reduce ROM, cause ankyloses, and complicate pressure area care. Treatment is difficult, with indomethacin and etidronate disodium probably the most useful treatments. Bone maturation is usually completed within 6–18 months of onset, at which time surgical intervention may be considered.

Hypopituitarism

Neuroendocrine dysfunction in is very common in patients with TBI. In the acute post-injury period, up to 50–70% of people with severe TBI will show neuroendocrine disruption, while 15–20% of hospitalized TBI patients will develop chronic hypopituitarism (not all of whom will require supplementation). The likelihood of neuroendocrine dysfunction increases with increasing injury severity, with up to a third of those with severe TBI having chronic neuroendocrine abnormalities. While a number of screening guidelines exist,[8] the general suggestion is that all people hospitalized for their TBI should be screened, weighted towards those with longer acute LOS and poorer outcome, or those with any clinical feature suggestive of abnormalities.

Life expectancy

On average, research has shown that life expectancy after severe TBI is reduced by 3–5 years even in the absence of severe physical disability. Factors that serve to further reduce post-TBI life expectancy can be divided into those that existed prior to the injury, and those resulting from the effects of the injury. For example:

Pre-injury factors:
- Lower socioeconomic status
- Pre-injury psychiatric illness or alcohol/drug dependence
- Pre-injury epilepsy.

Injury related factors:
- Poorer functional status at discharge, especially immobility, dependence in ADLs, and so on (this is partly determined by injury severity).
- Impaired swallow (even where the need for early NG or PEG tube feeding resolves).
- Late post-traumatic epilepsy (whether controlled or uncontrolled).

Minor head injury and post-concussive syndrome

A person is said to have had a mild TBI if they have had a traumatically in-duced physiological disruption of brain function, observed as at least one of the following:

- Any loss of consciousness.
- Any loss of memory for events immediately before or after the accident.
- Any alteration in mental state at the time of the accident (e.g. feeling dazed, disoriented, or confused).

Neurological deficit/s may or may not be observed, but where present cannot exceed:

- a loss of consciousness of 30 minutes or more
- an initial GCS score below 13/15
- a PTA duration of 24 hours.

Furthermore, mild TBI tends to be divided into uncomplicated and compli-cated categories based on the absence or presence of CT changes, respect-ively. It is currently being debated whether 'concussion' is a functionally relevant subdivision of the mild TBI category.

The symptom complex seen after mild TBI is reminiscent of that occurring in more severe injury, however, the natural history can be quite different. The common symptoms and complaints are often labelled together as post-concussive syndrome (PCS) and can include:

- generic symptoms—headache, insomnia/heightened fatigue, and light headedness
- brainstem features—nausea, vomiting, dizziness, or vertigo
- visual changes—photophobia, impaired accommodation, and reduced visual acuity
- hearing changes—hyperacusis and tinnitus
- cognitive symptoms—impaired attention and concentration, mild memory disturbance/forgetfulness, slowed information processing, reduced new learning, word-finding problems, and difficulty completing tasks that were easily done
- behavioural changes—anxiety/depressed mood, irritability, and low frustration tolerance
- motor features—impaired high level balance, slowed reaction times, and reduced coordination.

The duration of PCS is generally short, with the symptoms resolving within 3 months for three-quarters of affected people. For the remainder, PCS can produce significant long-term disability. The reasons for the different time courses within the syndrome are unclear, although both premorbid and post-injury factors appear to influence both the likelihood of developing PCS and its time course.[9] PCS is more likely to be observed in females and people having a previous affective or anxiety disorder. Post injury, experi-encing pain or acute stress also increases the incidence. These associations become stronger over time.

Furthermore, the symptoms underlying PCS are not unique to minor head injury, having been found equally likely following trauma, with or without minor TBI, in a number of studies (e.g. Meares et al.[9]). This is not to say that PCS is evidence of psychological overlay or malingering, as there is clear evidence that both concussion and mild TBI produce organic cerebral injury.

Clinical interventions for mild TBI have been based around excluding significant disease and reassurance. This approach is thought to help manage anxiety in vulnerable individuals. Best rehabilitation practice would include access to a mild TBI clinic, particularly to provide follow-up for the group who appear to be following a more prolonged symptom trajectory. Where available, this group are likely to benefit from longer-term counselling and support or perhaps specific interventions, such as full neuropsychological assessment and a cognitive remediation programme. However, simply providing easily accessible written information will decrease the likelihood of ongoing sequelae. These resources are widely available on the Internet.

Second impact syndrome

Second impact syndrome (SIS) provides evidence of the significance of structural damage associated with minor TBI. SIS occurs when a person suffers two concussions or minor TBIs in 'quick succession', usually considered to be before symptoms from the earlier injury have subsided. The second injury can produce rapid brain swelling and associated intracerebral pressure and has resulted in death from what would normally be considered a relatively minor injury. SIS is a major reason that many sporting codes have developed formal protocols dealing with return to sport after minor head injury.

Chronic traumatic encephalopathy

Chronic traumatic encephalopathy (CTE) has been most commonly reported in professional athletes, particularly in American football, but cases are recognized in most sports where repetitive concussions or subconcussive events (even such as heading the ball in soccer/football) occur. CTE is also recognized in military veterans who have been exposed to blast injury. Neuropsychiatric symptoms often first appear around 8–10 years after the initiating event/s

Recovery from traumatic brain injury

There are a number of stages to the proper care of individuals following a TBI which largely parallel the patterns of recovery seen in clinical practice. Which pattern predominates is largely determined by the amount of energy absorbed by the brain in the injury. Conceptually, the stages of recovery can be thought of as follows:

• Days: a very fast initial phase where there is temporary functional derangement within systems without significant structural damage. Normal behaviour re-establishes once the neurological milieu is regained.

• Weeks to months: function is impaired due to the results of incomplete structural damage that can be repaired over a number of weeks (e.g. as may occur in neurons within a healing ischaemic penumbra following blood vessel damage).

• At 6–24 months: in deafferentation injuries (e.g. resulting from DAI), intact neurons rearborize and regain connections with other neurons over weeks and months. This plasticity reshapes function within the damaged brain and can be either adaptive or maladaptive depending on the circumstances.

• Long term: the reafferentation phase transitions into the neuronal/ synaptic behaviours consistent with normal learning. In the absence of a coincident degenerative process, this form of new learning continues lifelong.

Although conceptual, these processes can be used to explain to family members the reasons behind often-quoted advice that people show their most rapid phase of recovery over the first 6 months followed by a slower phase of neurological recovery over 2 or so years. However, survivors of TBI continue to improve over the rest of their lives, depending on structural limitations and their perseverance. Of course, no two individuals will have identical patterns of injury, and in the early period the mechanisms underlying these recovery phases are indistinguishable from each other, particularly as they will be occurring simultaneously. Nett recovery is observed as thresholds are passed back towards normal function, limited by individual variations in damage, genetics, and cognitive reserve. The speed of clinical improvement for any given individual gives clues as to which of these processes is the rate-limiting step for their pattern of injury.

Stages of rehabilitation

Following an injury, speed of recovery is broadly linked to injury severity. A number of phases of treatment are recognized, which often align with the various settings used for TBI rehabilitation. Service models for how optimal rehabilitation can be organized for this population are discussed in ➔ Chapter 3; however, basic considerations for each stage of TBI rehabilitation are given in the following sections.

Stage 1: immediate trauma care

Fast and appropriate road-side treatment followed by rapid transfer to the nearest trauma centre is of paramount importance. Trauma centres will have specialized surgical services (e.g. orthopaedic, neurosurgical, and vascular surgeons) with ready access to CT/MRI scanning and often a dedicated neurointensive care unit. As discussed in ➔ Chapter 3, the rehabilitation team should work closely with the acute neurosurgical team to help avoid unnecessary and predictable complications in the early days and weeks post injury, thereby preventing major rehabilitation difficulties later. Examples include maintaining adequate oxygenation, early swallowing assessment with appropriate initiation of gastrostomy feeding, pressure area management, and DVT prophylaxis.

Stage 2: hyperacute and post-acute rehabilitation

Optimal rehabilitation of TBI involves a specialized MDT or transdisciplinary rehabilitation team, with access to transitional living services and a community reintegration/maintenance programme. Several models of care are used, from rehabilitation being implanted into the acute surgical hospital through to specialist brain injury rehabilitation centres, whether co-located or remote. There is clear evidence that post-acute brain injury rehabilitation produces better functional outcome. The sooner the transfer is made to the rehabilitation unit, the better the outcome is likely to be.

Behavioural problems in the early stages of recovery from TBI are very common, particularly while the person is in PTA. During this period, people are often confused, agitated, and exhibit lack of control over their emotional drivers. In combination, these factors can lead to antisocial behaviours including violence and aggression. The rehabilitation management of agitation involves environmental modification (e.g. providing separate rooms with quiet surroundings) and behavioural approaches to avoid overstimulation and to de-escalate situations that could otherwise lead to verbal and/or physical aggression. These approaches usually require specialist units with highly trained staff. Behavioural outbursts can be monitored using tools such as the Overt Aggression Scale[10] or its broadened version (the Overt Behaviour Scale)[11]. Sedative and psychotropic medication should be avoided if at all possible. Animal research suggests that dopamine blockers (in particular) permanently and adversely impact recovery. Carbamazepine and propranolol are safer options, often used as 'mood stabilizers' in this context. Formal behavioural modification programmes may be necessary for people with persistent socially inappropriate irritability and/or aggression.

Cognitive assessments, ideally performed by a clinical neuropsychologist, document areas of impairment but can also highlight the areas of relatively intact function which can form the basis of an appropriate therapeutic strategy. The timing of assessment is not fixed, with some units preferring neuropsychology review once a person is out of PTA, while others will assess later when there are specific questions of capacity that need to be addressed (e.g. work readiness and capacity to drive). Various cognitive strategies can be taught to improve function and quality of life. Occasionally, profound psychiatric problems can emerge such as psychosis, mania, or obsessive–compulsive disorder, either in a previously predisposed individual or perhaps as a result of organic brain damage. The involvement of a neuropsychiatrist is important in such cases.

Stage 3: longer-term inpatient rehabilitation

In some systems, 'slow to recover' or 'intermediate' patients may be transferred to a 'step-down' rehabilitation unit. This is a system-based decision and is linked to the concept that some people recovering from severe TBI may display considerable disability while continuing to make slow change in areas such as ADL. Where available, these units are seen as a step towards discharge home, along with slower stream rehabilitation, examine issues such as a smooth, staged discharge back into the home environment. Such a unit is also appropriate when there are delays to being transferred home, for example, where there is a need for major home modifications or extensive equipment must be funded and acquired.

Alternatively, individuals with severe cognitive and intellectual damage or behavioural disturbance may need a much more prolonged period of rehabilitation in a less acute environment. Another group of TBI survivors are sufficiently physically independent to go home but have cognitive or behavioural issues that make a discharge to home problematic. Some services will manage this patient population in residential care or transitional living units (TLUs) where the focus is on independent living and social skills. The usual TLU set up is akin to a group home, where a small number of 'residents' live in accommodation under the supervision of case workers. In the commonest format, the residents are responsible for normal day-to-day activities of the house (e.g. shopping, food preparation, washing, cleaning, finances, and community mobility) with guidance or hands-on assistance available depending on their individual strengths and weaknesses. TLUs also teach a wide range of social skills, such as initiating and carrying on a conversation, retaining friends, finding appropriate social outlets, interests, and hobbies, and so on.

Stage 4: community-based rehabilitation

While situations exist where this is not possible, maximizing quality of life following TBI means attempting to return the person back to their home and family. However, discharge from inpatient rehabilitation often occurs a few months post injury and while there is still the expectation of ongoing recovery. There is good evidence that the most significant challenges for the family and carers often occur after discharge home, sometimes occurring many years post injury. For example, the most common interval for the development of depression in 18–24 months post injury in the case of severe TBI. Long-term support is also desirable to detect the emergence of avoidable physical, cognitive, intellectual, behavioural, and/or emotional complications. At other times, the focus may be to ameliorate difficulties by providing counselling or psychotherapy to support the family.

Such a programme ideally involves ongoing home-based rehabilitation undertaken by a MDT and coordinated by a case manager. In the early period following return to home, physiotherapists, occupational therapists, speech and language therapists, clinical psychologists, medical staff, and social service staff may need to be involved. Some individuals will need referral back to a specialist centre for management of particular problems, such as PEG feeding, spasticity management, or tracheostomy care. For many people, the need for community rehabilitation will cease after a period of time. For others, the mix of therapies will evolve to include a wider range of health, social service, and employment professionals. Accessing and coordinating these different professionals can be a major problem for the injured person and their family. It is therefore becoming increasingly common for a case manager to be appointed to assist with such coordination and who can often act as an advocate for the disabled person and their family.

Vocational rehabilitation

The cognitive, behavioural, and emotional issues that can follow severe TBI can make it difficult for people to return to work. Of those who are able to return to work, some will not be successful in sustaining employment in the longer term. The successful return to employment for an injured worker often requires access to a skilled vocational counsellor working with the brain-injured person and slowly reintroducing them to the work environment. In the concept of a 'job coach', the counsellor works alongside the person, helping them to adapt to the work itself as well as the necessary social and interpersonal skills that go with the job. This approach also focuses on education and training for colleagues, as well as more senior managers and employers. The process and advantages of returning to productive employment are covered in more detail in ⊃ Chapter 20.

References

1. Wijdicks EFM (2016). Traumatic brain injury. In: *The Practice of Emergency and Critical Care Neurology*, pp. 566–586. Oxford University Press, Oxford.
2. Andrews PJD, Rhodes JKJ (2016). Assessment of traumatic brain injury. In: Webb A, Angus D, Finfer S, et al. (eds), *Oxford Textbook of Critical Care*, 2nd edn, pp. 1630–1634. Oxford University Press, Oxford.
3. Teasdale G, Jennett B (1974). Assessment of coma and impaired consciousness. A practical scale. *Lancet* 2, 81–83.
4. Shores EA, Marosszeky JE, Sandanam J, et al. (1986). Preliminary validation of a clinical scale for measuring the duration of post-traumatic amnesia. *Medical Journal of Australia* 144, 569–572.
5. Kahn F, Baguley IJ, Cameron ID (2003). Rehabilitation after traumatic brain injury. *Medical Journal of Australia* 178, 290–295.
6. Meyfroidt G, Baguley IJ, Menon DK (2017). Paroxysmal sympathetic hyperactivity: the storm after acute brain injury. *Lancet Neurology* 16, 721–729.
7. Hendricks HT, Guerts ACH, van Ginneken BC, et al. (2007). Brain injury severity and autonomic dysregulation accurately predict heterotopic ossification in patients with traumatic brain injury. *Clinical Rehabilitation* 21, 545–553.
8. Tanriverdi F, Kelestimur F (2015). Pituitary dysfunction following traumatic brain injury: clinical perspectives. *Neuropsychiatric Disease and Treatment* 11, 1835–1843.
9. Meares S, Shores EA, Taylor AJ, et al. (2008). Mild traumatic brain injury does not predict acute postconcussion syndrome. *Journal of Neurology, Neurosurgery, and Psychiatry* 79, 300–306
10. Yudofsky SC, Silver JM, Jackson W, et al. (1986). The Overt Aggression Scale for the objective rating of verbal and physical aggression. *American Journal of Psychiatry* 143, 35–39.
11. Kelly G, Todd J, Simpson G, et al. (2006). The overt behaviour scale (OBS): a tool for measuring challenging behaviours following ABI in community settings. *Brain Injury* 20, 307–319.

Further reading

Plantier D, Luaute J (2016). Drugs for behavior disorders after traumatic brain injury: Systematic review and expert consensus leading to French recommendations for good practice. *Annals of Physical and Rehabilitation Medicine* 59, 42–57.

Wiart L, Laurent J, Stefan A, et al. (2016). Non pharmacological treatments for psychological and behavioural disorders following traumatic brain injury (TBI). A systematic literature review and expert opinion leading to recommendations. *Annals of Physical and Rehabilitation Medicine* 59, 31–41.

Zasler ND, Katz DI, Zafonte DO (eds) (2012). *Brain Injury Medicine*, 2nd edn. Demos Publishing, New York.

Useful websites

🔖 https://acrm.org/resources/professional/—American Congress of Rehabilitation Medicine guidelines for mild TBI.

🔖 http://www.headway.org.uk—Headway, the traumatic brain injury charity in the UK.

Spinal cord injury

Introduction

The term spinal cord injury (SCI) is often taken to denote damage to the spinal cord following trauma, with non-traumatic SCI treated as a separate condition in some services. The annual global incidence of traumatic SCI is estimated at 10–80 cases per million population, with developed countries having lower incidence figures of around 10–15 cases per million per annum. In developed countries and in those with ageing populations, however, non-traumatic SCI is around twice as common as traumatic SCI.

The issues that underpin the management of SCI are similar whatever the cause, although there can be differences in terms of prognosis and epidemiology. For example, while traumatic SCI is more common in males than females (average ratio 4:1) and can occur at any age, peak incidence occurs in those aged 20–40, with another small peak in the elderly. Conversely, non-traumatic SCI affects males and females equally, occurring more frequently in middle age and beyond (e.g. 50–70s). The proportion of people developing paraplegia is greater in non-traumatic SCI compared to traumatic injuries. Common SCI aetiologies are given in Table 27.1 (Fig. 27.1).

The prognosis for SCI varies depending on aetiology. Often, survival for those with non-traumatic SCI is determined by the underlying diagnosis. In traumatic SCI, life expectancy has improved dramatically, going from 10% 1-year survival in 1900 to current values of around 75% and 85% of normal life expectancy for quadriplegia and paraplegia respectively. The improvements in life expectancy are linked to better secondary prevention of predictable complications, particularly in terms of renal function.

Individuals with SCI have great capacity to maintain a good quality of life. Helping to make this a reality is one of the multiple challenges that SCI poses to the MDT. Following inpatient rehabilitation, the key to independence and participation in previous life roles is access to good-quality information. Individuals should be kept informed of developments at all times and put in touch with the necessary range of professionals, not only with regard to their health, but also in social services, employment, and other spheres. Information and support can be obtained from local and international spinal injuries associations, many of whom are also accessible via the internet.

Table 27.1 Common causes of SCI

Traumatic	Non-traumatic
Motor vehicle crash (either occupants or pedestrians)	Arthritis
	Tumours
Falls (e.g. from height or minimal trauma in osteoporosis)	Vascular (e.g. acute intraspinal bleed or ischaemia)
Sporting-related accidents (e.g. diving into shallow water)	Infection (e.g. abscess formation, acute discitis)
Assault (e.g. gunshot, blunt trauma)	Inflammatory (e.g. transverse myelitis)

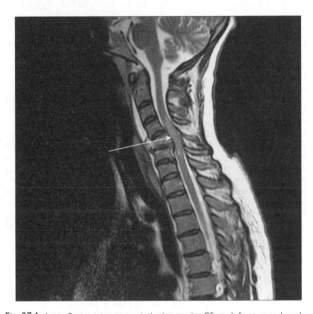

Fig. 27.1 Acute flexion injury to cervical spine causing C5 crush fracture and cord compression (arrowed). There is high signal in the cord indicating oedema.

Early acute management

Early recognition of spinal cord involvement in an injury is paramount, whether by emergency response personnel or in hospital. Immediate interventions are aimed at avoiding unnecessary worsening of the injury, whether through immobilization in a semi-rigid collar or rapid investigation to define the cause.

The level of spinal injury cannot be determined solely by examination (for dermatomes, myotomes, and associated reflexes, ⊃ see Chapter 5). The initial presentation may alter over time due to bruising, tenderness, or deformity which limit the value of early clinical evaluation. Radiographic investigations (± MRI) are critical in planning intervention. Methylprednisolone remains controversial in traumatic SCI but may possibly reduce inflammatory damage to nerve cells if used in the early stages (within 8 hours of injury). It also presents risks such as infection and GI haemorrhage. Similarly, early surgical decompression and stabilization of the spine (within 24 hours) has variably been associated with improved neurological outcome. However, even with the best management, only 10–15% of patients who present with a complete lesion on initial assessment will become incomplete over time.

Spinal shock is a common early presentation. In this self-limiting phase, the loss of supraspinal inputs to the distal cord inactivates normal cord functions such as sensorimotor and autonomic reflexes. Not all patients develop spinal shock and the duration of changes are also variable. Polysynaptic reflexes tend to return earliest, followed by the monosynaptic deep tendon reflexes. Central cord syndrome, seen in hyperextension injuries of the cervical spine, presents a mixed picture with greater damage to areas subserving the upper limbs compared to lower limbs.

While many people with SCI can be managed conservatively in the acute hospital system, early surgery offers the advantage of more rapid mobilization. If a conservative approach is adopted, mobilization can be limited during the first 6 or so weeks. This is particularly the case where cervical spine traction is utilized. It is not uncommon for extended periods of bed rest (e.g. 8–12 weeks) to be necessary to allow fracture stabilization, before bracing can be applied.

Post-acute management

Many people with traumatic SCI will have other injuries to other body systems occurring at the time of the injury that can complicate rehabilitation. For example, concomitant TBI is common, reported to occur in 16–59% of people in various case series. Orthopaedic or other trauma is also common and needs to be factored in to early intervention. Improvement in rehabilitation is associated with lesser injury severity at presentation, more distal lesions and incomplete injury. Older age, spinal cord oedema, and bleeding are all associated with poorer outcome. Individuals with SCI benefit from treatment in a dedicated, specialist spinal rehabilitation unit, as data suggest better outcomes with specialist as opposed to general rehabilitation. However, this depends on local availability, and any form of rehabilitation is preferable to none. Whether traumatic or non-traumatic, there are a range of predictable issues that require careful monitoring to avoid unnecessary morbidity or mortality. These issues include the followinh:

Respiratory difficulties

Cervical cord injuries can produce acute respiratory insufficiency from paralysis of the breathing muscles. Intercostal muscle paralysis will be present in complete lesions of the thoracic or cervical cord, and people with high cervical lesions may also have paralysis of the diaphragm. Respiratory function can decline quickly and careful monitoring and chest physiotherapy are important interventions. Hypostatic pneumonia, from shallow breathing and retained secretions, and the risk of aspiration pneumonia are higher in this group compared to people with lower-level SCI.

Pressure areas

The development of skin breakdown represents both an immediate and long-term issue in the management of people with SCI. Pressure areas form from prolonged direct pressure (e.g. between a bony prominence and a weight-bearing surface) or from shear forces which distort blood vessels in adipose tissue (discussed in ➔ Chapters 14 and 25). Individuals need to be nursed on a pressure-relieving mattress and/or seating, avoid pressure from folded clothing or bedclothes, and ensure that they have regular position changes. The skin should be kept clean and dry. Pressure areas are nearly always preventable. If they occur they can be very slow to heal and can sometimes require skin grafting. Septicaemia from pressure areas remains a leading cause of death in people with SCI.

Bladder dysfunction

Immediately post injury, the loss of supraspinal inputs leads to a non-contractile bladder. At this early stage, catheterization may be necessary to prevent incontinence and potential skin breakdown. Once spinal shock has worn off, the three most frequent issues are detrusor hyporeflexia (associated with S2–S4 nerve damage), detrusor hyperreflexia (from lack of inhibition of spinal reflex arcs), and detrusor sphincter dyssynergia (where detrusor hyperreflexia is associated with external urethral sphincter contraction). The management of bladder dysfunction is covered in detail in ➔ Chapter 12.

Bowel management

Initially, spinal shock leads to decreased peristalsis and prolonged bowel transit times. This can necessitate modification to feeding regimens to avoid over-distention. Defecation is often difficult due to disorganization of normal bowel reflexes and reduced ability to perform the Valsalva manoeuvre. This means that manual evacuation is usually needed. In later stages, the combination of bowel training, a modified high-fibre diet, and use of anal digital stimulation or glycerine suppositories can allow for continence and conveniently timed bowel movements (➤ see also Chapter 12).

Spasticity and contractures

Neuroplastic remodelling of dendritic fields in the disconnected spinal cord results in a number of the complications seen in SCI, including autonomic dysreflexia, neuropathic pain, and spasticity. The severity of spasticity is variable and is sometimes more problematic in incomplete lesions, depending on the pattern of damage to the cord. Contractures are nearly always preventable through careful positioning, physiotherapy, and antispastic treatments such as BoNT. The management of spasticity is covered in further detail in ➤ Chapter 10.

Heterotopic ossification

The development of ectopic bone in the soft tissues is quite common after SCI, with prevalence estimates ranging between 10% and 50%. It is most commonly seen around the hips, although (in decreasing incidence) the knees, elbow, shoulder, hand, and spine can also be involved. Early signs include a localized inflammatory response, swelling, pain and a decrease in range of movement. Heterotopic ossification can permanently reduce ROM, cause ankyloses, and complicate pressure area care. Treatment is difficult, with indomethacin and etidronate disodium probably the most useful treatments. Bone maturation is usually completed within 6–18 months of onset, at which time surgical intervention may be helpful to improve range of movement or remove bony prominences affecting skin care.

Deep venous thrombosis/pulmonary embolus

Clinically apparent DVT occurs in around 15% of people with SCI; however, the true incidence is likely to be two to three times higher. A small minority of people with DVT will develop PE, with the greatest risk occurring during the first 2 weeks post injury. Mechanical prophylaxis (compression (TED) stockings, external pneumatic calf compression) or anticoagulation with low-molecular-weight heparin is therefore recommended in the early post injury period. The risk of DVT/PE reduces with increasing time post injury and many protocols consider 8–12 weeks of anticoagulation adequate. Long-term thromboprophylaxis is not required unless there is a history of thromboembolic disease.

Pain and dysaesthesia

The experience of pain is very common in the early post-injury period. This can be mechanical in nature, for example, from musculoskeletal (in areas at or above the level of the lesion) or neuropathic sources. Neuropathic pain can be experienced below the level of the injury (more likely in incomplete lesions), at the level of the injury (through central sensitization processes), or above the lesion. The pain may be continuous, intermittent, and/or evoked by peripheral inputs. It is often associated with features of allodynia (pain from non-noxious stimulation) and wind-up (from repeated stimulation of receptors). Pain can continue for 6 months or more in 40–70% of people with SCI. The neuropathic pain can be difficult to manage, particularly in those with poor coping mechanisms and/or a tendency to catastrophize. A discussion of pain treatment can be found in ➲ Chapter 11.

Orthostatic hypotension

In the initial stages of spinal shock, loss of sympathetic tone can produce hypotension and bradycardia which improve over time with return of sympathetic reflex activity. In high-level lesions and complete lesions, the sympathetic control return is delayed resulting in reduction of blood pressure with position changes from supine to upright (orthostatic hypotension). The associated symptoms are light headedness, dizziness, or syncope in extreme cases. Management involves using abdominal binders while standing, adequate hydration, tilt-table training, and use of medications (such as ephedrine, midodrine, or fludrocortisone) in selective cases. These symptoms generally improve during the neurological recovery process.

Autonomic dysreflexia

This potentially fatal condition occurs as a result of maladaptive neuroplasticity in the disconnected spinal cord. It is seen in cord injuries above the sympathetic outflow to the gastrointestinal tract at T6, and is effectively an exaggerated sympathetic response to stimuli arising from below the level of the lesion. These stimuli can include:
• distension of the pelvic organs, such as bladder, colon, and rectum
• catheterization
• infections (e.g. urinary tract, ingrown toenails)
• sexual intercourse
• pressure sores
• tight clothing
• surgical procedures.

Autonomic dysreflexia (AD) is categorized by a range of symptoms and signs consistent with excessive sympathetic drive. Not all people with AD will experience all symptoms, and some may experience other idiosyncratic symptoms. Common symptoms include the following:
• Sudden-onset hypertension. This can be significant, with systolic pressures reaching 250–300 mmHg, although relative hypertension in a patient with quadriplegia (i.e. an increase to 140 mmHg systolic in a person whose blood pressure is usually 90 mmHg) can be just as indicative.
• Headaches, often described as pounding.
• Skin pallor and piloerection below the level of the spinal injury.
• Blurred vision (from pupillary dilatation).
• Nasal congestion.
• Anxiety or apprehension, and perceived shortness of breath.
• Paraesthesia.

During an AD crisis, the person's brainstem increases parasympathetic drive in an attempt to maintain homeostasis. This produces the other half of the recognized symptoms of the syndrome:

• Bradycardia.
• Vasodilatation, potentially with profuse sweating above the spinal injury level.
• Flushing/blotching of the skin above the level of the spinal injury.

AD should be treated as a medical emergency. The first step of intervention is clinical assessment to remove any identifiable nociceptive stimuli that may be driving the crisis (e.g. a kinked catheter or tight clothing). In some people, removing nociception and elevating the person's head will be enough to control the episode. In others, medical intervention will be necessary particularly where systolic blood pressure remains above 150 mmHg. A number of protocols are available, most of which suggest increasing levels of intervention depending on the initial response. Interventions include sublingual nitrates (except in men with recent phosphodiesterase 5 (PDE5) medication usage), oral nifedipine, and/or parenteral narcotics. Intravesical lidocaine has occasionally been used to resolve persistent AD. It is worth remembering that people with a recent episode of AD remain at increased risk of another episode for 48–72 hours.

Early rehabilitation issues

As always, the processes used in rehabilitation of people with SCIs need to be individualized to the situation that the person finds themselves in. Central to this will be the physical difficulties related to the degree of completeness and the level of injury to the cord. Rating the degree of completeness of a lesion has been standardized by using the American Spinal Injury Association (ASIA) Impairment Scale. This scale is presented in Table 27.2 (see Fig. 27.2 for the ASIA score sheet).

For complete lesions, the maximum level of functional improvement from rehabilitation follows a predictable pattern (Table 27.3). For incomplete lesions, the degree of predicted impairment can only be identified following a full functional assessment to see how any retained neurological innervation can be turned into function.

In addition to the neurological impairment from the cord injury, the injured person needs to be assessed with consideration (and potentially treatment) of any co-morbidities, their social situation, psychological coping skills, and their personal wishes and goals. These concepts are covered elsewhere in this handbook. Rehabilitation interventions that are relatively more common following SCI include the following:

Physiotherapy interventions

- Maintenance and improvement of respiratory function.
- Muscle strengthening.
- Stretching programmes to maintain/increase muscle length, including serial casting/splinting.
- Spasticity management.
- Bed mobility and transfer techniques.
- Standing practice using tilt tables, standing frames, and calipers.
- Gait re-education dependent on the level of the lesion.
- Provision of lower limb orthoses (e.g. calipers and AFO).

Table 27.2 ASIA Impairment Scale

A	Complete	No motor or sensory function is preserved in the sacral segments S4–S5
B	Incomplete	Sensory but not motor function is preserved below the neurological level and includes sacral segments S4–S5
C	Incomplete	Motor function is preserved below the neurological level and >half of key muscles below the neurological level have a muscle grade of <3
D	Incomplete	Motor function is preserved below the neurological level and >half of key muscles below the neurological level have a muscle grade of >3
E	Normal	Motor and sensory function is normal

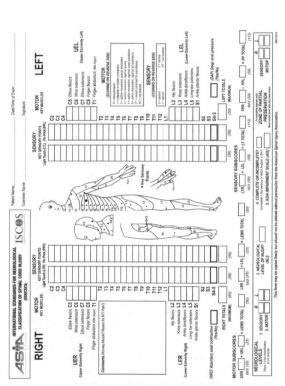

Fig. 27.2 The American Spinal Injury Association (ASIA) score sheet.

Table 27.3 Expected residual functional ability according to the level of lesion

Level of injury	Complete lesions
Lesion below C3	Dependent on others for all care
	Diaphragm paralysed, needs permanent ventilation or diaphragm pacing
	Chin-, head-, or breath-controlled electric wheelchair
Lesion below C4	Dependent on others for all care
	Can breathe independently using diaphragm
	Can shrug shoulders
	Can use electric wheelchair with chin control
	Can type/use computer with a mouth stick
	Environmental control system operated by shoulder shrug or mouthpiece
Lesion below C5	Can move shoulders and flex elbows
	Can eat with a feeding strap/universal cuff
	Can wash face, comb hair, clean teeth using feeding strap/universal cuff
	Can write using individually designed splint and wrist support
	Can help in dressing upper half of body
	Can push manual wheelchair short distances on the flat provided that pushing gloves are used with capstan rims on the wheels
	May be able to transfer across level surfaces using sliding board and a helper
	Electric wheelchair needed for functional mobility
Lesion below C6	Can extend wrists, still needs strap to eat and for self-care
	Can write using individually designed splint but may not need wrist support
	Can dress upper half of body unaided
	Can help in dressing lower half of body
	Can propel wheelchair up gentle slopes
	Can be independent in bed, car, and toilet transfers
	Can drive with hand controls
Lesion below C7	Full wrist movement and some hand function, but no finger flexion or fine hand movements
	Can do all transfers, eat, and dress independently
	Can drive with hand controls
Lesion below C8	All hand muscles except intrinsics preserved
	Wheelchair independent, but difficulty, but difficulty in going up and down kerbs
	Can drive with hand controls
Lesion below T1	Complete innervation of arms
	Totally independent wheelchair life
	Can drive with hand controls

Occupational therapy interventions
- Maximizing hand function (including tenodesis training).
- Splinting (resting and functional).
- ADL training such as dressing practice.
- Provision of aids, equipment, and adaptations to facilitate independent living (e.g. self-propelling or power wheelchairs).
- Environmental assessment regarding return to home and advice and recommendation on adaptations to property.
- Assistive technology including voice activation software and switch activated devices.
- Community activities including leisure.
- Facilitating return to work.

Nursing interventions
- Skin care
- Bowel and bladder management
- Sexual function.

Long-term rehabilitation issues

Discharge home

The transition from hospital to home is best undertaken following a series of trial home visits and/or day leave. Occupational therapy assessments of the home are vital to assess the suitability of the house for independence. It is common for structural alternations to be required to provide access to the house, both externally and internally. Houses may need to have hoisting equipment installed, along with major adaptations to the toilet, bathroom, and kitchen. Environmental control equipment may also be needed for those with quadriplegia. It is normal for the injured person and their family to feel a degree of anxiety on first returning home. As a consequence, an increased focus on psychological support can be useful over this period.

Depending on service arrangements, a transition in care may also be needed when the person first returns home. This will usually involve establishing a team of attendant care workers to assist the person with self-care and other tasks. The education and training of such community staff most commonly occurs via a case conferencing system between the hospital and the new staff. While contact with specialist spinal unit staff should be maintained for the long term, home-based therapy or other case workers may work with the person outside of the rehabilitation service. Many centres employ outreach workers who can monitor the situation and refer the individual back to the specialist care in the centre as necessary.

Psychological issues

Dealing with any life-altering or acutely disabling event is a stressful time that draws on the internal and external resources of the injured person, their spouse/partner, family, and friends. SCI can be particularly difficult for those with permanent changes in function, as it places a considerable strain on the individual and their relationships, with the potential of long-term change or even loss of relationships for some people. Clinical depression is common and occurs at some point in at least 50% of people with a SCI. There is an increased risk of suicide in people with SCI compared to the general population. Counselling and psychological support are vital and sometimes medication is needed.

Sexual life

The rehabilitation of conditions affecting sexual function is covered in ➔ Chapter 13. In SCI, sexual ability depends on the level and completeness of the spinal lesion. Men with complete UMN lesions have the capacity to have reflex but not psychogenic erections. Reflex erections are usually impossible in those with parasympathetic lesions. Attaining an erection that is satisfactory for penetration may require a PDE5 inhibitor such as sildenafil, tadalafil, and vardenafil. Intracavernosal injections are preferred by some men. Mechanical erection aids (e.g. vacuum erection and compressive retainer rings or intracavernosal implants) can be used where other interventions are nor suitable or have failed. Ejaculation remains possible but can be more difficult for those with complete spinal cord lesions. In these circumstances, direct stimulation or electro-ejaculation may be required. In women, problems commonly arise from decreased sensation and lack of vaginal lubrication.

Aside from sexual function, the person with SCI may experience changes in self-image and self-confidence which can severely affect their expression of sexuality. Where appropriate, it is ideal for counselling to explore the full expression of sexuality and how changes within relationships may impact this. It is important for sexual counselling to cover the entire range of issues around sexuality, as there is a tendency for discussions to focus on fertility and penetrative sexual intercourse.

Fertility

The influence of SCI on fertility varies between the sexes. Women rarely have reduced fertility as a result of their injury, as ovulation and uterine receptivity are predominantly under hormonal control and remain unaffected. For men, however, overall fertility is significantly affected by SCI. Viable sperm counts and sperm motility are both reduced by increased scrotal temperatures from prolonged sitting, and potentially less frequent ejaculation. Women with SCI who experience autonomic dysreflexia are at increased risk of complications during labour, although these risks can be minimized through good-quality obstetric care.

Late medical complications

Pathological fractures

People with SCI who are either unable to, or have restricted capacity for, undertaking weight-bearing exercise are at increased risk of osteoporosis and pathological fractures in affected limbs. Monitoring and replacing vitamin D may be of advantage where levels are found to be low.

Post-traumatic syringomyelia

Post-traumatic syringomyelia is an ascending myelopathy due to secondary cavitation of the central part of the cord. It occurs in about 4% of people with a SCI and is more commonly identified in quadriplegia compared to paraplegia. In the cervical spinal cord it usually presents with pain in the arm with characteristic dissociated sensory loss (reduced pain and temperature sensation but preservation of proprioception). It is also associated with progressive loss of motor function which can be of the LMN type. It is known as syringobulbia where the ascending syrinx goes on to affect the face. A small or non-progressive syrinx may be treated conservatively. Larger or progressive cases may benefit for surgery such as decompression and drainage of the CSF filled central cavity.

Respiratory management

Chronic hypoventilation represents a significant health risk for those with high cervical cord lesions, whether from the time of the initial injury or developing later, for example, from syringomyelia. Ventilatory assistance is most often provided by wheelchair-mounted positive pressure ventilators. Speech is possible with an uncuffed tracheostomy tube that allows air to escape through the larynx. For some people, particularly those with an intact phrenic nerve and injuries above C3, another alternative for long-term ventilatory support is the implantation of a phrenic nerve stimulator.

Forced expiration and coughing are impaired in those with lower cervical and thoracic lesions due to weakness of intercostal and abdominal muscles. Various techniques of cough augmentation and respiratory muscle training can assist with this (→ see Chapter 17).

Issues of participation

Driving

Driving a motor vehicle should be possible for all levels of spinal injury except perhaps for those with very high cervical cord lesions. Depending on the level and completeness of the injury, a range of vehicle modifications are available that allow safe driving. Automatic transmission is important and hand controls are usually essential. A variety of infrared devices can be used to control secondary function, such as windscreen wipers, lights, and horn. Very light powered steering simplifies steering the vehicle for those with a weak grip. Individuals with cervical lesions who retain useful shoulder and upper limb function can also drive a car using a variety of devices attached to the steering wheel. There are a number of devices that can allow the driver to stow a wheelchair safely and independently. There are also a range of vehicles available that allow a person to drive the vehicle while seated in their wheelchair. Specialist driving assessment centres that adapt and approve vehicles and provide licensing and/or training of people with SCI are available in most jurisdictions.

Employment

Many people who experience a SCI will be of working age, and returning to productive employment is a common life goal after injury. While returning to work is associated with improved health and quality of life, success rates can be poor with figures of 21–67% reported in the literature. Many factors affect return to work prospects, some of which are intrinsic to the person (e.g. the person's pre-injury capabilities and the nature of their SCI), while others relate to environmental factors (such as social attitudes, and physical characteristics like access, climate, and terrain). Attributes that enhance the likelihood of work include:

• younger age
• high personal motivation
• personal support (family and/or friends)
• having a flexible/supportive employer
• the type of industry the person is re/engaging with.

The chance of returning to work can be maximized by encouraging links with employment advisors or job retraining services. In some situations, affected individuals may be eligible for financial assistance to help achieve this goal.

Leisure pursuits

Alongside employment, an active participation in hobbies and sport adds meaning to people's lives. After injury, such leisure pursuits offer an important opportunity for social reintegration, increased self-worth, and better general health. These activities are also seen to decrease the adverse effects of life stressors. The physical constraints that occur with SCI may clearly modify how a person undertakes an activity, however, advice and assistance on becoming involved in wheelchair and other sports are freely available through support groups and the Internet (e.g. ➔ see 'Further reading').

Further reading

American Spinal Injury Association (2000). *International Standards for Neurological Classification of Spinal Cord Injury*. American Spinal Injury Association, Chicago IL.

Bates D (2011). Spinal cord disorders. In: *Brain's Diseases of the Nervous System*, 12th edn, pp. 809–846. Oxford University Press, Oxford.

Royal College of Physicians (2008). *Chronic Spinal Cord Injury: Management of Patients in Acute Hospital Settings*. Concise Guidance to Good Practice Series, No. 9. Royal College of Physicians, London.

Singh A, Tetreault L, Kalsi-Ryan S, et al. (2014). Global prevalence and incidence of traumatic spinal cord injury. *Clinical Epidemiology* 6, 309–331.

Wilson JR, Cho N, Fehlings MG (2016). Traumatic spinal cord injury. In: *Oxford Textbook of Neurocritical Care*, pp. 271–281. Oxford University Press, Oxford.

Witiw CD, Fehlings MG (2015). Acute spinal cord injury. *Journal of Spinal Disorders and Techniques* 28, 202–210.

Useful websites

International Spinal Cord Society (ISCOS): ℘ http://www.iscos.org.uk.

Quadriplegic, paraplegic and caregiver resources: ℘ http://www.sci-info-pages.com.

Spinal Injuries Association (UK): ℘ http://www.spinal.co.uk.

Spinal injury support groups: ℘ http://www.aspire.org.uk; ℘ http://www.spire.org.au.

Stroke

Introduction

The WHO defines stroke as: 'Rapidly developing signs of focal (or global) disturbance of cerebral function, lasting more than 24 hours or leading to death, with no apparent cause other than that of vascular origin'. This definition may be a little outdated with modern imaging techniques commonly diagnosing pathology at a very early stage or diagnosing old 'silent' infarcts.

Epidemiology

- *Incidence*: 16.9 million strokes worldwide in 2010.
- *Prevalence*: around 33 million survivors worldwide.
- *Mortality*: one in eight in first month, 20–25% die within 1 year. MI, bronchopneumonia, and further stroke are the commonest causes.
- *Acute impairments*: 77% weakness, 45% dysphagia, 23% dysphasia, 44% cognitive impairment, 26% visual field defect, and 20% neglect.

Types of stroke

- Transient ischaemic attack (TIA): full resolution of symptoms within 24 hours.
- Cerebral infarction: a focal infarction of a vascular territory (sometimes territories). Other conditions (i.e. hypoxia) may cause more global infarction and are not stroke.
- Intracerebral haemorrhage.
- Spontaneous subarachnoid haemorrhage.
- Cerebral venous thrombosis: may be classed as stroke if local parenchymal damage leads to focal neurological signs.

Oxford (Bamford) ischaemic stroke classification

- *Total anterior circulation stroke* (TACS): higher cerebral dysfunction plus homonymous visual field defect plus ipsilateral motor with or without sensory deficit. Mortality: 39% at 1 month, 60% at 1 year. Recurrence: low risk.
- *Partial anterior circulation stroke* (PACS): two out of three of TACS symptoms *or* higher cerebral dysfunction alone *or* monoparesis. Mortality: 4% at 1 month, 16% at 1 year. Recurrence: very high risk.
- *Lacunar stroke* (LACS): motor stroke *or* sensory stroke *or* sensorimotor stroke *or* ataxic hemiparesis. Mortality: 2% at 1 month, 11% at 1 year. Recurrence: low risk.
- *Posterior circulation stroke* (POCS): ipsilateral cranial nerve palsy with contralateral motor deficit *or* bilateral deficit *or* disorder of conjugate eye movement *or* cerebellar dysfunction *or* isolated homonymous hemianopia. Mortality: 7% at 1 month, 19% at 1 year. Recurrence: high risk

Anatomy and localizing features of stroke

Visual loss in stroke is shown in Fig. 28.1.

There are a large number of classical brainstem syndromes relating to strokes in specific anatomical locations which can be viewed in greater detail in a neurology textbook (Table 28.1).

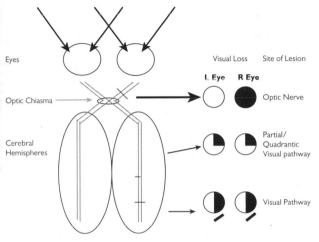

Fig. 28.1 Visual loss in stroke.

Table 28.1 Possible impairments by infarcted arterial territory

Site	Impairments/deficits
Anterior cerebral artery	Contralateral weakness ± sensory loss (often leg affected more than arm)
	Reduced initiation/aboulia/executive problems
	Expressive/motor aphasia[a]
	Gait apraxia
Middle cerebral artery	Contralateral weakness ± sensory loss (often arm affected more than leg)
	Contralateral hemianopia or contralateral superior quadrantanopia
	Aphasia[a]
	Unilateral spatial neglect[b]
	Apraxia[a]
Posterior cerebral artery	Contralateral hemianopia
	Memory impairment
	Alexia
	Contralateral hemisensory loss
	Cranial nerve palsies
Vertebrobasilar	Ataxia/vertigo
	Dysphagia
	Unilateral or bilateral paresis and/or sensory loss
	Drop attacks
	Horner's syndrome
	Dysphonia
	Gaze palsies
Retinal artery	Unilateral visual loss

[a] More common in dominant hemisphere stroke.

[b] More common in non-dominant hemisphere stroke.

Transient ischaemic attack

Transient ischaemic attack (TIA) is commonly said to be an ischaemic stroke, the symptoms and signs of which fully resolve within 24 hours. Diffusion-weighted imaging (DWI) MRI if performed will demonstrate completed infarcts in a significant number of TIAs. In reality, a spectrum of ischaemic syndromes exists from TIA to large vessel completed infarcts, the majority of which have the same underlying pathology of atherosclerosis and thromboembolism.

A TIA is a potent harbinger of a pending stroke, and rapid identification and treatment is essential. Between 2004 and 2012, as rapid access TIA clinics came into being in the UK, the number of people with TIA who went on to complete a stroke fell from 10% to 5%.

Someone with a suspected TIA (or non disabling stroke) should be reviewed urgently in a dedicated clinic. High-risk TIAs (ABCD² score >3, two or more episodes within 1 week, or TIA with atrial fibrillation (AF)) should be reviewed and investigated within 24 hours of first medical contact and lower-risk TIAs within a week. Anyone with complete resolution of symptoms should be given aspirin 300 mg daily prior to specialist review.

The ABCD² score

A = Age greater than 60 years (1 point).

B = Blood pressure (BP) higher than 140/90 mmHg (1 point).

C = Clinical symptoms—unilateral weakness (2 points) or speech disturbance alone (1 point).

D = Duration longer than 60 minutes (2 points) or 10–59 minutes (1 point).

D = Diabetes (1 point).

The first key function of the TIA clinic is to confirm or refute the diagnosis of TIA or minor stroke. Clear history (and collateral history) taking is essential and may alone give the diagnosis—for instance, where focal neurological deficits of sudden onset are clearly described by a patient with significant risk factors.

Remediable risk factors such as AF or carotid stenosis in anterior circulation TIA should be screened for and treated (anticoagulation and evaluation for carotid intervention respectively). Antiplatelet therapy should be given to anyone else with confirmed TIA. Confirmed TIA in someone with very low vascular risk should be investigated more extensively for conditions such as thrombophilia, patent foramen ovale, connective tissue disorders, and so on. Common vascular risk factors such as hypertension, diabetes, and hypercholesterolaemia should be screened for and aggressively treated and finally all patients with TIA or significant vascular risk should receive advice on smoking, alcohol, diet, and exercise as appropriate. People with TIA may not drive for 1 month.

Acute completed stroke

Thrombolysis or intra-arterial revascularization should be offered to appropriate patients within local or regional protocols.

Anyone suspected of having an acute stroke should be transferred directly to a monitored bed on an acute stroke unit (i.e. a hyperacute stroke unit), unless requiring immediate neurosurgical assessment or a critical care admission. Urgent brain imaging (usually CT) should be performed to exclude intracerebral haemorrhage before starting antiplatelets and to look for signs of raised intracranial pressure or an intracranial mass.

The hyperacute stroke unit

All patients on a hyperacute stroke unit should receive:

- urgent stroke consultant evaluation
- full diagnosis of stroke and the underlying causes
- medical optimization, and consideration of DVT prophylaxis
- early swallow assessment and nutritional/hydration management plan
- early detection of neurological deterioration and re-evaluation
- early detection and treatment of secondary complications
- early MDT assessment and acute rehabilitation plan (e.g. for seating)
- plan for secondary prevention
- prognosis and clear communication with patient and family
- antiplatelet therapy according to local guidelines.

Diagnostics

Initial CT has high sensitivity for intracerebral haemorrhage. Someone with clear clinical evidence of stroke and a normal CT may well be diagnosed with ischaemic stroke without need for further imaging (Fig. 28.2). MRI DWI has excellent sensitivity for acute infarction if performed within 10–14 days and may help if diagnostic uncertainty remains. CT angiography/magnetic resonance angiography may help if vasculitis or subarachnoid haemorrhage is suspected. Lumbar puncture is also useful in diagnosing subarachnoid haemorrhage, though if the patient has in fact had an ischaemic stroke, could theoretically reduce intracerebral pressure and extend the infarct.

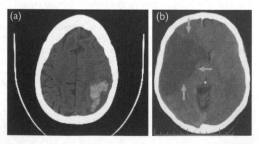

Fig. 28.2 CT scans showing acute intracerebral haemorrhage (left) and established infarct (right).

Anyone with intracerebral haemorrhage and evidence of mass effect (on CT or clinically, i.e. reduced GCS score), or anyone with subarachnoid haemorrhage, should be discussed urgently with neurosurgery. Hypertensive patients with lobar or deep white matter haemorrhage are unlikely to need intervention or neurosurgical follow-up. Patients aged less than 65 years with large vessel stroke and secondary oedema should be discussed with neurosurgery for consideration of decompression.

Anyone with anterior circulation stroke deemed to have a good prognosis of recovery should have carotid imaging. If carotid stenosis on the symptomatic side is present, vascular opinion should be obtained.

All patients should receive an ECG and if AF is diagnosed, anticoagulation should be offered in most circumstances. Anticoagulation is usually started after an interval especially in larger strokes, according to local guidelines. Anyone with suspected cardioembolic (i.e. large vessel) stroke should have further cardiac evaluation considered, such as prolonged cardiac monitoring and echocardiography.

Deteriorating neurology

Any patient with declining GCS score or new focal neurological signs should be urgently re-evaluated including brain imaging. Patients with symptoms and CT appearances of high intracerebral pressure from malignant middle cerebral artery syndrome or expanding intracerebral haemorrhage should be discussed with neurosurgery.

Patients having a second ischaemic stroke are unlikely to be candidates for thrombolysis because of the risk of bleeding from the first infarct, but they may be candidates for clot retrieval.

Medical optimization and prevention of medical complications

All patients with ischaemic stroke should receive aspirin 300 mg by mouth, rectum, or NG tube as soon as haemorrhage is ruled out, and daily thereafter until definitive secondary prevention is agreed.

Cardiorespiratory optimization is important to prevent worsening of ischaemic insult to the brain:

- Oxygen therapy only if oxygen saturations less than 95%.
- Rate control AF with appropriate agent.
- Treat chest infection or pulmonary oedema if diagnosed.
- Consider IV insulin by sliding scale in type 1 diabetes or if sugars are very high. Otherwise optimize glycaemic control medically.
- Avoid instituting BP control in the first 2–3 days unless there are serious concomitant medical issues.
- Avoid introducing or changing statin therapy acutely.

The CLOTS3 trial[1] demonstrated efficacy for intermittent pneumatic compression (IPC) stockings reducing rates of DVT (predominantly asymptomatic DVT) following stroke. It is important that, if IPC stockings are used, that this does not interfere with early mobilization or other therapies for the patient. The skin underneath the stockings should be monitored closely. Prophylactic low-molecular-weight heparin should be considered acutely in people at particularly high risk of DVT/PE according to local protocols. All patients who are still immobile 2 weeks post stroke should be considered for low-molecular-weight heparin prophylaxis. CLOTS1 and CLOTS2 demonstrated no benefit from knee-length or full-length compression stockings in preventing DVT/PE.

All patients with stroke should have a formal assessment of swallow as soon as possible. Patients with an unsafe swallow should have NG feeding and/or artificial hydration considered.

Meticulous food and fluid charts should be kept and people falling behind in fluid or nutritional intake should have supplementation considered—this may take the form of high-energy oral supplements, top-up NG feed, or artificial IV or subcutaneous fluids.

Early mobilization is widely thought to be a key component of the efficacy of modern acute stroke care in preventing death and reducing disability, and has been proven safe. As part of the initial MDT assessment, plans should be made to seat and/or mobilize patients as quickly as possible in the context of their impairments. It should be noted, however, that the AVERT trial[2] showed that intensive very early rehabilitation may be associated with a poorer outcome than a gentler 'out of bed' early mobilization commenced within 24 hours.

It is commonly believed that patients with intracerebral haemorrhage should have an initial period of bed rest, but this idea is not supported by any high-quality evidence.

Prognosis after stroke

There should be clear communication of professional assessments, medical and rehabilitation plans, and possible future outcomes with patients and families from the outset. This is particularly important when a patient has had a life-threatening or disabling stroke. Efforts should be made to gain insight into what a person might want if their outcome is likely to be poor. Ask the family if a patient has made any advance directives or has specifically expressed any wishes.

Indicators that a person is at high risk of death or poor functional outcome include:

- extensive deficits (i.e. total anterior circulation infarcts or reduced GCS score)
- multiple co-morbidities, especially organ failure, advanced cancer, or dementia
- premorbid care needs
- advanced age
- lack of progress, or decline over time.

In instances where clinicians agree that a poor prognosis is likely, it is reasonable to have early discussions about resuscitation and ceilings of care. It may be appropriate for instance, to decide not to place an NG tube if death is highly likely regardless, or to trial NG feeding for a defined period to allow a better assessment of prognosis to be made.

Secondary prevention of stroke

A single TIA or stroke is a potent risk factor for another and timely secondary prevention can reduce risk substantially. In stroke, it is particularly important to marry the evidence base with individual factors. One should never prescribe a number of new medications to a patient without consideration of their cognition, ability to swallow, and support network and without proper counselling of side effects and arrangements for follow-up and monitoring.

This section is not meant as an exhaustive guide to stroke secondary prevention. The evidence base is complex and there is a striking lack of comparator trials between similar medications. Recommendations vary between guidelines and practice differs between clinicians and there will be nuances to treating every patient. Treatment programmes should certainly be individualized—particularly as many patients will present who are already taking antiplatelets, antihypertensives, and lipid-lowering medicines. Every team involved in stroke care should regularly compare prescribing practice between their own clinicians and with other trusts and should review new evidence as it is published.

Oestrogen-containing contraceptives and hormone replacement therapies are a risk factor for stroke and should always be reviewed.

The specific situations of carotid artery stenosis and cardioembolic stroke are covered earlier in this chapter.

• *Antiplatelets*—aspirin 300 mg should usually be given as soon as haemorrhage has been excluded and continued daily for 2 weeks or until discharge. Anticoagulation should only be prescribed in defined high-risk circumstances (cardioembolic stroke, but not usually antiphospholipid syndrome) and certainly not routinely combined with an antiplatelet. Definitive antiplatelet therapy should be decided at discharge or after 2 weeks—usually clopidogrel monotherapy.

• *Antihypertensives* should usually only be commenced after a least a few days post stroke. The usual first-line recommendation is an ACE inhibitor in non-African/Caribbean patients under 55 years and a calcium channel blocker or thiazide diuretic in everyone else—with a target BP of 130/80 mmHg or less. Evidence does seem to support combination therapy over single-agent therapy.

• *Lipid-lowering drugs* should also usually only be commenced after an interval. A common regimen for a first stroke is to commence simvastatin 40 mg at night and intensify treatment if total cholesterol level less than 4.0 mmol/L and low-density lipoprotein less than 2.0 mmol/L are not achieved (i.e. simvastatin 80 mg or atorvastatin 80 mg). Note that atorvastatin can be given in the morning which can be useful in discharge planning. Be aware that statins may increase the risk of intracerebral haemorrhage and caution should be exercised in people with a history of this condition.

• *Advice on lifestyle alteration* should be offered to all patients. There are a wide range of smoking and alcohol cessation medications and services available which should be discussed with all appropriate patients. All patients should be advised to take regular exercise to increase their cardiovascular fitness (in line with their physical ability). Patients should be advised to reduce fat and salt consumption, increase fruit and vegetable consumption, and to eat two portions of oily fish per week. Community services to support lifestyle modification will vary widely and the rehabilitation clinician is advised to familiarize themselves with what is available locally.

Stroke rehabilitation

Rehabilitation settings

Most people who have a stroke will initially be cared for on an acute stroke unit. Patients with ongoing rehabilitation needs may move on to a range of settings including specialist neurorehabilitation units, stroke rehabilitation units, generic inpatient settings (such as care in community beds), and home with early supported discharge or community stroke team support. Tools such as the Rehabilitation Complexity Scale (RCS) or Patient Categorisation Tool (PCAT) may help define how complex the rehabilitation needs are for a particular patient.

All inpatient rehabilitation services caring for substantial amounts of people with stroke should have:

* a suitable rehabilitation environment
* a MDT with stroke expertise—usually medical consultant/rehabilitation medicine consultant, nursing, psychology, physiotherapy, occupational therapy, speech and language therapy/swallowing therapy and social worker
* access to other services such as orthoptics/optometry, audiology, continence team, dietetics, orthotics, electronic aids, dietetics, liaison psychiatry, pharmacy, podiatry, and wheelchair/specialist seating services.

Initial MDT assessment

A comprehensive history/collateral history should be taken and initial examination and assessments made to ascertain the person's past medical history, premorbid functional level, and pertinent social, personal, and environmental factors. The immediate admission MDT assessment should then focus on:

* ability to swallow
* ability to transfer/mobilize and move in bed
* skin and pressure areas
* nutrition and hydration status
* ability to understand information and express needs and choices
* ability to see and hear
* continence.

Over the following few days, the patient should have a comprehensive assessment of their risks, impairments, and activity limitations, using validated and standardized assessment tools where possible (➔ see Chapter 6). This should be clearly documented and communicated with patients and their families or carers, along with a realistic assessment of their possible functional outcomes.

Principles of stroke rehabilitation

The multidisciplinary rehabilitation team should meet regularly to review the overall status of each patient, to review and set rehabilitation goals, and make specific treatment plans that are appropriate to the overall rehabilitation plan. Rehabilitation goals should:

- be generated in collaboration with patients and families where possible
- be meaningful and relevant to the patient and their overall plan
- focus on activities and participation rather than individual impairments
- be challenging but achievable
- include short- and long-term goals
- be reviewed and modified regularly
- be clearly communicated with receiving teams on referral and transfer
- be clearly communicated with patients and families ideally in written form.

The MDT should collect appropriate outcome measures to measure progress through the rehabilitation programme—at least one of which should be a measure of function (Barthel Index or Functional Independence Measure are commonly used).

For those that can tolerate it and are making progress towards defined goals, patients should receive a minimum of 45 minutes of therapy, 5 days per week, from each relevant therapy discipline. More should be considered if appropriate. Short, frequent sessions are usually preferred for patients who have less endurance for therapy, and clear thought should be given to rehabilitation priorities at multidisciplinary review meetings in order to optimize therapy. The fundamental principle should be that rehabilitation programmes are tailored to each individual patient and their needs at a particular time.

It may be appropriate for families or carers to be involved in therapy sessions. Consideration should also be given to giving patients and/or their family or carers some therapeutic activities to do during 'down time' between therapy sessions.

Predictors of poorer functional prognosis

See Table 28.2.

Table 28.2 Prognostic indicators

Poor signs at 1 week	MRC grade 0 power in upper limb
	Unable to locate affected thumb with eyes closed
	Cannot maintain sitting balance
	Incontinence
	Loss of consciousness at onset
Prognosticators of poor functional outcome at 4 weeks post stroke	Low scores in the Barthel scale of ADLs
	Pre-existing and post-stroke incontinence
Adverse factors	Inability to walk
	Loss of arm function
	Loss of postural control
	Hemianopia
	Proprioceptive sensory loss
	Spatial neglect
	Impaired cognition
Rate limiting barriers in rehabilitation	Pre-existing physical disability (e.g. joint or cardiopulmonary disease)
	Multiple pathology (e.g. loss of limb)
	Sensory impairment
	Complications of disabling disease
	Incontinence
	Pressure sores
	Impairment of intellect, memory, perception, communication, mood

Stroke rehabilitation by impairment

Upper limb impairment

Impairments of arm function are probably the most common deficit experienced after stroke. Neuroplasticity is the ability of brain to reorganize and remodel after injury and can be maximized using rehabilitation approaches. The standard rehabilitation therapy is targeted not only at practising basic movement patterns but also real-life activities that incorporate use of the arm such as personal ADLs. Patients should also be offered repetitive task training of tasks such as manipulating objects, reaching, and grasping. Strength training may also be useful, but beware of encouraging a spastic limb into a more flexed position—extension strengthening may be more appropriate. Other specific therapies may be indicated in some patients:

- *Constraint therapy* involves constraining the good arm and performing repetitive task practice with the affected arm. Evidence would support its use in people with sufficient range and function of the affected arm and particularly those with learned disuse of the affected arm.
- *Bilateral therapy* is repetitive training of tasks requiring the coordinated activity of both arms. It is believed to stimulate the affected hemisphere via the interhemisphere connections. It may be used in people with moderate to severe deficits in the chronic stage of recovery.
- *Electrical stimulation* may be considered in people with flickers of UL movement but no activity against gravity or resistance—ideally as part of a research trial as improvements in functional outcomes are yet to be demonstrated.
- *Hand and wrist orthoses* should only be considered in people with spasticity or complete paralysis, in order to maintain or improve range, prevent deformity, improve comfort, aid hygiene, or improve function.
- *Robot-aided therapy* provides repetitive, non-fatiguable, and meaningful therapeutic movements to the UL. It has been shown to be equally effective as conventional hands on therapy, and hence has the potential of enabling therapists to work on multiple patients at the same time. This modality is, however, in its experimental stages and not widely available.

Shoulder pain is very common after stroke and in many cases associated with subluxation. The reported causes are multifactorial and hence it is difficult to have a standard treatment protocol. Neuropathic or central pain may be amenable to pharmacological treatment (gabapentin/pregabalin). Shoulder–hand syndrome or CRPS needs treatment as highlighted in
Chapter 11. True joint inflammation or impingement syndrome may benefit from mobilization exercises, simple analgesia, and steroid injections or shoulder block. True subluxation may benefit from electrical stimulation and/or shoulder brace.

Lower limb impairment

Repetitive task practice (such as walking or sit to standing), balance training, and practising activities that require LL movement (such as dressing) are the mainstay of treatment. Aids to bed mobility, transfers, and walking should be introduced as appropriate by the MDT in line with rehabilitation goals:

- *Splinting* may be considered to maintain range of paralysed or spastic muscle groups.
- *Functional electrical stimulation, using either external or implantable electrodes* can improve gait pattern in foot drop.
- *AFOs or foot-up splint* should be considered in people whose walking is significantly impaired by foot drop.
- *Treadmill training with or without a harness* may be considered as part of walking practice, though good-quality evidence is lacking.
- *Fitness training* should be offered to appropriate patients.

Dysphagia and nutrition

Swallowing is frequently impaired after stroke because of muscle weakness, problems with coordinating the swallowing movement, and problems with attention and cognition—commonly for a combination of these reasons. Assessment of swallow is a vital component of initial assessment (➔ see Chapter 9). Anyone with swallowing problems should be given specific recommendations around what consistencies of food and fluids they can most safely take and should receive regular support from a therapist with swallow expertise, as well as a dietician with stroke expertise. NG feeding should be considered within 24 hours of admission and regularly reviewed. Swallowing therapy and nutrition is described in detail in ➔ Chapter 9.

Using mittens and/or nasal bridles as well as using one-to-one nursing may help to protect a NG tube *in situ* from being removed by the patient. If such measures are instituted this should be done in conjunction with a Deprivation of Liberty Safeguards (DOLS) order if the patient lacks capacity to decline artificial feeding.

Decisions to place a long-term gastrostomy tube (such as a PEG or radiologically inserted gastrostomy) should also be carefully considered by the MDT and involve patients, families, and carers. The risks, benefits, and long-term prognosis of the patient should be given due consideration, along with the nutritional vulnerability of the patient (i.e. losing weight, needing frequent resiting of NG tube). Many studies show a mortality rate of 20–50% within 3–6 months after PEG insertion (the variation reflecting differences in patient selection), the majority of whom will have succumbed to stroke complications unrelated to the PEG. In frailer people with larger strokes, it may be wise to delay decisions on long-term feeding where possible in order to assess prognosis more accurately.

Speech impairments

Common subtypes:
- *Dysarthria*—poor articulation leading to reduction in speech clarity.
- *Receptive (fluent) aphasia*—reduced understanding of language. Speech may be fluent and nonsensical (jargon).
- *Expressive (non-fluent) aphasia*—reduced production of language. Speech lacks fluency, naming of objects is commonly impaired. Paraphasia may occur ('toothspooth' for toothbrush).
- *Conduction aphasia*—reduced ability to repeat language.
- *Speech apraxia*—reduced ability to plan and execute the orofacial motor tasks required to produce speech.

Speech and language therapy and communication strategies are detailed in ➔ Chapter 8.

Visual impairments

Nystagmus, diplopia, and visual field defects may all occur following stroke and may be compounded by ocular conditions such as long sightedness, glaucoma, or cataract.

- *Assessment*—patients with new visual impairment should receive full ophthalmology and optometry assessment. Consider registering patients as partially sighted if appropriate.
- *Prism glasses for hemianopia*—should only be trialled by someone with expertise and with proper evaluation of effects.
- *Compensatory eye movement training for hemianopia* can be considered if available.

Unilateral spatial neglect

The cardinal deficit of spatial neglect is that a person fails to report, orientate towards, or make responses to meaningful stimuli on the affected side. It is more common and often more severe on the left side, though more subtle right-sided neglect is not uncommon. It is a highly heterogeneous entity and quite separate from hemianopia, though the two deficits may well coexist. When persistent, it is highly disabling and refractory to treatment:

- *Education*—patients and families should have the deficit explained.
- *Diagnosis*—requires a battery of tests (such as the Rivermead Behavioural Inattention Test).
- *Environmental cues*—such as bright marks on the left side of doorways or the dinner plate may help with specific tasks.

The mainstay of treatment is to try and compensate for the deficit during specific tasks practice (e.g. teaching patients to deliberately scan left during a task and give regular prompts to attend to the affected side). There is commonly little carry-over of improvements between individual tasks, however, and there will always be risks associated with not noticing novel hazards in the real world as long as neglect persists.

Mental capacity and deprivation of liberty

Cognitive and communication impairments after stroke frequently impair a person's capacity to make choices regarding their medical care. This can commonly complicate decision-making about artificial feeding, discharge planning (especially discharge destination), and setting ceilings of care or making 'do not attempt resuscitation' orders. It is vital that capacity is assessed for each specific decision, by appropriate members of the MDT, in strict accordance with the Mental Capacity Act. Where restraint is being considered (e.g. using a one-to-one nursing special to prevent a patient from leaving the ward), a DOLS order should always be applied for.

Other rehabilitation issues

The following issues should be reviewed regularly by the MDT:

- Skin integrity (➲ see Chapter 14)
- Bowels and bladder (➲ see Chapter 12)
- Cognition, mood, and behaviour (➲ see Chapter 7)
- Self-care ability
- Pain (➲ see Chapter 11)
- Spasticity and contractures (➲ see Chapter 10)
- Nutritional status.

Discharge planning

Discharge planning should be considered from the very start of someone's admission. The home circumstances, pre-existing functional status, care needs, and support network of the patient should be assessed early in the admission as they will be highly relevant to discharge planning. Social work referrals and continuing health assessment referrals should be made as soon as care needs on discharge are known.

Rehabilitation in hospital is often geared towards enabling people to self-care, mobilize, meet nutritional needs, and so on and to minimizing the risks of adverse events occurring. However, discharge planning should consider the wider participation issues that are ultimately the key to returning to a high quality of life after stroke:

• Relationships and sexual functioning
• Social reintegration
• Driving and community mobility
• Working
• Leisure activities.

Various rehabilitation options post discharge may exist depending on the area. Long-term rehabilitation goals such those previously listed, rehabilitation potential, and individual social and environmental circumstances should be considered to help marry up the patient with the correct service to meet their goals. Services may include:

• community stroke team
• stroke early supported discharge team
• other community rehabilitation teams with stroke expertise
• generic rehabilitation such as intermediate care team
• community rehabilitation beds
• outpatient therapy
• voluntary sector services
• local council provided services.

Prior to discharge, medications should be reviewed in line with the patient's needs and wishes. Warfarin in particular is problematic to take for people who would to attend clinics or deal with a fluctuating dosing regimen. Alternatives such as low-molecular-weight heparin or off-licence use of a novel oral anticoagulant may be considered. Common side effects of medications (dizziness, nausea, cough, muscle pains, reflux) should be warned about and patients advised to speak to their GP about medication changes.

References

1. Dennis M, Sandercock P, Reid J, et al. (2013). Effectiveness of intermittent pneumatic compression in reduction of risk of deep vein thrombosis in patients who have had a stroke (CLOTS 3): a multicentre randomised controlled trial. *Lancet* 382, 516–524.
2. AVERT Trial Collaboration Group (2015). Efficacy and safety of very early mobilisation within 24 h of stroke onset (AVERT): a randomised controlled trial. *Lancet* 386, 46–55.

Multiple sclerosis

Background and epidemiology

Multiple sclerosis (MS) is the commonest of the demyelinating CNS conditions and is the most frequent condition causing neurological disability in younger adults. It causes a combination of physical and cognitive disabilities, which, when combined with starting in young adult life and with an uncertain rate of progression, make it both challenging and responsive to rehabilitation.

MS is well known for having a variable incidence and prevalence, both of which were thought to increase in latitudes towards the poles. We now know that the picture is not as straightforward: in the Northern hemisphere the increase with northerly latitude is less clear, although it still holds in the Southern hemisphere. This is probably due to MS being secondary to a number of interacting factors, including human leucocyte antigen (HLA) type, other genetic influences, previous infections (e.g. Epstein–Barr virus), and vitamin D.

MS affects approximately 2.5 million people worldwide. Prevalence in the UK, estimated in 2010, is 285.8 per 100,000 in women and 113.1 per 100,000 in men. Overall prevalence in Australia estimated in 2009 is about 100 per 100,000. The mean age of onset is 32 years, but the range is wide. There is a female-to-male predominance which is thought to be increasing and is currently 2:1.

Disability in MS can be estimated in various ways. For instance, 66.7% of Australians with MS require assistance with at least one of ten everyday activities. MS affects employment rates, for instance, in Australia in 2009 there were 20,400 people with MS aged 15–64 years, of whom 9800 were employed.

Diagnosis and prognosis

Patients are usually referred for rehabilitation having already received a diagnosis and having developed disability due to the condition. There may be exceptions where a person has presented with a very severe clinically isolated syndrome that requires rehabilitation. Diagnosis may occur several years after first symptoms. The revised 2010 McDonald criteria are used to define the diagnosis, based on:

- clinical symptoms and signs of an MS attack
- MRI lesions that are typical of MS—periventricular, juxtacortical, infratentorial, and spinal
- dissemination of the previously listed criteria in time and space.

Examination of CSF for oligoclonal bands and increased immunoglobulin G is supportive.

Information at the point of diagnosis affects a person's ability to adapt to the challenges of the condition. The concept of rehabilitation and management of the disease is as important as information about disease-modifying therapy (DMT). Prognosis for a person diagnosed now with MS is different from a person diagnosed in previous years due to present and future changes in DMT and in rehabilitation. During rehabilitation, patients will be seen at different stages of disease and having had different DMT, so it can be very difficult to discuss prognosis accurately with them.

It is important to understand the criteria for diagnosis, both to be able to discuss prognosis with patients and because symptoms may become apparent later which affect the diagnosis—for instance, evidence may arise of a person thought to have primary progressive MS having had a distinct earlier relapse or a clear Mendelian inheritance pattern may become apparent in the person's family which indicates the diagnosis is not MS, but an inherited condition similar to MS. Conversely, a patient receiving rehabilitation for a segmental transverse myelitis may develop separate neurological symptoms and signs that suggest they have MS. Some of the possible conditions or groups of conditions that may have overlap with symptoms and signs of MS are listed in Box 29.1.

There is uncertainty over which initial factors are associated with later disability; those which are consistently shown to have an effect are shown in Table 29.1.

Box 29.1 Conditions with similar symptoms and signs to MS
- Neuromyelitis optica
- Spinocerebellar ataxia
- Acute disseminated encephalomyelitis
- Hereditary spastic paraparesis
- Sarcoidosis
- Late-onset Krabbe disease
- Cerebral vasculitis secondary to conditions such as systemic lupus erythematosus
- Fabry disease
- Cerebral malignancy
- Mitochondrial disease
- CADASIL (cerebral autosomal dominant arteriopathy with subcortical infarcts and leucoencephalopathy)
- Leucodystrophies
- Tropical spastic paraparesis (human T-lymphotropic virus 1 (HTLV-1))
- Lyme disease
- Tertiary syphilis
- Vitamin B_{12} deficiency

Table 29.1 Factors affecting disability in MS

	Worse prognosis	Better prognosis
Age at onset	>40 years	
Initial optic neuritis		√
Initial polysymptomatic onset	√	
Shorter time to second relapse	√	
Shorter time to secondary progressive MS	√	

Types of multiple sclerosis

About 85% of patients have relapsing–remitting MS at initial onset and 15% have primary progressive MS. Relapsing–remitting MS transitions to secondary progressive MS after a variable time period (Figs. 29.1 and 29.2), with that transition thought to be due to the cumulative effect of axonal loss. These three main forms of MS are described in Table 29.2. Other subtypes of MS are described, for instance, relapsing progressive MS and tumefactive/malignant (incidence 1 in 1000 people with MS per year).

It is more likely that rehabilitation medicine clinicians will see those with primary or secondary progressive MS than relapsing–remitting because the impact of disability tends to be greater and the current benefits from DMTs less in progressive MS. An important consequence of this for patients with secondary progressive MS is they may first see a rehabilitation physician at a particularly difficult phase in their condition as they undergo the transition to secondary progressive MS. The recognition that the person is going into this phase can be almost like receiving the diagnosis again, due to its associations with progressive disability and with lack of efficacy of DMT. However, it is also the point at which a good rehabilitation approach becomes relatively more important and where the emphasis on managing disability can assist the person during this time.

Table 29.2 Forms of MS

Type of MS	Characteristics
Relapsing–remitting MS	Discrete relapses, initially with no residual disability. 50% later develop secondary progressive MS
Secondary progressive MS	Occurs a mean 10 years after onset of relapsing-remitting MS, with transition occurring over a 2-year period. For the patient, this phase can be like receiving the diagnosis again
	Due to progressive axonal loss
Primary progressive MS	Progressive impairment with no relapses

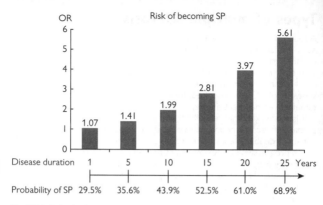

Fig. 29.1 Risk of relapsing–remitting MS converting to secondary progressive (SP) MS over time. OR, odds ratio.

Reproduced with permission from Scalfari A. et al. Onset of secondary progressive phase and long-term evolution of multiple sclerosis. *J Neurol Neurosurg Psychiatry*, 2013(00):1–9. Copyright © 2014, British Medical Journal. doi:10.1136/jnnp-2012-304333.

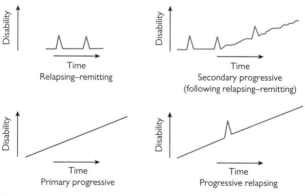

Fig. 29.2 Time course of different forms of MS.

Adapted with permission from Lublin F.D. et al. Defining the clinical course of multiple sclerosis: results of an international survey. *Neurology*, 46(4):907–911. Copyright © 1996, American Academy of Neurology. https://doi.org/10.1212/WNL.46.4.907.

Relapses

Relapses are not always straightforward to diagnose. It is recognized that relapses can occur in any form of MS. They are defined by:
- occurring at least 30 days since the start of a previous relapse
- onset over hours to days
- lasting at least 24 hours—this includes paroxysmal symptoms that continue recurring over a 24-hour period
- absence of infection or fever.

About 74% of relapses are monofocal. The commonest are sensory, but they may also be motor, cognitive, visual, or autonomic.

There are several factors associated with an increased risk of relapses, including:
- infections
- stress
- postpartum.

A reduced risk of relapses is associated with:
- pregnancy
- breastfeeding
- sunlight
- higher vitamin D levels.

There is no association between vaccinations or epidural anaesthesia and relapses. The influence of hormonal contraceptives is uncertain.

Worsening symptoms associated with infections can be particularly difficult to diagnose as they may cause a pseudo-relapse or a true relapse. A pseudo-relapse is an exacerbation of previous symptoms that occurs when body temperature is increased or when there is a systemic inflammatory response. It will resolve alongside the pyrexia or inflammatory response.

In addition to relapses, people with MS will experience fluctuations in their symptoms from day to day, especially associated with fatigue.

Good communication between rehabilitation and neurology services is important in managing relapses, as the latter will usually have a system for managing these. The decision to use methylprednisolone to speed up natural recovery from a relapse is an individual decision. Use of steroids does not affect disease progression or accumulation of disability but it may allow a person to resume their normal activities at an earlier stage and thus help the person with MS to return to their normal roles at an earlier stage than they otherwise would have done. However, repeated steroids may have a detrimental effect on the person's long-term health. Potential weight gain and risk to bone health need to be weighed against the short-term benefits of the treatment, especially if the person is receiving repeated courses of steroids.

There is evidence that multidisciplinary rehabilitation following an MS relapse can improve impairment and disability-related outcomes but the length of and types of rehabilitation for optimal outcomes are not known.

Disease-modifying treatment

DMTs for MS have advanced over the last decade, but it is still uncertain exactly how these affect prognosis and progression of disability. From the point of view of the rehabilitation physician it is important to recognize when to refer a patient for DMT. At the time of going to press, there were no DMTs known to be effective in primary or secondary progressive MS without relapses, but the field is rapidly changing. If a person who has not had a relapse for a number of years starts to develop relapses again, this indicates an increase in disease activity; such patients should be referred to the neurologist in order to assess the use of DMT. The long-term effect of DMT on progression of disability is still uncertain.

Evidence regarding DMT is frequently changing, so it is not described here. Guidelines and summaries of evidence can be found in several places (e.g. the 2015 Association of British Neurologists guidelines are published in Scolding et al.[1]).

Multiple sclerosis-associated impairments and their management

There are a wide range of impairments associated with MS, and some of the more frequent ones are described in this section. The general principles of rehabilitation for these impairments, as described in other chapters, are also relevant.

The majority of patients with MS seen within a rehabilitation medicine service will have a progressive form of MS; however, it is important to re-member that patients will have been experiencing significant impairments from the beginning of their MS, even though those impairments will have been more variable initially. For instance, one study showed that 85% of patients reported sensory symptoms, 81% unexplained fatigue, and 50% cognitive impairment within the first year after onset.[2]

Bladder and bowel-related problems

For full details regarding neurogenic bladder and bowel management, ➔ see Chapter 12. The following is a summary of the issues for those with MS.

Bladder

Up to 80% of people with MS experience bladder problems, and they have a large effect on disability and health-related quality of life in MS. Lesions at the level of the spinal cord, pons, and suprapontine can all have an effect on bladder function affecting storage, voiding, or both. Patients present with symptoms of detrusor hyper-reflexia, detrusor sphincter dyssynergia, and, less commonly, a flaccid bladder. The commonest symptoms are:

- urgency
- urge incontinence
- frequency
- nocturia.

Less common symptoms, occurring in about a quarter of those who have urinary symptoms, are those often associated with bladder hypoactivity, including:

- hesitancy
- overflow incontinence
- use of abdominal pressure when voiding
- episodes of retention.

Risks of urinary tract dysfunction include:

- UTIs
- urosepsis
- hydronephrosis
- renal failure
- renal and bladder calculi
- negative effect on mood and well-being
- interference with daily activities
- pressure sores.

Management of bladder impairment in MS follows the same principles as for those with other brain and spinal cord conditions affecting bladder function, and can be divided into measures to assist in reducing bladder overactivity, reduce risk of infections, and assist in bladder emptying. ➲ See Chapter 12 for further details.

Bowel-related problems

Constipation occurs in many people with MS. Management includes:
- keeping a diary in order to link bowel movements and stool consistency with diet, fluid intake, medication, and daily schedule
- attention to both timing and amount of time spent in defecation
- maximal use of gastrocolic reflex
- appropriate use of mechanical factors, such as hip flexion during defecation
- abdominal pressure or digital stimulation can be helpful
- a diet high in fibre, sometimes with use of supplementary fibre.

If these measures fail then medication can be used, such as sodium docusate, senna, macrogols, suppositories, and enemas.

Cognitive function

Cognitive impairment occurs in approximately 50% of the MS population. There is wide variation from patient to patient in the specific type of cognitive impairment, which probably relates to the variation in sites of demyelination and axonal loss. The commonest problems are:
- memory, with the main problems being in working memory and long-term memory
- switching attention
- rate of information processing, and the effect of this on learning
- visuoperceptual skills
- executive function
- word finding.

These cognitive impairments can have wide ranging effects, especially on self-esteem, employment, and driving. They can be compensated for to some extent, which can assist in employment and other roles, but it is harder to compensate with regard to driving and it is important to consider this when patients are reviewed.

Fatigue

MS-related fatigue can be due to several reasons, many of which have overlap with other progressive neurological conditions. Factors may include:
- mood
- cognitive fatigue—use of different and greater cortical areas in compensation for axonal loss
- increased effort required for daily activities due to the various physical disabilities associated with MS
- medication (e.g. for pain or spasticity)
- cytokine activation
- disrupted sleep secondary to spasms, pain, or urinary frequency
- sleep disorders.

About 75% of people with MS experience fatigue at some point over a 2-year period and in 55% it is their worst MS-related symptom. Assessment of fatigue requires a detailed history of both fatigue and sleep, as the two are closely inter-related. Variation in fatigue levels, exacerbating and relieving factors, drug history, strategies the patient has used, assessment of non-MS causes of fatigue, and drug history are important.

Therapeutic approaches for which there is some evidence include:
- pacing
- CBT
- exercise, both endurance and strength training.

There are varying degrees of evidence for combining these therapeutic approaches using individualized, group, or Internet-based sessions.

Pharmacological approaches include:
- amantadine helps approximately 50% of those with MS-related fatigue
- modafinil.

Mobility

Difficulty walking is the most common symptom in MS. It is often due to a combination of different factors including:
- pyramidal weakness
- spasticity
- fatigue
- disuse
- pain
- ataxia
- proprioceptive impairment.

A structured exercise programme, planned and supervised by a physiotherapist, can be of benefit. It has been recommended that the elements of such a programme should include the following:
- Specific strengthening exercises for identified muscle weakness.
- Exercises and advice on postural correction and control.
- Passive stretching to reduce spasticity, improve the range of movement, and prevent contractures.
- Exercises utilizing ADLs to improve dexterity and coordination.
- Gait training using mobility aids as necessary.
- Hydrotherapy to increase activity and range of movement dependent on the individual's reaction to heat as the hydrotherapy pool is kept at a higher temperature (30–36°C) and this can induce fatigue.
- Various exercise modalities can be used, including gym-based endurance and strength-based programmes, robot-assisted training, and other forms of exercise such as tai-chi, yoga, and Pilates.

The types of exercise that are most beneficial to the person with MS will change over time as their goals and physical impairments and abilities change, so it is important for them to be able to access a physiotherapist to review their exercise.

Aids to mobility and adaptions to improve the accessibility of the environment are important, and covered in ➲ Chapters 22 and 23.

There is evidence that prolonged release (PR) fampridine (acetylcholine release enhancer) can have effects on mobility in some people with MS. It is approved in Europe for use to approve walking in patients with an Expanded Disability Status Scale (EDSS) score of 4.0–7.0, in Canada an EDSS score of 3.5–7.0, and with no EDSS score specified in Australia, at a dose of 10 mg twice daily. As only some patients respond, it is recommended that an initial 2-week trial combined with measurement of walking velocity is used.

Mood disorders and psychosis

Anxiety and depression each occur in approximately 50% of the MS population[3] and are more prevalent in secondary progressive than other forms of MS.

Suicidality, psychosis, and bipolar disorder are also commoner in the MS population. Both the brain pathology of MS and the effects of having a long-term neurological condition contribute to these mood disorders in MS, with prevalence being higher than in some other neurological long-term conditions. Depression and anxiety can be both a primary effect of MS and a secondary complication. There is also debate as to whether depression can be exacerbated by beta-interferon.

Assessment of mood disorders can be difficult due to overlap with other MS-associated symptoms and because of the negative effects of these conditions, so depression may go unrecognized and patients may not bring up the issue unless prompted to do so. Treatment is similar to depression in other contexts, and both pharmacological and psychological interventions for depression have been shown to be beneficial in MS. Some people develop emotionalism/pseudobulbar affect which responds well to a SSRI.

Aside from treating people with MS who have mood disorders, it is important for any clinician seeing people with MS to appreciate the psychological effects of having the condition and to integrate this into rehabilitation and condition management.

Dependent oedema

LL oedema occurs readily in MS. It is thought to be due to a combination of reduced mobility, increased time spent with LLs dependent, and vascular autonomic changes. It increases the risk of venous thromboembolism and cellulitis and affects mobility. Advice regarding elevation of legs when at rest and use of compression hosiery can help. Some patients also use static pedals to exercise their legs when sitting. Gabapentin and pregabalin can also increase the risk of LL oedema.

Pain

Pain is common in MS, an overall estimate from a meta-analysis being 63%.[4] Both musculoskeletal and neurogenic pain can occur, and interact with each other and with the psychological aspects of having a long-term progressive condition. There are specific types of pain that are more frequent in MS:

- Trigeminal neuralgia
- Lhermitte's phenomenon
- Pain related to spasticity
- Optic neuritis-related pain
- Migraine and headache
- Neuropathic extremity pain.

Postural changes and decreased mobility lead to musculoskeletal pain.

The general principles of pain management are the same as for other conditions (➲ see Chapter 11), with a combined approach using psychological interventions, exercise modalities and pharmacological interventions.

Posture

Muscle weakness, spasticity, ataxia, and impaired sensation all affect posture in the person with MS. Poor posture can lead onto contractures, pressure sores, respiratory infections, pain, and LL oedema. Specialized seating, both in wheelchairs and static chairs, is very important. In those with more advanced MS who have trunk and pelvis affected, adaptations to bed positioning also become important, with mattresses of appropriate pressure-relieving grade and hospital type beds usually being useful as well as positioning using pillows, T rolls, and even a sleep system being of help. Treatment of spasticity using BoNT and oral medications (➲ see Chapter 10) is important.

Adaptive equipment is not only useful for passive aspects of posture, it also helps to stabilize the person in a position where they may optimize their abilities—whether using ULs in a functional way, eating, or enabling communication.

Respiratory function

Respiratory function becomes progressively impaired and is a major cause of mortality and morbidity in MS. The principles of respiratory impairment, its rehabilitation, and its management are similar to other conditions, as described in ➲ Chapter 17.

Respiratory muscle training has been shown to improve both inspiratory and expiratory muscle strength, although it is less effective in those with more advanced MS. The effects of respiratory muscle training on mortality, morbidity, and participation are uncertain at present. Use of NIV and cough assist devices is a poorly studied area, but benefit is certainly seen for some individuals. Cognitive function will be more often affected in MS than in other neurological conditions where NIV and cough assist devices are considered. It will have an effect on the success of both of these methods, and is an important aspect to note when considering use of these.

Sexual function

(➲ See also Chapter 13.)

MS generally affects people at an age when they are more likely to be sexually active. With potentially so many symptoms to be dealt with, difficulty maintaining sexual function may not be addressed. Yet the number of patients experiencing problems is high. Studies indicate that 80% of women and 50–90% of men will have sexual problems related to their MS at some point. There is no reason for neurorehabilitation clinicians to shy away from problems regarding sexual functions as there is much within the skill set that can help.

The problems people experience may be:
• primary (impairment of an aspect of sexual function)
• secondary (associated with other symptoms such as spasticity)
• tertiary (linked to feelings of sexual attractiveness)

with these differing problems interacting.

Male-specific problems are regarding having and maintaining an erection. Usual treatment is with sildenafil. The longer-acting options of tadalafil or vardenafil may be more acceptable, especially if there is a tertiary component to the dysfunction. Patients who do not respond to these treatments should be referred to a specialist service as there are other options available.

Female-specific problems are regarding lubrication and orgasm, for which no drug treatments are available. Improvements are possible with lubricating agents and increased time given for arousal.

Problems common to both include the following:
• Decreased libido, which sexual counselling may help with.
• Decreased sensation.
• Fatigue affecting sexual function. It may help to include time for intimacy within an overall fatigue management plan.
• Incontinence and continence care should be sensitive to sexual activity.
• Spasticity can be a significant secondary problem. A little well-timed extra antispasticity medication can be effective.
• Positioning.
• Fitting within a care plan, so care plans of patients who require hoisting should be sensitive to sexual activity.

Spasticity and contractures
Spasticity and contractures can cause major problems for people with MS. The same principles apply as for other conditions (for more details, ➔ see Chapter 10).

Speech problems and communication
(➔ See also Chapter 8.)

Dysarthria can lead to problems with communication, and is a spastic or ataxic dysarthria, or a combination of the two. Fatigue, poor breath control, and low respiratory volumes can also have an adverse effect on speech. Measures such as reducing the rate of speech, concentrating on articulation of important words, identifying times of day when less fatigued, and training family and carers as communication partners can help, especially if these methods become habitual, so early referral to a speech and language therapist is important.

Augmentative communication aids, both paper based and electronic, can help in those whose communication does not improve using these initial measures.

Swallowing impairment
Dysphagia affects nutrition, hydration, risk of aspiration pneumonia, and control of saliva, and develops as MS progresses. Details of screening questions for, and management of, dysphagia are given in ➔ Chapter 9, with the principles being the same in MS.

Tremor and cerebellar dysfunction
Cerebellar involvement is common and difficult to treat, with little convincing evidence of a reliable improvement using any treatment. Table 29.3 shows the impairments that can occur.

Table 29.3 Terminology and impairments associated with cerebellar ataxia

Term	Description
Ataxic gait	A gait with a wide base and poor balance that includes the other disorders of movement described in this table
Cerebellar dysarthria	Equal and excessive stress placed on syllables (sometimes called 'scanning'), accompanied by slurring of speech
Dysdiadochokinesia	Difficulty in performing rapid alternating movements with effects on rhythm and force
Dysmetria	Inability to accurately reach the intended end position of a movement, either undershooting (hypometria) or overshooting (hypermetria) due to incoordination of force and rate of movement
Dysrhythmia	An incoordinated rhythm of movement due to cerebellar dysfunction
Dyssynergia	Contractions of different muscle groups in an action not occurring in a coordinated way, such as not in the correct sequence or with agonists and antagonists contracting at the same time
Intention tremor	A low-frequency tremor occurring with and worsening towards the end of movement
Postural tremor	A tremor occurring while trying to maintain posture in trunk or limb
Titubation	A tremor affecting the head leading to a 'nodding' action

Adaptive equipment that may help includes:
- large-handled implements
- plate guards
- Velcro® fastenings for buttons and shoelaces
- electric toothbrushes
- electric page turners
- powered mobile arm supports.

Stabilizing the trunk can assist in reducing ataxia, either using appropriate seating or Lycra® garments. Other physical approaches such as use of weight wrist bands to dampen the movements, visual and verbal cues when walking, biofeedback, and altering the pattern of movement may help.

Specific drugs are sometimes used but with very limited success, including:
- isoniazid (given with pyridoxine)
- cannabinoids
- benzodiazepines.

Surgical treatment is sometimes used, but there is uncertainty over the long-term benefits. Deep brain stimulation of the ventralis intermedius (VIM) thalamic nucleus and thalamotomy are both used, with the former being the least invasive option.

Use of upper limbs

The same combination of impairments found in problems with mobility contributes to problems with UL function. Use of adaptations and equipment is the main method by which a person can optimize their abilities, but there is also evidence that training, again using various modalities as for mobility, can improve function. There is emerging evidence that fampridine PR also improves UL function.

Ataxia can sometimes be relatively more problematic with regard to UL function. Equipment that can help includes mobile arm supports, Lycra® garments and weighted wrist bands. There is a lot of variation as to how effective these are but they provide various treatment options for individual patients.

Visual impairment

Optic neuritis is one of the main presenting symptoms of MS and will often respond well to corticosteroid therapy. However, there are a range of other problems including:

- residual scotomas
- diplopia
- oscillopsia
- colour vision
- binocular vision
- motion perception (Pulfrich phenomenon)
- intermittent visual impairment associated with heat (a sometimes forgotten manifestation of the Uthoff phenomenon)
- low-contrast vision—this has been increasingly recognized in recent years as a cause of visual impairment, not just for reading but for driving and facial recognition.

Many such symptoms are difficult to treat. Stable diplopia can be helped by converging prisms or BoNT therapy. Referral to low-vision clinics can sometimes be necessary and helpful.

Overall impact of impairments on activity and participation

All the previously described impairments progress and interact with activity and participation, secondary complications (Table 29.4), and non-MS aspects of health. In addition, MS usually starts between the ages of 20 and 40 years meaning that roles at work, in education, and in parenting are prominent aspects of participation. Therefore, it is important that rehabilitation is individualized, that an interprofessional approach is used, and that changing needs are reviewed. As with any aspect of rehabilitation, enabling the patient to be an active participant in the rehabilitation process is vital. The multiplicity of problems that can occur in MS means that helping the patient to understand their causes and impact, and weigh up decisions regarding them can be challenging. The impact of MS on communication and cognition requires that information is imparted in a way and with the time that is needed for an individual patient. This will maximize their ability to make decisions and assist them and significant others to understand as much as possible, if they have lost the capacity to make specific decisions.

The unpredictability of MS is a further challenge to the person's emotional and psychological approaches to the condition and to the ability of healthcare professionals to work with the person with MS to optimize their participation.

In addition to health-related complications, the effects on activity and participation have a social impact. In common with many other disabling conditions, having MS has a negative effect on finances due to decreasing income and increasing outgoings. It has an effect on employment, maintaining relationships, and inclusion in leisure activities.

Table 29.4 Important secondary health complications in MS and non-pharmacological factors that can be modified to decrease or increase risk of complication

Secondary complication	Factors influencing complication
Constipation	Mobility, nutrition, hydration, bladder and bowel management
Contractures	Mobility, stretches, seating, pain, spasticity
Obesity	Mobility, loss of muscle mass, mood, nutrition
Osteoporosis and fractures	Mobility, nutrition, time spent indoors, genetics
Pressure sores	Spasticity, sensation, mobility, incontinence, nutrition, hydration, seating, mattress
Respiratory tract infections	Respiratory management, nutrition, oral hygiene, posture, bowel management, mobility
Urinary tract infections and urosepsis	Bladder and bowel management, hydration, mobility, UL and trunk function
Venous thromboembolism	Mobility, dependent oedema

MS affects those involved with the individual. In a consultation with a person with MS it is important to consider significant others, particularly if they are adopting a caring role. Ways in which this can be done include the following:

- Gaining permission of the person with MS to include the significant other in the consultation.
- Informing both of sources of help—practical such as care and equipment, and supportive such as carer organizations and support groups.
- Including discussion of and planning about respite as part of rehabilitation management.
- It is important not to get drawn into aspects of the carer's health, but where this is a concern they can be advised to seek help themselves.

References

1. Scolding N, Barnes D, Cader S, et al. (2015). Association of British Neurologists: revised (2015) guidelines for prescribing disease-modifying treatments in multiple sclerosis. *Pract Neurol* 15, 273–279.
2. Kister I, Bacon TE, Chamot E, et al. (2013). Natural history of MS symptoms. *International Journal of MS Care* 15, 146–158.
3. Jones KH. A large scale study of anxiety and depression in people with multiple sclrosis. *PLoS One* 7, e41910.
4. Foley PL, Vesterinen I IM, Laird BJ, et al. (2013). Prevalence and natural history of pain in adults with multiple sclerosis: systematic review and meta-analysis. *Pain* 154, 632–642.

Further reading

Feinstein A, Freeman J, Lo AC (2015). Treatment of progressive multiple sclerosis: what works, what does not and what is needed. *Lancet Neurology* 14, 194–207.

Rieckmann P, Boyko A, Centonze D, et al. (2015). Achieving patient engagement in multiple sclerosis: a perspective from the multiple sclerosis in the 21st Century Steering Group. *Multiple Sclerosis and Related Disorders* 4, 202–218.

Support groups

MS Australia: ℘ https://www.msaustralia.org.au/.
MS Society of New Zealand: ℘ https://www.msnz.org.nz.
MS Society: ℘ https://mssociety.org.uk/.
MS Trust: ℘ https://www.mstrust.org.uk/.

Cerebral palsy

Background

This chapter concerns rehabilitation for adults with cerebral palsy (CP). It will begin with aspects of CP in childhood as the definition, aetiology, and classification of CP are all based on its origins preterm or in infancy.

The current definition of cerebral palsy, derived from an international workshop in 2004, is: 'a group of permanent disorders of the development of movement and posture, causing activity limitation, that are attributed to non-progressive disturbances that occurred in the developing foetal or infant brain. The motor disorders of cerebral palsy are often accompanied by disturbances of sensation, perception, cognition, communication and behavior, by epilepsy and by secondary musculoskeletal problems.'[1] This definition has developed as knowledge has grown regarding the importance of factors other than those affecting movement and posture, the aetiology of CP, and recognition of the initial similarity of some progressive conditions that mimic CP.

Information about epidemiology comes from national registers, such as the Surveillance of Cerebral Palsy in Europe (SCPE) database, the CP Register in Australia and New Zealand, and the Canadian Cerebral Palsy Registry. The prevalence of CP is about 2 per 1000 live births, with some evidence that it is reducing. In the Australian cohort, the prevalence in pre- and perinatal CP, accounting for approximately 95% of CP, was decreasing between 1993 and 2006 (the latest years analysed). The SCPE database showed a fall from 1.9–1.77 live births between 1980 and 2003, most marked in the very low birthweight cohort. These registers are based in high-income countries, and prevalence in low- and middle-income countries is uncertain.

Risk factors for CP are those that will affect the developing brain. Examples of risk factors are shown in Box 30.1 and a diagram of how these relate to preterm brain development is shown in Fig. 30.1.[2] There may also be a genetic component and some children with CP will have no risk factors. There is a slightly higher proportion of males with CP than in the non-CP population.

> **Box 30.1 Risk factors for cerebral palsy**
> - Pre-and post-term birth, multiple births, and low birthweight
> - Infections preterm and in infancy
> - Birth asphyxia
> - Congenital abnormalities
> - Fetal growth restriction
> - Untreated maternal hypothyroidism
> - Perinatal stroke

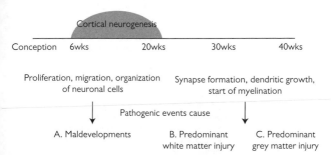

Fig. 30.1 Pathogenic patterns seen on brain MRI in relation to timing of insult during brain development.

Reproduced with permission from Himmelmann K. et al. MRI classification system (MRICS) for children with cerebral palsy: development, reliability, and recommendations. *Developmental Medicine & Child Neurology*, 59(1):57–64. Copyright © 2016, John Wiley and Sons. https://doi.org/10.1111/dmcn.13166.

Classification

There are various classifications for CP, probably because of the different factors included in its definition and the different causes. The classification system summarized in Table 30.1 is derived from the working party that proposed the CP definition given in the ⊃ 'Background' section and from the SCPE classification.

Motor function in cerebral palsy is usually described by the Gross Motor Function Classification System (GMFCS) (Table 30.2).

The GMFCS was originally developed for young children, in whom it has been shown to be a good predictor of functional physical ability, and has been modified to be applied to various ages up to 18 years. Studies have shown the level remains stable into early adulthood, but longer-term follow-up studies show a deterioration in levels as middle adult life is reached. More detailed information can be found at the CanChild GMFCS page (⊃ see 'Further reading'). Reading the descriptors, it is easy to see how an adult may change category, especially from level II to III, as muscle strength decreases with age, osteoarthritis develops, and weight increases.

Table 30.1 Classification of cerebral palsy

Components of CP classification	Description
Nature and typology of the motor disorder	• Spastic (hypertonia with hyperreflexia) • Ataxic (lack of coordination) • Dyskinetic: dystonic or choreoathetotic (involuntary movements) • Non-classifiable
Functional motor abilities	Extent to which motor function is limited, can use scales validated for CP to describe this (e.g. GMFCS; Table 30.2)
Anatomical distribution	Impairments in trunk, each limb and oropharynx should be described. The terms 'diplegia' and 'quadriplegia' are discouraged due to ambiguity
Neuroimaging results	Divided into five categories[2] (Fig. 30.1): • Maldevelopments • Predominant white matter injury • Predominant grey matter injury • Miscellaneous (e.g. cerebral or cerebellar atrophy, calcifications) • Normal
Causation and timing	The cause should be stated if known Timing of the event that caused CP should only be given if there is good evidence that a definite cause of CP occurred at that specific time In order to be classified as CP the causative event must have occurred before the affected function has developed

Table 30.2 GMFCS classification system, descriptors for age 12–18 years

Level	Descriptor
I	Walks without limitations, can also run, jump, etc. Balance and coordination can be limited
II	Walks with limitations. Environmental factors, (e.g. uneven surfaces, steps) influence walking; may use handrails on steps/stairs; may use wheeled mobility for longer distances
III	Walks using a handheld mobility device. Environment affects mobility more than in levels I and II. Sit to stand, floor to stand requires assistive device or other person; uses a wheelchair, manual or powered, at school and in community; may be able to walk up and downstairs using a hand rail
IV	Self-mobility with limitations; may use powered mobility. Uses wheeled mobility in most settings, and requires adaptive seating to control trunk and pelvis. Can perform standing transfers, possibly with assistance; may walk short distances indoors
V	Transported in a manual wheelchair. No mobility without using a wheelchair; limited ability to maintain head, neck, and trunk alignment or control movement of limbs. Assistive technology helps but does not fully compensate for impairments. May be able to control a powered wheelchair unaided if it is adapted

The Manual Ability Classification System (MACS) is an ordinal scale of hand function and can be used alongside the GMFCS. It is of a similar format to the GMFCS and was also validated in children. ➜ See 'Further reading' for the website concerning this scale.

Transition to adulthood

Adolescence is a time of great change for any person as they develop an autonomous existence and learn to take responsibility for various aspects of life. Having a disability such as CP brings additional challenges. Table 30.3 shows the developmental tasks occurring during transition to adulthood and how those can be further affected by the physical and cognitive impairments associated with CP.

Transition does not just affect the young person but also affects their family, particularly parents who are still helping in ways that are not traditionally expected for a young adult, such as assisting with dressing and hygiene. The process of transition takes place across all the systems that a young person is involved with: their family, friends, education, social care and healthcare. It is well recognized that a smooth transition is difficult to achieve, with several documents and recommendations having been written on transition for those with physical disabilities, including CP.

The common features of current best practice recommendations include:
- involvement of the young person
- early planning, from at least the age of 14
- individualized planning
- involvement of key stakeholders in health, social, and education systems and coordination between them
- use of a transition record held by the young person
- using a key worker or case manager
- availability of adult services for the young person to transition into
- training for those involved in the young person's care
- understanding of changing needs.

The impairments described in the following section, concerning adults, are relevant to adolescents with CP, but there are some important aspects during adolescence that are worth emphasizing. There is often a combination of needs that had been met under paediatric services and newer ones that will continue to be relevant throughout adulthood. It is important that healthcare services for adults understand this combination of needs, some of which will be different from those usually met by adult services. The young person may not see the importance of health maintenance and may rebel against some aspects of healthcare. Important physical aspects in a state of flux in adolescence include the following:
- Screening for hip dislocation. This is recommended up until the young person reaches skeletal maturity for GMFCS levels III and IV.[3] This should occur every 6 months for GMFCS IV if there is pelvic obliquity or scoliosis, otherwise it is every 12 months. Any young person with CP who develops new hip pain or worsening scoliosis or pelvic obliquity should also be screened. Screening is by migration percentage on hip X-ray.

Table 30.3 Developmental tasks during adolescence in relation to CP

Tasks	Further challenges for young person with CP
Ability to look after own health	More healthcare needs compared with others
	Extra time investment required for preventative healthcare needs, e.g. physical activity
	Accepting role of managing healthcare needs from parents
	May not know the details of their condition
	May have less opportunity to adapt to new challenges to health, such as alcohol and drugs
Ability to look after personal ADLs and domestic affairs independently	Further learning, aids, and adaptations needed to carry out such tasks
	May require at least one other person to assist with care needs
Ability to look after financial affairs independently	Extra financial demands
	Navigation of the benefits system
	Role as employer in some benefit systems (e.g. direct payment system in UK and the NDIS in Australia)
Consolidation of identity and emotional separation from parents	Developing an independent identity can be difficult if having to depend on others, often parents, for practical help and companionship
	Will be alone less often and thus have less opportunity to manage situations alone
	May adversely compare themselves with siblings who do not have CP
Development of social and intimate relationships	May have less opportunity to meet others outside of family, e.g. due to mobility needs or access issues
	Dependence in personal ADLs may dissuade young person from socializing with peers
	Disabilities may affect sexual relationships
Development of abstract thinking, beliefs, and ideology	May have less opportunity to explore ideas with peers
	May think about health condition and its impact differently from when a child
Discerning vocation in life	May have reduced expectations
	Lack of role models
	Physical and intellectual limiting factors
	Practicalities regarding higher education, work placements, apprenticeships, parenting, etc.

- Avoidance of increasing obesity and adipose tissue deposition. Eating and exercise habits are developing at this age, and there is often a preference for nutritionally poor food. Obesity can develop, but with less impact on health and well-being than in older age groups, so the need to avoid it is less obvious to the young person.
- Possible instability of seizure control. This can occur for several reasons: as body weight increases to that of adulthood, the dose of anticonvulsants (antiepileptic drugs (AEDs)) needed increases; seizures can vary in frequency according to the menstrual cycle; sleep can be more irregular; recreational drugs and alcohol may be used for the first time; and the young person may be reluctant to take prescribed medication. In addition, the potential teratogenic effects of AEDs and interference with oral contraceptives become important for young women.
- Continuing exercises, stretches, and wearing of splints. These all rely on habitual activities which can be difficult to maintain during the environmental, behavioural, cognitive, and psychological changes of adolescence and young adult life.

Important aspects of cerebral palsy in adults

The dominant issues affecting health for an adult with CP are understandably different from those during childhood. Factors that affect this include the following:

- Adulthood covers a long period of time, with many transitions other than that from childhood, such as into employment, living away from parents, into married life, and into old age.
- Peak muscle and bone mass occur in the mid 20s. It is likely that these are lower in the CP population, with consequences for earlier onset of sarcopenia and osteoporosis.
- The long-term effects of abnormal forces affecting joints can lead to earlier onset of degenerative joint disease.
- The long term metabolic effects of both reduced physical activity and time spent in sedentary behaviour will have secondary health consequences. The amount of time spent in physical activity and sedentary behaviour is illustrated by Fig. 30.2.[4]

The following impairments, activities, and aspects of participation may be relevant in an adult with CP (➲ see the chapters in Section 1 for more detail on management):

- *Cervical myelopathy*. The risk of this is increased in athetoid CP.
- *Cognitive function*. Between 40% and 60% of children with CP have an associated intellectual disability. When they reach adulthood, this may lead to ongoing effects on participation and autonomy.
- *Dysphagia*. Some adults with CP will have had gastrostomy insertion as a child, requiring long-term follow-up. New dysphagia should not occur as an adult, and is likely to be due to another co-morbidity.
- *Epilepsy*. Data from the SCPE register suggests that about 35% of children with CP have epilepsy, with a greater likelihood in those with intellectual disability. Childhood epilepsy can stabilize, and some children can be weaned from AEDs, so the adult prevalence is less, for example, a recent survey of adults with CP found 28.7% were taking AEDs.[5] Epilepsy affects aspects such as employment, driving, exercise, pregnancy, and child rearing.
- *Fatigue*. Fatigue is a common issue for adults with CP, with a higher prevalence than the general population. It is associated with greater BMI and less physical activity. It has been shown to respond to rehabilitation programmes that include physical activity.
- *Gastro-oesophageal reflux*. This is common in children with CP, and many of the precipitating factors will remain in adulthood, in addition to possible new factors such as obesity and reduced mobility.
- *Mobility*. There is a high risk of mobility deteriorating during adult life (Fig. 30.3),[6] being associated with bilateral motor impairment, older age, initially worse gait, pain, and fatigue. Evidence is emerging that increasing physical activity and decreasing sedentary activities can assist in maintaining mobility.
- *Pain*. Pain, mostly of a musculoskeletal nature, affects 60–80% of adults with CP, and interacts with fatigue and depression.

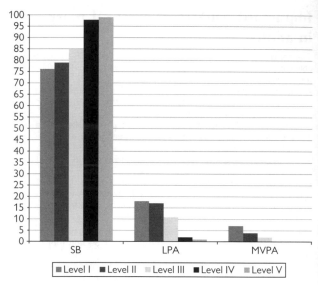

Fig. 30.2 Percentage of time spent in physical activities across all GMFCS levels. LPA, light physical activity; MVPA, moderate to vigorous physical activity; SB, sedentary behaviour.

Reproduced with permission from Verschuren O. et al. Exercise and physical activity recommendations for people with cerebral palsy. *Developmental Medicine & Child Neurology*, 58(8): 798–808. Copyright © 2016, John Wiley and Sons. https://doi.org/10.1111/dmcn.13053.

- *Respiratory function*. This does not deteriorate, but will be compromised by factors such as kyphoscoliosis, dysphagia, and gastro-oesophageal reflux.
- *Relationships*. There is a later development of intimate relationships by people with CP and fewer in a relationship compared with peers without CP.
- *Speech and communication*. These can remain significant issues during adult life, having an impact on many areas of life, such as relationships, employment, and education.
- *Spasticity*. Problems associated with spasticity persist or increase into adult life. Secondary complications, such as secondary musculotendinous changes and contractures, become relatively more prominent.
- *Visual impairment*. This is common in children with CP, and will affect needs in adult life.
- *Work*. Training for, finding work, and staying in work will present difficulties for adults with CP. There is evidence from vocational rehabilitation programmes for young physically disabled people that targeted vocational rehabilitation can improve employment rates.

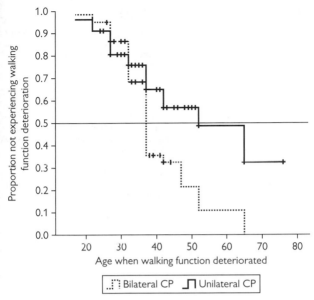

Fig. 30.3 Kaplan–Meier survival curve of the proportion of adults with CP not experiencing a deterioration in walking.

Reproduced with permission from Opheim A. et al. Walking function, pain, and fatigue in adults with cerebral palsy: a 7-year follow-up study. *Developmental Medicine & Child Neurology*, 51(5):381–8. Copyright © 2009, John Wiley and Sons. https://doi.org/10.1111/j.1469-8749.2008.03250.x.

Overall, many of these factors combine to affect general health. Hospital admissions are higher than the population without CP—in one study, 19.3% of a young adult population with CP were hospitalized over a 4-year period,[7] with the two commonest reasons being pneumonia and epilepsy.

Rehabilitation programmes

There have been several trials of single discipline and multidisciplinary rehabilitation interventions aiming to increase activity and participation. Specific interventions that have shown effect in improving mobility[8] include:

- gait training with rhythmic auditory stimulus
- treadmill training
- BoNT and physiotherapy
- LL strengthening exercises.

Physical activity is recommended for adults with CP based on current literature and expert opinion[9] with the purpose of improving health and cardiovascular fitness (Table 30.4). An important aspect of these guidelines is to aim for both increasing physical activity and reducing sedentary behaviour.

Although there has been limited research on multidisciplinary rehabilitation interventions for adults with CP, from the results of individual research programmes and expert recommendations it is likely that programmes that promote physical activity and understanding of the condition are beneficial. An example of a multidisciplinary programme is that explored by the 'LEARN 2 MOVE 16–24' study in the Netherlands.[10] This consisted of a supervised physical fitness training at home designed to improve both cardiorespiratory fitness and strength. The programme lasts 3 months with a motivational interviewing-based approach (with regard to physical activity) and counselling (with regard to sports participation that included identifying suitable local sports facilities), both over a 6-month period. The programme has shown benefits for aerobic conditioning, waist circumference, blood pressure, fatigue, pain, and social support.

Table 30.4 Recommendations for exercise and physical activity prescription for people with cerebral palsy

Exercise—cardiorespiratory (aerobic)	
Frequency	Start with 1–2 sessions/week, gradually progress to 3/week
Intensity	>60% peak HR, or >40% of HR reserve, or 46–90% VO_{2peak}
Time	>20 min per session, for at least 8–16 consecutive weeks, depending on frequency (2 or 3 times/week)
Type	Regular, purposeful exercise that involves major muscle groups and is continuous and rhythmic in nature
Exercise—resistance	
Frequency	2–4 times/week on non-consecutive days
Intensity	1–3 sets of 6–15 reps of 50–85% repetition maximum
Time	Training period for at least 12–16 consecutive weeks
Type	Progression in mode from primarily single joint, machine-based resistance exercises to machine plus free-weight, multijoint (and closed kinetic chain) resistance exercises. Single-joint resistance training may be more effective for very weak muscles, or for those who tend to compensate when performing multijoint exercises, or at the beginning of training
Daily physical activity—moderate to vigorous	
Frequency	≥5 days/week
Intensity	Moderate to vigorous physical activity
Time	60 min
Type	A variety of activities
Daily physical activity—sedentary	
Frequency	7 days/week
Intensity	Sedentary (<1.5 METs)
Time	<2 h/day, or break up sitting for 2 min every 30–60 min
Type	Non-occupational, leisure-time sedentary activities, e.g. watching TV, using computer, playing video games

HR, heart rate; METS, metabolic equivalents.

Reproduced with permission from Van der Slot W.M.A et al. Chronic pain, fatigue, and depressive symptoms in adults with spastic bilateral cerebral palsy. *Developmental Medicine & Child Neurology*, 54(9):836–42. Copyright © 2012, John Wiley and Sons. https://doi.org/10.1111/j.1469-8749.2012.04371.x.

References

1. Rosenbaum P, Paneth N, Leviton A, et al. A report: the definition and classification of cerebral palsy April 2006. *Developmental Medicine and Child Neurology Supplement* 1, 8–14.
2. Himmelmann K, Horber V, De La Cruz J, et al. (2017). MRI classification system (MRICS) for children with cerebral palsy: development, reliability, and recommendations. *Developmental Medicine & Child Neurology* 59, 57–64.
3. Wynter M, Gibson N, Kentish M, et al. (2011). Consensus Statement on Hip Surveillance for Children with Cerebral Palsy: Australian Standards of Care. *Journal of Pediatric Rehabilitation Medicine* 4, 183–195.
4. Verschuren O, Peterson MD, Balemans AC, et al. (2016). Exercise and physical activity recommendations for people with cerebral palsy. *Developmental Medicine & Child Neurology* 58, 798–808.
5. Pons C, Brochard S, Gallien P, et al. (2017). Medication, rehabilitation and health care consumption in adults with cerebral palsy: a population based study. *Clinical Rehabilitation* 31, 957–965.
6. Opheim A, Jahnsen R, Olsson E, et al. (2009). Walking function, pain, and fatigue in adults with cerebral palsy: a 7-year follow-up study. *Developmental Medicine & Child Neurology* 51, 381–388.
7. Young NL, McCormick AM, Gilbert T, et al. (2011). Reasons for hospital admissions among youth and young adults with cerebral palsy. *Archives of Physical Medicine and Rehabilitation* 92, 46–50.
8. Morgan P, Dobson FL, McGinley JL (2014). A systematic review of the efficacy of conservative interventions on the gait of ambulant adults with cerebral palsy. *Journal of Developmental and Physical Disabilities* 26, 633–654.
9. Verschuren O, Peterson MD, Balemans AC, et al. (2016). Exercise and physical activity recommendations for people with cerebral palsy. *Developmental Medicine & Child Neurology* 58, 798–808.
10. Slaman J, Roebroeck ME, van Meeteren J, et al. (2010). Learn 2 Move 16–24: effectiveness of an intervention to stimulate physical activity and improve physical fitness of adolescents and young adults with spastic cerebral palsy; a randomized controlled trial. *BMC Pediatrics* 10, 79.

Further reading

Useful websites

CanChild website, McMaster University: ✍ https://www.canchild.ca/en/resources/42-gross-motor-function-classification-system-expanded-revised-gmfcs-e-r—gross motor classification system, expanded and revised.
Manual Ability Classification System: ✍ http://www.macs.nu/download-content.php.

Neurodegenerative conditions

Introduction

The neurodegenerative conditions (NDGCs) encompass a wide variety of neurological conditions, with varying signs, symptoms, age of onset, prognoses, and underlying pathologies. However, they share a number of challenging features:

- Progressive accumulation of disability.
- Progressive dependence.
- The majority do not have treatments that will affect progression.
- They can induce feelings of nihilism in healthcare professionals.

Many people with NDGCs will have read extensively about the conditions and possible treatments. They will have been living with the uncertainty and concern about the future that such conditions bring, and, in those which are hereditary, may have had experience of family members affected by the condition.

Rehabilitative approaches can offer a great deal to people with NDGCs. While there may be no 'magic bullet', the rehabilitation ethos of promoting autonomy and maximizing participation can make huge differences to the way people adapt to their diagnosis, manage their symptoms, and continue to lead a full, minimally dependent, and rewarding life for as long as possible, while making informed preparations for the future.

The NDGCs can be divided into early, middle, and late stages, with varying needs at each. Typically, in the early stages, patients are fairly independent; in the middle stage, some assistance may be needed for ADLs; in the later stages, the patient is dependent for many aspects of care, with or without cognitive impairment.

The aims of this chapter are to describe the essentials of some of the more frequent NDGCs that are not covered elsewhere in this book, to indicate symptoms that are common features, and to provide an overview of some of the strategies that may be useful. The individual conditions are not described in depth; a textbook of neurology is recommended for this. Naturally, some of the areas outlined will be more relevant to some conditions than others (e.g. genetic testing in the setting of Huntington's disease (HD), and non-invasive ventilation in the setting of motor neuron disease (MND)). Some of the other NDGCs are dealt with separately in their own chapters (e.g. MS and certain of the neuromuscular conditions).

Parkinson's disease

- Parkinson's disease (PD) affects 0.15% of the population but is more frequent with age, affecting 1% over the age of 65 years; average age of onset is the mid 50s (15% present before the age of 45 years). Average duration is 15 years.
- First described by James Parkinson in 1817.
- Increased risk in non-smokers; slight male predominance.
- Classical clinical triad:
  - Bradykinesia
  - Rigidity
  - Tremor (low frequency, 4–7 Hz, 'pill-rolling').
- Onset usually asymmetrical.
- Up to one-fifth of patients may not have tremor.
- Around 40% have cognitive problems, dementia increases in frequency over time; around 40% also have peripheral polyneuropathy.
- Hypo/anosmia may precede diagnosis.
- GI and bladder symptoms common.
- Underlying pathology—degeneration of dopamine containing neurons in the substantia nigra and Lewy body α-synuclein aggregates.
- Clinical diagnosis; imaging may help to rule out alternative diagnoses.
- Mainstay of treatment is augmenting or replacing dopamine—patients will often respond to levodopa for two decades but it may become increasingly difficult to control motor fluctuations (e.g. on/off phenomena; peak dose dyskinesias—seen in nearly half at 5 years).
- Anticholinergics can help with tremor but lots of side effects, especially in elderly people.
- Postural hypotension and instability, sleep disorders can be disabling.
- Dopamine agonists/replacement are also associated with impulsive and compulsive behaviour as well as 'punding'—repetitive, stereotyped behaviours or 'compulsive hobbyism', all of which can be socially disabling.
- Surgical treatment (including pallidotomy or deep brain stimulation) may be useful in selected cases.

Parkinsonian syndromes

In approximately 80% of cases Parkinsonism is caused by PD. However, Parkinsonian signs and symptoms may be seen following insults to the basal ganglia. Causes can include drugs (including amiodarone and lithium), diffuse subcortical white matter ischaemia, traumatic brain injury, normal pressure hydrocephalus, and Hallervorden–Spatz syndrome. Some of these may respond to dopamine therapy.

The 'Parkinson's plus' syndromes are more characteristically neurodegenerative. Both have similar age of onset to PD, lower prevalence rates (<0.004%), and shorter duration (8–10 years).

Progressive supranuclear palsy

(Also known as Steele–Richardson syndrome.)
- Clinical features:
  - Parkinsonian
  - Akinesis, rigidity
  - Downgaze impairment
  - Frontal lobe dementia
  - High falls risk (particularly falling backwards early in disease course).
- Pathology of neurofibrillary tangles with frontal cortical involvement.
- Poor response to levodopa.
- More symmetrical than idiopathic PD.

Multisystem atrophy

- Clinical features:
  - Parkinsonian
  - Autonomic disturbance
  - Cerebellar signs
  - Bulbar and pyramidal involvement.
- Widespread neuronal degeneration in brain and spinal cord with neuronal inclusions.
- Up to 50% may show some response to levodopa.
- Cognitive impairment not usually a feature (unlike progressive supranuclear palsy).

Huntington's disease

- Affects 0.005% of the population, with average age of onset between 25 and 45 years (i.e. often after reproduction). Average duration is 17 years.
- Clinical features include movement disorders (choreiform classically but also dystonias), cognitive impairment, and psychiatric manifestations.
- Depression in over half; may precede other symptoms as part of a prodromal phase.
- Underlying mutation is a highly penetrant trinucleotide repeat disorder on chromosome 4 which is inherited in an autosomal dominant fashion, resulting in neuronal degeneration and death.
- Around 30–35 repeats may be unstable; 40 repeats or more cause clinical disease.
- Earlier onset and more rapid progression tend to be associated with higher triplet repeat number.
- Neuroimaging may show caudate nucleus atrophy.
- Treatment is symptomatic only.
- Juvenile phenotype (approximately 5%) onset at less than 21 years.

Friedreich's ataxia

- Affects 0.002% of the population; average age of onset less than 20 years; approximately 25 years of disease duration.
- Degeneration of dorsal root ganglia, spinocerebellar tracts, corticospinal tracts, and cerebellar Purkinje cells.
- Ambulation lost 10–15 years after onset.
- Clinical features include cerebellar and pyramidal signs with peripheral neuropathy (absent ankle jerks and upgoing plantars) and cardiomyopathy.
- Associated skeletal abnormalities (pes cavus, scoliosis).
- Dorsal column involvement—loss of vibration sense/proprioception.
- Optic atrophy and abnormal eye movements; deafness.
- Trinucleotide repeat expansion in the Frataxin gene (small percentage have point mutation).
- Autosomal dominant inheritance.
- No treatments available.
- About 90% have abnormalities on ECG; 50% on echocardiography; cause of death usually cardiac.
- About 20% have diabetes mellitus.

Motor neuron disease

- Affects 0.005% of the population with average age of onset in mid 50s and average disease duration of 3–5 years.
- About 10% have onset at less than 40 years of age.
- Majority are sporadic; less than 10% are inherited.
- Progressive degeneration of lower and UMNs in spinal cord, cranial nerve nuclei, and cortex.
- Different subtypes:
  - Amyotrophic lateral sclerosis—most common (70%); UMN and LMN signs.
  - Progressive bulbar palsy—10–20% of cases, starts with speech/swallowing problems; may progress to involve limbs (worst prognosis).
  - Progressive muscular atrophy—10% of cases, LMN signs in limbs, often followed by bulbar involvement.
  - Primary lateral sclerosis—least common, UMN signs in limbs, longest survival (up to 20 years).
- About 5% also have signs of frontotemporal dementia.
- Due to loss of motor neurons in anterior horn cells; majority are acquired but a small amount (<10%) are familial.
- Signs include muscle weakness, wasting, fasciculations, and bulbar involvement.
- Typically asymmetrical, insidious, and focal onset.
- Diagnosis is clinical—neurophysiology can support; neuroimaging can exclude myelopathy/radiculopathy.
- Progressive tongue wasting and fasciculation almost pathognomonic.
- Most common cause of death is ventilatory failure.
- Riluzole may prolong life expectancy by a few months (side effects include nausea, GI upset, and deranged liver function tests; need monitoring). Supportive care (NIV, PEG feeding) may also be life-prolonging.
- Multidisciplinary rehabilitation approaches are vital in a rapidly evolving condition to maximize function and participation.
- Differentials include degenerative cervical spine disease (UMN signs from myelopathy; LMN signs from radiculopathy).

Dementia

Dementia of any type causes a progressive cognitive loss and thus increasing dependence on others. It is increasing in prevalence, primarily because of the ageing population (Fig. 31.1).

The four main types of dementia are as follows:

- *Alzheimer's dementia*. This affects about 0.7% of the population aged over 60 years. The pathology includes amyloid plaques and intraneuronal tangles associated with cortical atrophy. The dominant clinical feature is memory loss, and there are also language, visuospatial, praxis, and neuropsychiatric disturbances.
- *Vascular dementia*. This affects about 0.2% of the population over 60 years. It is associated with other conditions linked with vascular disease such as hypertension, diabetes mellitus, smoking, and hyperlipidaemia. There are multiple small white matter infarcts, especially in cortical and subcortical regions. Progression tends to be stepwise and there may be associated pyramidal signs.

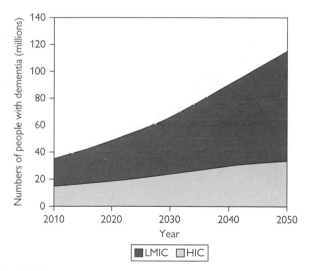

Fig. 31.1 The growth in numbers of people with dementia in high-income countries (HIC) and low- to moderate-income countries (LMIC).

Reproduced with permission from Prince M. et al. The global prevalence of dementia: a systematic review and meta-analysis. *Alzheimer's & Dementia*, 9(1): 63–75. Copyright © 2013 The Alzheimer's Association. Published by Elsevier B.V. All rights reserved. https://doi.org/10.1016/j.jalz.2012.11.007.

- *Dementia with Lewy bodies.* This also affects about 0.2% of the
population over 60 years. It is associated with accumulation of the
α-synuclein protein in Lewy bodies within cortical neurons. There is
an overlap with PD, and about 80% of people with PD will eventually
develop a Lewy body-like dementia. Features include Parkinsonism, a
fluctuating mental state, executive dysfunction, visuospatial impairment,
visual hallucinations, REM sleep behaviour disorder, and autonomic
dysfunction. Importantly, people with Lewy body dementia are very
sensitive to antipsychotics and develop adverse effects easily. They
may also develop side effects such as visual hallucinations easily from
dopaminergic drugs.
- *Frontotemporal dementia.* This affects about 0.1% of the population over
65 years. It is associated with several conditions, including MND and
corticobasal degeneration. There is an accumulation of tau protein,
and atrophy of the frontal and temporal lobes. There are three broad
types of onset which merge as the condition progresses. These are
behavioural (disinhibition, apathy, food cravings, repetitive behaviours,
dysexecutive problems), semantic, or a progressive non-fluent aphasia.

Disease-modifying drugs
Anticholinesterase inhibitors have been shown to be efficacious in Lewy
body and Alzheimer's dementia.

Traumatic brain injury and dementia
There is increasing evidence that not only repeated trauma (e.g. 'dementia pugilistica') but even single episodes of brain injury may have
neurodegenerative consequences, causing a chronic traumatic encephalopathy. The public health implications of this are not insignificant.

Treatment approaches

Multidisciplinary working

Many different individuals (Table 31.1) are likely to be involved in the care of a person with an NDGC. Where available, case managers are valuable in enabling coordinated delivery of multiple services which can otherwise be overwhelming for patients and family.

Treatment essentials

Aim to maximize independence and QOL throughout disease, so frequent reassessment with or without alteration of input may be required.

Treatment can be:

- preventative, for example, good seating (skin integrity)/influenza vaccination/physical therapy to minimize deterioration or atrophy and maximize lung function; advice on energy conservation strategies
- restorative, for example, antibiotics for infection, physiotherapy or BoNT to improve flexibility and reduce spasticity
- compensatory, for example, environmental adaptations/NIV

Rehabilitation encompasses the whole person:

- Physical aspects—regarding tone, strength, balance, coordination, sensation; treatment of intercurrent infections and so on
- Cognitive aspects—memory, awareness, attention, processing, and so on
- Psychological well-being—helping patients optimise this in the context of diagnosis, evolving issues, and prognosis.

Table 31.1 Examples of individuals involved in care of a patient with a neurodegenerative condition

Patient and immediate support network	Medical professionals	Allied health professionals
Patient	Neurologist	PT
Family	Geneticist	OT
Friends	RM physician	Dietician
Carers	Palliative care physician	Orthotist
	Interventional radiologist	Social worker
	Respiratory physician	Care coordinator
	Pain physician	SLT
	Paediatrician	Specialist nurses
	Geriatrician	Respiratory physiologist
	Psychiatrist	Psychologist

OT, occupational therapist; PT, physiotherapist; RM, rehabilitation medicine; SLT, speech and language therapist.

Symptom management

Patients with NDGCs may believe that there is 'nothing to be done' and so avoid mentioning potentially remediable symptoms. Medications should not be used in isolation; holistic care is the aim.

Pain

Multifactorial—muscle cramps, spasticity and contractures, oedema, musculoskeletal, neuropathic, postural, skin sensitivity, difficult transfers, and so on. Early (with or without anticipatory) intervention can avoid significant pain and distress, including review of seating and postural management, as well as medications. ➔ See Chapter 11.

Spasticity

While some spasticity may be useful in the context of weakness (e.g. aiding with transfers), spasticity can be troublesome, painful, and interfere with care. For details, ➔ see Chapter 10.

Weakness and exercise

Weakness leads to specific disabilities which will vary according to the pattern of weakness associated with the neurodegenerative condition, so knowledge regarding individual conditions combined with a detailed history and examination are crucial. Weakness will also be associated with muscle fatigue.

There is increasing evidence in individual conditions that muscle strengthening and aerobic exercise may be beneficial, including PD and Alzheimer's dementia, where cognitive, as well as physical, benefits have been seen. Moderate exercise appears to be of benefit in MND, although overexertion may be detrimental.

Movement disorders

- Chorea (HD)—may not be disabling—can be partially treated by neuroleptics and benzodiazepines.
- Impairment of voluntary movement—often more disabling; in Parkinsonian syndromes can be helped by dopamine agonists/ replacement.
- Rigidity/dystonia—benzodiazepines, baclofen, anti-Parkinsonian medications.
- Myoclonus, tics, epilepsy—clonazepam, antiepileptic medications.

Falls/impaired balance/ataxia

Consider environment (including uneven surfaces, lighting, etc.), medications, vision, sensation, fatigue, insight, and awareness.

Ataxia may be a part of many of the NDGCs and contribute to falls risk, reduced mobility, impaired confidence, and reduced coordination. There is evidence that coordination training and home- or outpatient-based exercise programmes may be of benefit.

Balance and gait have been improved by targeted physiotherapy interventions in patients with HD and degenerative cerebellar disorders.

Respiration

Many individuals with NGDCs will experience a progressive decline in respiratory muscle strength, often alongside a progressive dysphagia, that puts them at risk of atelectasis, pneumonia, and restrictive respiratory failure. Details regarding this are given in ➲ Chapter 17. Management depends on which prophylactic and treatment interventions are required following an assessment of respiratory pathology, balancing these against the patient's wishes regarding interventions and the overall effect on QOL.

Autonomic dysfunction

Orthostatic hypotension is seen most commonly in PD, but can occur in any NDGC with autonomic involvement, including MSA. It can significantly impair mobility and thus participation and is an independent risk factor for mortality. Interventions range from simple (e.g. compression stockings, timing and composition of meals, and medications) to specific medical therapy. Patient education and self-monitoring, where appropriate, may be of benefit.

Speech

Early involvement of speech and language therapists may anticipate problems and help the patient, family, and carers in maximizing communication throughout the course of disease. NDGCs may have different vocal consequences, including dysphasia in the dementias, speech ataxia or apraxia in HD, and hypophonia in PD.

Simple compensatory strategies for the early/mid stages of disease include:
- quiet environment
- time to speak
- choices rather than open-ended questions
- repetition.

Later on, assistive devices can be helpful, ranging from simple (eye gaze/personalized book) to electronic aids with or without voice banking.

Even in later stages of, for example, HD, when verbal output may be greatly reduced, patients' understanding of language may remain.

Swallow/nutrition

Problems common in HD and MND with consequent risks of malnutrition and aspiration (adverse effects on prognosis). Early involvement of speech and language therapy and dietetics is essential, with regular monitoring of weight and nutritional status. Early strategies include attention to positioning (head tilt/chin tuck), timing, and food textures. For further detail regarding swallowing impairment see Chapter 9.

Caloric requirement is often higher in HD (chorea with or without increased metabolic rate). Fatigue in NDGC may make eating harder work, so calorie-dense food is required. Tastes may change, such as wanting dessert first. Discussions regarding PEG/radiologically inserted gastrostomy insertion should take place at an appropriate time (advice in MND is to insert when there is a 5% body weight reduction from time of diagnosis; earlier insertion = less risky; increased risk when forced vital capacity <50%).

It is important to be realistic regarding expectations around tube feeding—families may have inappropriately high expectations regarding prognosis and clinical benefit/improvement.

Sleep

Sleep is often disrupted in NDGC for many reasons, including:

- pain/discomfort
- muscle spasms
- inability to reposition
- mood disturbance
- urinary frequency/urgency
- breathing difficulties (including central/peripheral apnoeas)
- REM sleep parasomnias
- choreas (not always abolished in sleep).

Addressing these symptoms may help sleep quality. Good sleep hygiene is essential; melatonin may be helpful.

Depression and anxiety

It is important to screen for depression and anxiety; ask about suicidal thoughts if depression is identified. Treatment using psychotherapeutic strategies and antidepressants can help.

Fatigue

Extremely common and multifactorial. Advise patient and family/carer regarding pacing and energy conservation techniques.

Cognition

Different NDGCs are associated with different forms and severity of cognitive impairment. Thorough assessment is vital, with regular reassessment as cognition is likely to deteriorate and may affect engagement with rehabilitation or treatment, as well as the ability to make decisions. Initial studies have indicated a benefit of cognitive training ('cognitive rehabilitation') in patients with mild to moderate PD, mild cognitive impairment, and dementia and potential benefits for patients with HD, attenuating or delaying cognitive decline. Further details are in Chapter 7.

Other psychiatric manifestations

Obsessions/compulsions, psychoses, changes in personality and mood with HD and PD.

Behavioural management and psychological support

Many of the NDGCs have behavioural manifestations. They may initially be subtle, such as a person seeming selfish or self-obsessed, but can progress to include aggression, inappropriate behaviour, apathy, and fixation/perseveration. MND is associated with pseudobulbar affect (inappropriate laughing/crying). Recognition and appropriate staff training can help with management and prevent escalation.

NDGCs can be seen as a series of losses; psychological support may help with the continuous adaptation. Psychological distress is not always linked to functional capacity; QOL can be excellent despite physical limitations.

Intercurrent illness and inpatient episodes

Important to consider if new/worsening confusion or other symptoms. Consider drugs (prescription or other), infection, hypoxia, and intracranial bleed if patients are at risk of falling/injury.

Patients with NDGCs are at increased risk of being admitted to hospital for medical, surgical, or psychiatric problems. Hospital admissions come with a whole host of risks. Issues to consider include patients with PD being put on 'nil by mouth' or having finely tailored medication schedules disrupted; patients with reduced mobility being at extra risk of pressure ulcers or respiratory tract infection; and any patients with NDGC being more likely to struggle with deconditioning. Education and support of the patients and their inpatient team may allow risk reduction of in-hospital morbidity and mortality.

Assistive technology

AT and adaptive aids may be invaluable in NDGCs, transforming QOL and enabling participation in activities which would otherwise be impossible. It is important to be aware of the evolving nature of the underlying condition and to ensure that needs are anticipated as best as possible such that equipment is suited to the patient at that particular stage of their illness. ⊃ See Chapter 22 for further details.

Driving

In the UK, patients with NDGC have the responsibility of informing the Driver and Vehicle Licensing Agency of their condition, but can drive as long as they are safe to control the vehicle. Enquiring about driving is an important aspect of rehabilitation assessment. Doctors have a duty to report if the patient does not.

Ethical issues

Capacity to make decisions
➲ See Chapter 7. Disease progression may require reassessment.

Safeguarding and safety
People with physical or mental health needs, disability, incapacity, older age, or those in institutions are, sadly, at particular risk of abuse.

Safety issues to consider include smoking, falls, cooking, transport, and impulsive behaviour. Involve appropriate professionals to assess and discuss.

Alternative and complementary medicines
May be helpful for well-being, for example, aromatherapy, hydrotherapy, acupuncture, music, animal and reminiscence therapy, and so on; however, there are potential risks such as abandonment of conventional therapy, interactions and metabolic effects, and expense.

Genetic testing and insurance
Prenatal genetic testing is available for some genetic conditions. There are ethical issues regarding the testing of family members and the impact on different generations, for example, if caring for a parent and anticipating one's own inevitable deterioration, or testing in grandchildren of an affected patient before the parent who may have passed on the condition is tested or has symptoms.

Guidelines are available for insurance—essentially there is no need to disclose family members' predictive test results but companies can ask about family history, personal medical history, and (under certain conditions) personal predictive genetic tests.

Palliative care

Palliative care is defined as 'an approach that improves the quality of life of patients and their families facing the problem associated with life-threatening illness, through the prevention and relief of suffering by means of early identification and impeccable assessment and treatment of pain and other problems, physical, psychosocial and spiritual'.

End-of-life care is generally taken to refer to the last year of life and includes those with:

- advanced, progressive, incurable conditions
- general frailty and coexisting conditions, expected to die within 12 months
- existing conditions, at risk of dying from an acute crisis in their condition
- life-threatening acute conditions caused by sudden catastrophic events.

The holistic, palliative approach, particularly when implemented early in the course of a life-limiting disease, can make huge improvements to the QOL for a terminally ill person and their loved ones. It can be part of care in the rehabilitation follow-up of patients, or is sometimes specifically performed by palliative care teams.

Palliative care teams, usually have inpatient wards (often hospices), community support, hospital liaison teams, and day therapy. The team is multidisciplinary and includes spiritual leaders and psychological and complementary therapists.

Gold Standards Framework

Various tools have been developed to aid the care of those with life-limiting conditions. One of these in the UK is the Gold Standards Framework (GSF), a tool used by GPs, district nurses, and care homes, alongside other community care providers to *identify* those who are likely to die, *assess and record* their needs, and *plan* for their care. The approach uses the seven 'C's;

1. Communication
2. Coordination of care
3. Control of symptoms and ongoing assessment
4. Continuing support
5. Continued learning
6. Carer and family support
7. Care in the final days.

GSF-accredited practices have been shown to identify patients earlier in the last year of life, increased the number of non-cancer and care home patients on their register, shown significant increases in advanced care planning, greatly improved systematic carer support offered, and resulted in more patients dying in their preferred place of care, with some halving hospital deaths.

'Do not attempt cardio-pulmonary resuscitation' (DNACPR) order

As with every clinical decision, the benefits, burdens, and risks of attempting resuscitation should be considered. If it is felt that resuscitation would not be successful, consideration of the appropriateness of conveying the decision to the patient should be made. In most cases a sensitive discussion should be had, exploring if the patient is willing to talk about resuscitation. Some may find this discussion difficult or pointless. If they are willing to have a discussion about resuscitation the decision for DNACPR should be explained clearly. It is not a choice to be offered to the patient or relative. Consent should be sought to explain the decision to carers and relatives.

If the patient is unwilling or unable to enter DNACPR discussions, the decision should be explained to those closest to the patient.

Advanced care planning

Advanced care planning helps to ensure access to appropriate and timely care according to the patient's wishes. A patient cannot demand treatments, but can specify their preferences. Advanced care planning discussions can include:

- preferences for place and mode of care
- types of treatments they wish to avoid (DNACPR, admissions to hospital, etc.)
- views, values, and beliefs that may influence care
- people they wish to be involved with decisions about care.

Advanced care planning discussions should be recorded (currently this differs between regions). If the patient wishes for their preferences to be formalized, they may want to complete an advance decision to refuse treatment (ADRT) or appoint an attorney for health and welfare.

An ADRT is considered valid if:

- it has been completed by someone over 18 years with capacity
- it is signed
- it is witnessed
- it clearly specifies what is being refused and in what context (e.g. 'I do not want to have IV antibiotics if I have an infection, even if this may result in my death')
- there is no indication of a change of mind since the ADRT was made.

Anticipatory prescribing at the end of life

In order to avoid crises in the last days of life, remain in the preferred place of death and ensure good symptom control, a set of medication to be held in anticipation of end-of-life symptoms has been developed. In the home, this is available via a 'just in case' box. Medications, administered by mouth or injection, should be available to treat pain, nausea, agitation, delirium, seizures, noisy respiratory secretions, and breathlessness. Typical drugs include opiates (typically) morphine, diamorphine or oxycodone, levomepromazine, haloperidol, midazolam, and hyoscine butylbromide or glycopyrronium. Boxes may also include a larger 'crisis' dose of midazolam, rectal diazepam, syringe driver with water for injection, and other drugs as required.

Individualized care planning at the end of life

In the last days of life, care planning needs to be individualized with the dying person at the centre. The Leadership Alliance for the Care of Dying People identified five priorities:

1. The possibility that the person is dying is recognized and communicated clearly, decisions made and actions taken in accordance with the person's needs and wishes, and these are regularly reviewed and decisions revised accordingly.
2. Sensitive communication takes place between staff and the dying person, and those identified as important to them.
3. The dying person, and those identified as important to them, are involved in decisions about treatment and care to the extent that the dying person wants.
4. The needs of families and others identified as important to the dying person are actively explored, respected, and met as far as possible.
5. An individual plan of care, which includes food and drink, symptom control, and psychological, social, and spiritual support, is agreed, coordinated, and delivered with compassion.

Regions and hospitals have end-of-life individualized care plans available for healthcare teams.

Nutrition and hydration at the end of life

Good mouth care, food, and drinks should be given to a person in the last days of life as far as possible. Those close to the patient should be encouraged to participate in this, by giving sips of any fluid (including favourite tipple), mouthfuls of favourite foods, and moistening the mouth with sponges, gels, and sprays.

It is currently unclear if clinically assisted hydration (CAH) (IV or subcutaneous fluids) in the last days of life prolongs life, extends the dying process, or if not giving CAH hastens death. Although CAH is considered by law to be a medical treatment, it is often considered as a necessary aspect of care, and withdrawal of IV or subcutaneous fluids may be perceived as neglect.

Hydration should be reviewed regularly at the end of life and decisions discussed sensitively with the patient and those closest to them. The risks (fluid overload, worsening incontinence, etc.) and benefits should be clearly explained. If it is felt by the clinician that CAH may help symptoms such as thirst or delirium, a trial may be considered and assessed for benefit or harm after 12 hours.

The General Medical Council recommends that if the benefits and burdens of clinically assisted nutrition or CAH are finally balanced, the patient's preference will be the deciding factor. The clinician does not have to provide clinically assisted nutrition or CAH if they do not feel it is beneficial.

Future developments

A major area for hope is in the development of treatments to prevent, delay onset/progression, halt, and reverse NDGCs.

Stem cell therapy

Replacing neurons is a hugely attractive idea. There still remains a large amount of research to be done before this is clinically viable.

Gene therapy

Specific genetic mutations represent clear targets for gene therapy. As the knowledge and technology about bioinformatics continues to progress, genetic modification or manipulation may become feasible for the NDGCs.

Neurostimulation

An exciting development in recent years, with good evidence for use in PD, epilepsy, and chronic pain. New devices and systems are being developed which can be modulated according to need, to maximize effects while minimizing side effects and inconvenience. Such devices may be applicable to other conditions (e.g. HD).

Neuroprotection

Identifying compounds to modulate disease development/progression.

Drug delivery

Compounds which cross the blood–brain barrier to target affected areas.

Telemedicine/'telerehabilitation'

Provision of virtual clinics/monitoring and reducing time-consuming, inconvenient, and uncomfortable travel and clinic visits.

Further reading

Carey TS, Hanson L, Garrett JM, et al. (2006). Expectations and outcomes of gastric feeding tubes. *American Journal of Medicine* 199, 11–16.

Coyle H, Traynor V, Solowij N (2015). Computerize and virtual reality cognitive training for individuals at high risk of cognitive decline: systematic review of the literature. *American Journal of Geriatric Psychiatry* 23, 335–359.

Dal Bello-Haas V (2002). A framework for rehabilitation of neurodegenerative diseases: planning care and maximizing quality of life. *Journal of Neurologic Physical Therapy* 26, 115–129.

Department of Health and Social Care (2014). *Liverpool Care Pathway Review: Response to Recommendations*. ℗ https://www.gov.uk/government/publications/liverpool-care-pathway-review-response-to-recommendations.

Leung IH, Walton CC, Hallock H, et al. (2015). Cognitive training in Parkinson's disease—a systematic review and meta-analysis. *Neurology* 85, 1843–1851.

Majmudar S, Wu J, Paganoni S (2014). Rehabilitation in amyotrophic lateral sclerosis: why it matters. *Muscle & Nerve* 50, 4–13.

National Institute for Health and Care Excellence (NICE) (2015). *Care of Dying Adults in the Last Days of Life*. NICE Guideline [NG31]. NICE, London. ℗ https://www.nice.org.uk/guidance/ng31.

NHS England (2008, updated 2017). *Advance Decisions to Refuse Treatment: A Guide for Health and Social Care Professionals*. ℗ https://www.england.nhs.uk/improvement-hub/publication/advance-decisions-to-refuse-treatment-a-guide-for-health-and-social-care-professionals/.

Royal College of Physicians (2016). *End of Life Care Audit – Dying in Hospital: National report for England 2016*. ℗ https://www.rcplondon.ac.uk/projects/outputs/end-life-care-audit-dying-hospital-national-report-england-2016.

Twycross R, Wilcock A, Howard P (2017). *Palliative Care Formulary*, 6th edn. Pharmaceutical Press, London.

Useful websites

AgeUK: ℗ http://www.ageuk.org.uk.

Caring for Carers Hub: ℗ http://caringforcarers.info.

Cochrane Database of Systematic Reviews: ℗ http://www.cochranelibrary.com.

Driver and Vehicle Licensing Agency: ℗ https://www.gov.uk/guidance/current-medical-guidelines-dvla-guidance-for-professionals—guidance for doctors.

Dying Matters: ℗ http://dyingmatters.org—end of life care

Genetic alliance UK: ℗ http://www.geneticalliance.org.uk.

General Medical Council- ethical guidance on end of life care: ℗ http://www.gmc-uk.org/guidance/ethical_guidance/end_of_life_care.as; ℗ http://www.who.int/cancer/palliative/definition/en/; ℗ http://www.gmc-uk.org/static/documents/content/Treatment_and_care_towards_the_end_of_life_-_English_1015.pdf.

Gold Standards Framework: ℗ http://www.goldstandardsframework.org.uk.

Huntington's Disease Association: ℗ https://www.hda.org.uk—resources for healthcare professionals.

Motor Neuron Disease Association: ℗ http://www.mndassociation.org/—variety of guides available online:
- *Mental Illness and Mental Capacity in Huntington's disease—A Guide for Mental Health Workers*.
- *Motor Neuron Disease: A Guide for GPs and Primary Care Teams*.
- *A Professional's Guide to End of Life Care in Motor Neuron Disease*.
- *Cognitive Change, Frontotemporal Dementia and MND*.
- Also provides support grants and equipment loans.

National Institute for Health and Care Excellence: ℗ http://www.nice.org.uk—guidelines on MND, dementia, and intramuscular diaphragm stimulation for ventilator-dependent chronic respiratory failure due to neurological disease.

Prolonged disorders of consciousness

Introduction

The term 'consciousness' refers to our brain's capacity to provide an integrated, running commentary over our sensations and motivations for actions. It also provides for continuity of existence, so that your yesterdays are seamlessly integrated into an understanding of 'self' and are available to influence your likely behaviour today. Consciousness is a common feature of higher-order animals, although what it means to be conscious is thought to vary from one species to another.

The organic substrate underpinning 'consciousness' has not been identified. The connectivity and functional integrity of the frontoparietal network, subcortical nuclei, and brainstem nuclei play a critical role. There is some evidence that the claustrum (a thin band of grey matter encased within white matter in the human brain) may be instrumental in this role. It is highly unlikely that any one structure plays a dominant role, and consciousness is probably best thought of as a massively distributed system within the brain. It is therefore highly susceptible to widespread, diffuse injuries of any aetiology.

In reality, consciousness is not an on/off mechanism, but occurs across a spectrum of sophistication. Many altered states of consciousness are recognized, including temporary altered states of consciousness such as disorientation, delirium, and those resulting from some illicit drugs. These states present as misinterpretation of and/or response to stimuli. Some acute psychiatric disorders could also be considered to present with alterations in the expression of consciousness. Some of these temporary disorders of consciousness are discussed elsewhere in this handbook.

Another group of patients will present with prolonged disorders of consciousness (PDOCs). It is this group of patients who will be discussed in this chapter.

Arousal versus awareness

A number of systems are integral to consciousness. Consciousness is intimately tied up with arousal and the ability to recognize and/or maintain attention to stimuli. To effectively recognize external stimuli, one needs to have functional sensory systems to provide the raw data for interpretation. This raw data requires additional internal processing to extract meaning. The process of generating internal thoughts and stimuli responses requires an intact 'default mode network', an integrated series of anatomical structures in the brain engaged during wakeful rest, day dreaming, thinking about yourself or others, and planning.

In considering disorders of consciousness, it is helpful to consider the difference between arousal and awareness. Arousal networks consist of the reticular activating system in the brainstem along with complex feedback circuits into multiple cortical areas. Arousal is associated with increased sympathetic drive through links into the autonomic nervous system and is also associated with endocrine changes. Arousal levels determine a person's readiness to respond to incoming sensory signals as well as any internally generated thought process.

Awareness is the ability to appropriately perceive, monitor, interpret, and understand the impact of events, irrespective of whether they occur internally or external to the person. As a term, awareness is often used synonymously with 'consciousness' and is self-perceived as an integrated experience of being 'myself'. The interlinked concepts of arousal and awareness are commonly shown as a two-dimensional construct and are presented in Fig. 32.1. As can be seen, arousal underpins consciousness in the same way that you need to turn on your desktop computer before typing.

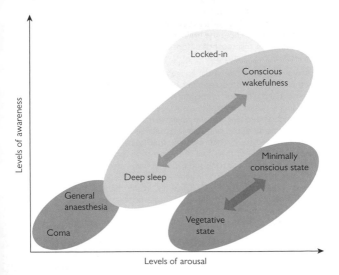

Fig. 32.1 The relationship between arousal and awareness.

Conscious versus subconscious versus unconscious

Much of the work of the brain is devoted to processing stimuli, whether they are visual, auditory, touch, taste, and/or olfactory. From the perspective of consciousness, stimulus interpretation happens at multiple levels:

- Unconscious—most processing of stimuli in the brain happen at an unconscious level. These background processes are completely hidden from conscious experience and are not accessible. Intuitive mental processing can also be unconscious, where you may arrive at a correct result but are not able to explain how you got there. Other examples include how you know an object is 'red', how adults complete simple arithmetic, the process of remembering someone's name when you see their face, and so on.

- Subconscious—traditionally, the term subconscious has been used interchangeably with unconscious, but the two concepts are quite different. Subconscious stimuli can be accessed by the conscious mind, but only once salience is achieved. While you are sitting in a chair, you will not notice the feel of weight of your body on your skin until it is mentioned or it becomes uncomfortable. The sensation of breathing is mostly subconscious, until highlighted for some reason (such as mentioning it in the text). Emotions are commonly subconscious drivers of your ongoing behaviour. Other conscious information can become blocked in some situations, such as the word-finding experience of having a word 'on the tip of your tongue'.

- Conscious—these processes can be thought of as being those that we are aware of and make the conscious choice to respond to. While we usually think that we are in charge of the decision-making process, in many circumstances the brain makes automatic reflex responses to stimuli tens of milliseconds before conscious awareness of the response generation has occurred.

As a working example, visual images are preprocessed by the retina before the occipital lobe determines basic features (e.g. edge determination, movement and direction of movement, basic shape, etc.). This unconscious processing is passed on to the associative cortex where further details are added, such as deciding that the object in front of you is a piece of fruit, can be labelled as an apple, and that it has started to go off. This information may not immediately reach salience, that point being when you become consciously aware of the smell of the overripe apple, rather than it merely forming part of the background. Conversely, small sudden movements within a relatively steady scene achieve salience quickly, such as a bird flying between trees against the sky. Clinically, in the medical condition of cortical blindness, much of the normal image processing occurs but without conscious awareness that it has taken place. A similar situation occurs in unawareness syndromes, for example, following a non-dominant stroke.

Assessment of level of consciousness

The sensation of being conscious is an entirely internal process. Medically, we infer a person's level of consciousness by observing their ability to display these internal processes to the external world. Most commonly, this is assessed by interpreting responsivity to stimuli given at the bedside. Depending on arousal level, we may ask the person to follow commands, or to evaluate movement in response to painful stimuli. Observation of these actions forms the basis of the GCS. To infer that a person is conscious, however, they must have the capacity for action, for example, through having adequate motor control or language processing. This is a significant limitation for a subgroup of patients following severe brain injury, who for various reasons, may not be able to provide interactions to allow us to determine whether or not they are 'conscious'. Thus, the concepts in Fig. 32.1 are more readily understood if a third dimension is added—that is, the person's ability to express information to an observer (Table 32.1). This structure allows various states of consciousness to be broken down into syndromes and conditions which will be discussed in turn.

- Wakefulness—this is the normal conscious state involving psychological and cognitive responses to external and internal events.
- Locked-in syndrome (LIS)—in classical LIS following a discrete brainstem lesion, the person is aware but lacks voluntary muscle movement other than vertical eye movements and blinking. This restricts the person to expressing their consciousness via communicating through eye movements. Non-classical LIS can occur in TBI where the net effect of structural damage simulates that seen in brainstem LIS. Individuals with paroxysmal sympathetic hyperactivity can also mimic LIS, particularly during storming episodes.
- Sleep—multiple cerebral processes occur during sleep such as restorative housekeeping, laying down of new memory, planning, and dreaming. Multiple (four to six) sleep cycles occur across each night, each consisting of REM and non-REM sleep (itself divided into three levels, the deepest of which is slow-wave sleep). Sleep is associated with reduced stimulus responsivity, although repetitive or intrusive stimuli

Table 32.1 Features and conditions affecting expression of consciousness and ability

	Arousal	Awareness	Ability
Wakefulness	++	++	++
Locked-in syndrome	+	+	−
Minimally conscious state	+/−	+/−	+/−
Sleep	+/−	+/−	−
Vegetative state	+/−	−	−
Coma/general anaesthesia	−	−	−

++, normal; +, present, possibly reduced; +/−, variably present; −, absent.

can lead to waking. During light sleep (dozing), arousal and awareness levels are higher than deep sleep, but remain lower than those seen during wakefulness. Muscle activity is usually limited, although complex behaviours are possible, such as in the parasomnias, where there may be a level of awareness at the time but no conscious recall after the event.

• Minimally conscious state (MCS)—MCS occurs where there is definitive evidence of consciousness (e.g. evidence of command following, verbalization, purposeful movements, etc.), however, the behaviour is less than consistent with the full expression of consciousness. While MCS is the accepted term for this syndrome, the diagnosis does not mean that the person *has* limited consciousness, only that they have limited ability to *display* consciousness. Some clinicians therefore prefer the older term of 'minimally responsive state', as this more accurately reflects what is being observed.

• Vegetative state (VS)—this term implies that the individual has preserved (or at least observable) arousal but there is no evidence of self- or environmental awareness. Thus the person may have a normal sleep–wake cycle and spontaneous eye opening but lacks purposeful movements or other responses to stimuli. Classically, persistent VS can be diagnosed a month post injury, becoming termed a 'permanent' VS after 6 months for non-TBI and 12 months for TBI.[1]

• Coma/general anaesthesia—in coma and general anaesthesia, basic physiological responses to stimuli do not occur. The person does not respond to pain, there is no eye opening, and no sleep–wake cycle. This differs from brain death where there is an irreversible loss of all brain function, including basic autonomic controls such as for breathing. Coma implies a breakdown of the reticular activating system, the cerebral cortex, and/or the white matter tracts between. Of note, patients who wake during anaesthesia can be aware but 'locked-in' due to the intercurrent use of muscle relaxants.

Prolonged disorders of consciousness following traumatic brain injury

Natural history

Coma results from a breakdown of cerebral processing and is associated with decreased oxygen utilization. Length of coma appears dependent on the extent of structural damage and functional impairment. In TBI, rotational shear forces exerted on the brain result in diffuse axonal injury (DAI). The more energy expended on the brain in this way, the greater its impact on deeper brain structures. As consciousness is a massively distributed system, it is particularly sensitive to severe DAI, with disruption of the reticular activating system and consequent damage to arousal pathway function. DAI in white matter tracts and the corpus callosum can also result in diaschisis (loss of function in an uninjured region secondary to deafferentation) producing a disconnection syndrome. Secondary compression and/or axonal shear resulting from cerebral oedema and/or uncontrolled seizure activity can contribute to a greater duration of coma, as can other influences such as cerebral hypoxia, metabolic disturbances, hypoglycaemia, inflammation, apoptotic cell death, blood vessel compromise, and so on.

Immediately post severe TBI, coma is a frequent and usually self-limiting clinical state. Around 99% of people rendered unconscious following a TBI will emerge from coma within 2 weeks of the injury. About half of those who remain in a coma at 1 month will have regained consciousness by 3 months. The longer an individual remains comatose, the poorer the outcome; however, there remains a tendency for people in coma to progress to VS and/or MCS over time (Table 32.2).

The extent of a person's recovery is dependent on their brain's capacity for ongoing repair of cognitive processes. PDOC is much more likely in those where there is extensive cortical neuron loss and extensive structural damage to the reticular activating system. Level of consciousness is associated with the integrity of the default mode and attentional networks. Functional imaging studies suggest that activation of the precuneus and posterior cingulate can be used to differentiate between the VS and MCS.

Table 32.2 Likelihood of recovery after coma of 1 month (% per category)

Status	At 3 months		At 6 months		At 12 months	
	TBI	NTBI	TBI	NTBI	TBI	NTBI
Death	15	24	24	40	33	53
VS	52	65	30	45	15	32
Regained consciousness	33	11	46	15	52	15

NTBI, non-traumatic brain injury; TBI, traumatic brain injury; VS, vegetative state.

Clinical data show that emergence from VS is more likely in younger patients and in those with TBI compared to those with hypoxic or other non-TBI causes. In turn, this suggests that people with extensive DAI may have a better overall prognosis for ongoing repair, presumed to be having intact neurons with the capacity for ongoing neuroplasticity and repair of diaschisis. However, even when people progress beyond a VS, they will usually show long-term and significant physical, cognitive, and social difficulties that necessitate high levels of support.

People remaining in a VS or MCS for long periods of time show an overall reduction in life expectancy, with the main risk factors being age at injury, male sex, and the degree of disability at discharge. Mortality in this group appears greatest in the first 5 years post trauma, while a less significant but still increased risk of death continues for those who survive longer than this. The most common cause of death is related to infection (e.g. aspiration pneumonia, pressure areas). Survival is usually dependent on continuing high-quality nursing care, maintaining nutrition (usually by PEG feeding), and the avoidance of and active treatment of infections.

Diagnosis and misdiagnosis

The crux of diagnosis hinges upon the person's capacity to respond in a timely and appropriate manner during assessment. Research has consistently shown a 40% misdiagnosis rate for VS, usually from assuming there is no consciousness when there is. Furthermore, a meta-analysis of 900 patients in a VS or MCS found that of those unambiguously diagnosed with VS, 10–24% had evidence of consciousness on quantitative EEG (qEEG), event-related potentials, or functional MRI.[2] It is therefore safest to assume that people have at least a rudimentary level of consciousness even if bedside testing suggests otherwise.

The reasons that bedside tests of awareness are not entirely accurate include:

- Evidence of responsivity may be limited to areas of relatively preserved function, and only discernible if all areas are assessed systematically.
- Arousal fluctuates, necessitating multiple assessments at various times of day, and/or picking the patient's 'best' times.
- There can be difficulty interpreting whether an observed movement is truly purposeful as opposed to being reflexive.
- Slowed speed of processing can lead to marked delays in understanding the instruction. The period of time required may be much longer than the examiner expects or greater than the injured person's ability to sustain attention to the requested task.
- Environmental load; noisy or busy ward environments are fatiguing and can produce prolonged performance impairment.
- Untreated pain/paroxysmal sympathetic hyperactivity will confound assessment of level of consciousness.
- Responses may be intermittent or inconsistent across assessments.

Assessment of PDOC

One approach to minimize misdiagnosis of PDOC is to use a standardized scale. Many different scales have been developed. The best performing scale from US based research is the Coma Recovery Scale—Revised (CRS-R). It consists of 6 subscales examining modalities of vision, hearing, oromotor/verbal, motor, communication and arousal to produce an ordinal scale with a range of 0 to 23. The CRS-R is considered the diagnostic gold standard for the bedside monitoring of people for differentiating and monitoring the emergence of PVS into MCS over time. However, it remains insensitive when compared to quantitative electroencephalography (EEG) or functional MRI.

In the UK, the Sensory Modality and Assessment Rehabilitation Technique (SMART) has been used in some specialist regional services for this patient group. It studies the patient's response to a multisensory programme including vision, hearing, taste, touch, and smell. Modalities of wakefulness/arousal and motor skills are assessed and the patient's functional and communication capabilities can be determined. The results are used to guide treatment and incorporate familiar and unfamiliar stimuli under the SMART programme.

Ethical issues

At times there will be complex ethical issues around appropriate care and end-of-life decisions for patients with PDOC. These are particularly apparent when the treating rehabilitation team and the patient's family begin to consider whether active treatment should be withdrawn. It is here that confidence in the accuracy of diagnosis is paramount, as is a firm understanding of the likelihood of any future recovery.

A common starting point for decision-making is evaluating what potential exists for a 'reasonable' quality of life (QOL) for the affected person. However, QOL is an internal process predicated on consciousness, and making decisions about how another person will perceive their own QOL can be fraught and misguided. On this basis, a person in a true VS has no capacity to determine their QOL, but this is markedly different for someone in a MCS. Good-quality research for people with severe disabilities and with LIS suggests a high self-perceived level of QOL for the majority, once a period of adjustment has taken place. However, because of the difficulties in communicating with people in a MCS, it can be extremely difficult to determine what the patient's wishes may be regarding treatment and end-of-life decisions.

In many countries, such ethical decisions are handled by the legal system. Ideally, the family and the treating physician will be in agreement. An independent medical expert is appointed both for the patient and also for the hospital and family. Solicitors are also appointed on both sides in order to make sure there is no undue financial advantage that would accrue to a third party following the patient's death. The expert reports are presented to a judge who will make a final decision. While euthanasia remains illegal in most countries, the withdrawal of active treatment (which includes the withdrawal of feeding or withholding of antibiotics) is often permitted after appropriate Court approval.

Treatment paradigms for prolonged disorders of consciousness

A number of treatment approaches have been put forward in an attempt to improve the outcome for people with PDOCs. Overall, evidence of efficacy remains poor other than for a few isolated pharmacological agents, and more research is required before it will be possible to determine whether a particular approach may be useful for any individual patient. The major limitation in all efficacy studies is that cerebral function will tend to improve over time; therefore, it can be difficult to prove that an intervention has produced sufficient functional improvement to allow arousal and awareness to become evident beyond what would have occurred due to natural recovery over time. The various approaches and evidence for efficacy are summarized as follows:

Sensory stimulation

This approach provides the person with a PDOC with varied sensory inputs, either singularly or together, with the aim of promoting recovery of processing pathways. The key to the success of this approach is that there is limited structural damage (in terms of disconnection, reticular activating system, and the cerebral cortex) and that the major deficit relates to inadequate processing of sensory inputs. This situation is likely to occur in a minority of patients with DOC. While there is no clear evidence that this approach is useful, there is also minimal risk of harm.

Physical approaches

These approaches involve the use of passive therapy, tilt tabling, stretching, and so on. This approach has similar limitations to sensory stimulation in terms of allowing a person to demonstrate awareness. Physical approaches are useful, however, in the secondary prevention of complications that could adversely impact future QOL if/when the DOC settles. Such issues include skin breakdown, spasticity management, contractures, etc. There is no confirmed link between physical rehabilitation strategies and restoration of consciousness.

Pharmaceutical

A number of drug classes have been used to modify arousal and potentially improve awareness. The most promising agents involve the off-label use of dopaminergic agonists (e.g. methylphenidate, amantadine, bromocriptine, or levodopa) and GABAergic drugs (e.g. baclofen or zolpidem). There is evidence for increased arousal and responsivity in the early recovery period for the dopaminergic medications, with less consistent evidence for the GABAergics. In both cases, the medications have the potential to improve the signal-to-noise ratio within the recovering brain, thereby allowing repairing circuits to function better while taking the medication.

Brain stimulation

Two approaches to brain stimulation have been reported. Non-invasive techniques utilize one of the various forms of transcranial stimulation (e.g. transcranial magnetic stimulation). Invasive techniques include implantation of spinal cord stimulators around the C2–C4 level or deep brain stimulation. At the present time there is preliminary evidence of effect, although larger and better designed studies are required to confirm the potential of these approaches.

References

1. Royal College of Physicians (RCP) (2013). *Prolonged Disorders of Consciousness: National Clinical Guidelines*. London, RCP.
2. Bender A, Jox RJ, Grill E, et al. (2015). Persistent vegetative state and minimally conscious state—a systematic review and meta-analysis of diagnostic procedures. *Deutsches Ärzteblatt International* 112, 235–242.

Further reading

Baguley IJ, Nott MT, Slewa-Younan S (2008). Long-term mortality trends in functionally-dependent adults following severe traumatic-brain injury. *Brain Injury* 22, 919–925.

Giacino JT, Kalmar K, Whyte J (2004). The JFK Coma Recovery Scale-Revised: measurement characteristics and diagnostic utility. *Archives of Physical Medicine and Rehabilitation* 85, 2020–2029.

Giacino JT, Katz DI, Whyte J (2013). Neurorehabilitation in disorders of consciousness. *Seminars in Neurology* 33, 142–156.

Gill-Thwaites H, Munday R (1999). The Sensory Modality and Assessment Rehabilitation Technique (SMART): a comprehensive and integrated assessment and treatment protocol of the vegetative state and minimally responsive patient. *Neuropsychological Rehabilitation* 9, 305–320.

The Multi-Society Task Force on PVS (1994). Medical aspects of the persistent vegetative state (part 1). *New England Journal of Medicine* 330, 1572–1579.

Disorders of the peripheral nerves

Background

Accurate diagnosis is important for the rehabilitation of people with disorders of the peripheral nerves. There are a small but increasing number of disorders that are now specifically treatable. Even in those disorders of peripheral nerves that do not currently have a specific treatment, accurate diagnosis remains important in order to determine natural history and prognosis. This will help to determine the rehabilitation strategy. Some conditions may recover—such as Guillain–Barré syndrome (GBS)—while others are progressive—such as the hereditary motor and sensory neuropathies. Some may require surgical intervention (e.g. the brachial plexus injuries).

This chapter will cover the following disorders of peripheral nerves in order to indicate the range and extent of rehabilitation techniques:
• Critical illness polyneuropathy
• Diabetic neuropathy
• GBS and chronic inflammatory demyelinating polyneuropathy
• Post-polio syndrome
• Hereditary motor and sensory neuropathies
• Nerve root, brachial plexus, and peripheral nerve injuries following trauma.

Disorders of peripheral nerves usually consist, in varying proportions, of the following problems:
• Weakness—LMN weakness
• Variable degrees of sensory disturbance
• Muscle fatigue
• Pain, directly as a result of the peripheral nerve damage and/or secondary to abnormal gait and posture
• Autonomic impairment.

Classification

Nerve injury

The Seddon and Sunderland classifications are useful in describing nerve injury and subsequent prognosis (Table 33.1 and Fig. 33.1)

Peripheral neuropathy

This can be classified in many ways, according to anatomical level and pattern, symmetry, fibre type, whether motor, sensory, or autonomic, and cause. Useful summaries are available.[1,2]

Table 33.1 The Seddon and Sunderland classifications of nerve injury

Seddon	Process	Sunderland
Neurapraxia	Segmental demyelination	First degree
Axonotmesis	Axon severed but endoneurium intact (optimal circumstances for regeneration)	Second degree
Axonotmesis	Axon discontinuity, endoneurial tube discontinuity, perineurium and fascicular arrangement preserved	Third degree
Axonotmesis	Loss of continuity of axons, endoneurial tubes, perineurium, and fasciculi; epineurium intact (neuroma in continuity)	Fourth degree
Neurotmesis	Loss of continuity of entire nerve trunk	Fifth degree

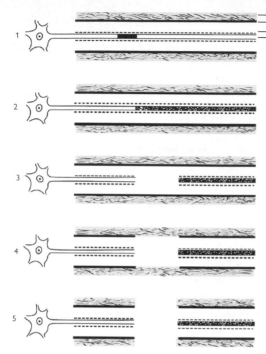

Fig. 33.1 Diagram of Sunderland's classification of nerve injury from (1) first-degree injury to (5) fifth-degree injury.

Reproduced with permission from Campbell WW. Evaluation and management of peripheral nerve injury. *Clin Neurophysiol*, 119(9):1951–1965. Published by Elsevier Ireland Ltd. https://doi.org/10.1016/j.clinph.2008.03.018.

Assessment

A detailed neurological examination with emphasis on testing myotomes, sensory dermatomes, and motor reflexes is recommended (➔ see Chapter 5).

Nerve conduction studies, electromyography (EMG), and sometimes nerve biopsy may all be necessary, not only to determine the diagnosis but also to determine the prognosis. There may, for example, be evidence of complete denervation (poor prognosis), partial denervation (better prognosis), or some denervation with evidence of reinnervation (good prognosis). Biochemical, haematological, genetic, and immunological investigations will add further information, chosen according to the differential diagnosis.

The remainder of this chapter covers impairments associated with different types of peripheral nerve disorders and examples of acute, severe, and reversible to chronic and steadily progressive conditions.

Weakness

Virtually all peripheral nerve lesions are associated with weakness. This not only includes weakness affecting the limbs which is obviously disabling, but also weakness of the trunk, swallowing, and neck muscles which bring additional rehabilitation challenges.

Weakness can cause activity limitations in the following areas:

Use of lower limbs, including:
- easy tripping over any obstacle, including rough ground, carpets, uneven pavements, kerbs
- reduced ability to walk upstairs and up slopes
- reduced ability to get up from sitting
- reduced speed of walking
- uneven gait
- difficulty turning in bed
- standing.

Use of upper limbs, including:
- difficulty in handling objects such as cutlery, work tools, phones, steering wheels, toilet paper, and so on.
- difficulty in getting objects to mouth or face
- difficulty in washing and grooming the face and head
- reduced ability to reach.

Use of trunk, including:
- respiration
- coughing
- opening bowels
- bending
- sitting
- provision of stable base for use of limbs
- turning in bed.

Use of cervical, pharyngeal and laryngeal muscles, including:
- maintaining a functional neck position
- swallowing
- talking.

Secondary problems resulting from weakness, including:
- pain
- contractures—it is often forgotten that contractures are associated with LMN and muscle conditions as well as UMN conditions; the basic mechanism is an agonist and antagonist muscle imbalance at rest, whatever the cause
- scoliosis
- pressure ulcers
- pneumonia
- malnutrition
- venous thromboembolism.

Interventions that can help to reduce the effects of weakness include:
- passive movements of the limbs, particularly in the acute phase
- orthoses to restore function and prevent contractures in both ULs and LLs (➲ see Chapter 21).

Exercise can improve muscle strength in some conditions, although it probably does not improve the rate of recovery from acute neuropathy. Isometric and isotonic exercises both increase muscle power and exercise tolerance but there is little information on the precise amount of such exercise required for maximum effect.

People with longer-term weakness may need adaptations to their immediate environment, such as ramps, lifts, wheelchairs, special utensils, and other hand adaptations (e.g. pen holder) as described in ➔ Chapters 22 and 23.

Other home and work adaptations, such as environmental control equipment, can also help to reduce the disability associated with chronic arm and leg weakness. These are described in ➔ Chapter 23.

Muscle fatigue

Muscle fatigue is an important and often overlooked contributor to muscle weakness and to reduced function in peripheral nerve disorders. It occurs due to abnormal recruitment of muscle fibres and a change in muscle fibre proportion, to aberrant peripheral feedback, and secondary central changes in response to the nerve injury and disuse.

This affects daily activities in several ways:
• Sustaining activity.
• Deterioration in movement as the day progresses, thus affecting quality of movement and affecting susceptibility to secondary injury such as falls and musculotendinous complex injury.
• Increasing central fatigue due to the increased effort required to sustain activity.

Autonomic impairment

Autonomic impairment will result from pathology affecting small nerve fibres.

The following impairments may occur:
• Orthostatic hypotension and LL oedema.
• Impaired temperature control, associated with sweating, abnormal vasodilatation or vasoconstriction, and heat or cold intolerance.
• GI symptoms, with impaired gastric emptying and GI motility, early satiety, constipation, and diarrhoea.
• Bladder symptoms resulting from impaired parasympathetic and sympathetic control of bladder (➔ see Chapter 12).
• Erectile dysfunction.
• Cranial parasympathetic impairment leading to dry eyes or dry mouth.
• Cardiac arrhythmia.

Autonomic neuropathy can occur in many neuropathies but is prominent in neuropathies due to the following:
• Diabetes
• Amyloid
• Autoimmune conditions
• Some paraneoplastic conditions
• Toxins such as vincristine and arsenic
• Storage disorders such as Fabry disease
• Sometimes in CMT
• Infections such as Lyme disease, HIV, and leprosy.

Sensory impairment and pain

Loss of normal sensation carries a significant risk of unnoticed trauma with the consequent dangers of pressure sores, neuropathic ulceration, and neuropathic arthropathy.

Involvement of sensory nerves can lead to severe neuropathic pain. For a detailed review, ➲ see Chapter 11. Neuropathic pain is variously described but words often used include constant, deep, and burning. The pharmacological treatment of neuropathic pain can be very difficult but may include:

- anticonvulsants—particularly carbamazepine, gabapentin, and pregabalin
- tricyclic antidepressants—such as amitriptyline or nortriptyline
- serotonin and noradrenaline reuptake inhibitors antidepressants—such as duloxetine
- tramadol
- cannabinoids
- local or regional sympathetic blockade
- capsaicin ointment.

It is also important to remember that some people with an abnormal gait or posture can develop secondary musculoskeletal pain. The most useful drugs for musculoskeletal pain are the NSAIDs, but these have to be used with caution due to their side effect profile, especially with regard to GI inflammation, renal impairment, and arterial thrombosis (➲ see Chapter 11).

Interventions that may help to reduce the effects of sensory loss and pain include the following:

- Education of the patient to look for any type of break in their skin in denervated areas.
- Education of patients with neuropathy affecting their feet to check the inside of shoes for stones, creases in socks, and so on, before and after putting them on.
- Chiropody for patients with neuropathy affecting their feet.
- Use of sensory cues to assist in motor control of denervated area (e.g. vision, use of various garments, orthoses etc.) that provide a greater stimulus or bridge over to an enervated area.
- Footwear.
- Psychological therapies, especially with regard to pain.

Intensive care unit-acquired weakness

This consists of an axonal peripheral neuropathy, a myopathy, or a combination of these that arises in the context of people admitted to intensive care. Causative factors are uncertain, but it is probably due to impairment of microcirculation, sodium channel dysfunction, and mitochondrial dysfunction. Various studies show between one-quarter and one-half of individuals on intensive care for more than 7 days had documented evidence of peripheral neuropathy or myopathy. The risk of it increases with:

* hyperglycaemia
* multiorgan failure
* sepsis
* persistent inflammation
* length of ICU stay
* possible association with use of glucocorticoids
* catabolic state
* female sex (4:1 risk)
* immobility.

There is evidence that the prognosis for a critical care myopathy is better than that for a neuropathy. Strategies to reduce the risk and severity are:

* early mobilization—this can include mobilization while still on mechanical ventilation (e.g. by use of a cycle ergometer)
* minimization and interruption of sedation
* good glycaemic control, but with caution not to cause hypoglycaemia
* resting orthoses and passive movements can be used to maintain position and range in the limbs.

Critical care weakness needing rehabilitation may present as a sole diagnosis, but may also be present in patients needing rehabilitation for other reasons, such as major trauma or head injuries.

Table 33.2 Clinical, electrophysiological, and histological features of intensive care unit-acquired weakness

Investigation	CIP	CIM	CINM
Physical examination	Distal muscle weakness	Proximal muscle weakness	Proximal and distal muscle weakness
	Distal sensory deficit	Normal sensory testing	Distal sensory deficit
	Normal or depressed deep tendon reflexes	Normal or depressed deep tendon reflexes	Depressed deep tendon reflexes
Electrophysiology studies	Decreased CMAP and decreased SNAP	Decreased CMAP and normal SNAP	Decreased CMAP and SNAP
	Normal MUAP	Decreased MUAP	Decreased MUAP
	Normal or near-normal conduction velocity	EMG shows short-duration, low-amplitude activity	EMG shows short-duration, low-amplitude activity
Histology	Axonal degeneration of distal motor and sensory nerves	Thick filament (myosin) loss, type II fibre (fast twitch) atrophy, necrosis	Axonal degeneration and evidence of loss in myosin, type II fibre atrophy, and necrosis

CIM, critical illness myopathy; CINM, critical illness neuromyopathy; CIP, critical illness polyneuropathy; CMAP, compound muscle action potential; EMG, electromyography; MUAP, muscle unit action potential; SNAP, sensory nerve action potential.

Diabetic neuropathy

Clinicians working in rehabilitation may see patients with diabetes in several different contexts. One major service area is in amputee rehabilitation, where most diabetic patients will also have evidence of a neuropathy. The global prevalence of diabetes in 2014 was 8.5%.[3] This will be at least the prevalence of diabetes in the population seen for specialist rehabilitation, so consideration of diabetes and its complications will need to be integrated into rehabilitation for a substantial minority of patients.

Diabetes mellitus is associated with several types of neuropathy, and is the commonest cause of neuropathy because of the high prevalence of diabetes. It can sometimes predate the diagnosis of diabetes. Prevalence is approximately a quarter in clinic-based populations of those with type 1 and type 2 diabetes. Neuropathy is associated with impaired glucose control, lipid levels, age, time since onset of diabetes, and height. Of these factors, glycaemic and lipid control are modifiable and there have been several studies suggesting this can reduce the development of neuropathy.

The following patterns of neuropathy can occur:
• A predominantly sensory symmetrical polyneuropathy. It is length dependent, so it occurs in a glove and stocking distribution and severity correlates with height. Increasing motor impairment also occurs over time.
• A predominantly small fibre neuropathy.
• Autonomic neuropathy.
• A radiculoplexopathy, such as neuralgic amyotrophy.
• Radiculopathy.
• Mononeuritis multiplex.
• Mononeuropathy.
• Treatment-induced neuropathy, if glycaemic control is too tight.

Potential complications include the following:
• Ulceration.
• Amputation.
• Charcot joints.
• Muscle weakness.
• Reduced balance.
• Impaired gait and mobility on flat and when climbing stairs.
• Falls risk is increased by two or three times compared to those with diabetes and no neuropathy.
• Neurogenic pain management is equivalent to other forms of neurogenic pain. Indeed, because of the frequency of diabetes, many of the trials of pharmacological management of neurogenic pain have been conducted in patients with diabetes.

Rehabilitation can focus on prevention or reduction of future complications alongside optimizing current participation:

- Diabetic neuropathy is frequently associated with vascular complications, so rehabilitation approaches should allow for both complications.
- Exercise is potentially beneficial in those with diabetic neuropathy, but precautions need to be taken in order to avoid tissue damage.
- Both acute trauma and repetitive minor trauma can lead to foot ulceration, with the latter also leading to a Charcot joint.
- Consistent levels of physical activity are associated with lower levels of diabetic foot ulceration and amputation. High levels of activity some days, and low levels on other days are associated with ulceration, but when levels of activity are kept consistent, then higher average activity levels are associated with less ulceration and amputation.
- There have been studies involving various exercise modalities, with increasing activity levels being protective whatever exercise modality is used. Resistance training can be helpful in improving several activities and is also associated with less foot trauma and falls risk. Choosing activities which reduce the risk of complications alongside the personal preferences of the patient may be the most beneficial.
- There are several physical treatments that may be used for treatment of foot ulceration, such as ultrasound, heat, and electrotherapy. The presence of neuropathy will need to be considered if using these.
- Use of diabetic shoes will help to reduce pressure in insensate areas at rest and when walking.

Guillain–Barré and Miller Fisher syndromes

GBS and Miller Fisher syndrome (MFS) are acute-onset autoimmune polyneuropathies. They affect 1–2 people per 100,000 population per year. The main clinical feature of GBS is a flaccid paralysis of all four limbs and trunk, whereas MFS consists of ophthalmoplegia and ataxia. Both have classic forms and various subtypes. Areflexia is a common feature to both, but does not occur in all patients. There is a relatively new classification system to which the reader is directed.[4]

The main aspects of note are the following:
- Often rapid onset, usually in a matter of days but sometimes a matter of hours.
- Maximum onset of 28 days, longer onsets suggest an alternative diagnosis, such as chronic inflammatory demyelinating polyneuropathy.
- Advancing weakness often starting in the feet but rapidly moving upwards to involve the muscles around the knees and hips and then the hands, wrists, elbows, and shoulders. The nadir of the condition is 2–4 weeks post onset. Fig. 33.2 shows the time course of GBS.
- Around 20% of people develop respiratory weakness requiring artificial ventilation.
- Can also be associated with bulbar weakness and autonomic failure.
- GBS can have demyelinating and axonal forms (acute inflammatory demyelinating polyneuropathy and acute motor axonal neuropathy respectively); MFS, paraparetic GBS, and pharyngo-cervical-brachial GBS are all axonal neuropathies.
- Examination of CSF reveals an increase in protein but not in white cells.

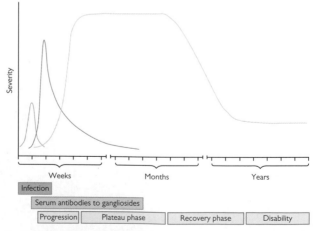

Fig. 33.2 Guillain-Barré syndrome time course.

Autoantibodies are associated with some forms:
- Pharyngo-cervical-brachial weakness with anti-GT1a or anti-GQ1b IgG antibodies
- Classical MFS and Bickerstaff brainstem encephalitis with anti-GQ1b antibodies
- AMAN with anti-GM1 or anti-GD1a antibodies.

Treatment involves plasmapheresis and/or intravenous immunoglobulin G infusion as soon as possible after the start of the illness.

About 10% of patients can experience a treatment-related fluctuation following treatment with plasma exchange and intravenous immunoglobulin as their effect wears off. This is most commonly reported in the first 8 weeks following treatment, potentially when the patient is in a rehabilitation unit. If symptoms recur, it is important to consider both a treatment-related fluctuation and reconsider diagnosis, in particular, whether the patient may have chronic inflammatory demyelinating polyneuropathy.

There are several possible complications during the initial illness and early rehabilitation, as seen in Table 33.3.

About 20% of patients will be unable to walk unaided 6 months after onset. Of those requiring inpatient neurological rehabilitation, many will have residual motor and sensory symptoms for at least several years, or long term, with recovery taking place over several years. Fatigue, both central and peripheral, can be a long-term issue. Later physical rehabilitation often focuses on endurance exercise and fatigue management. Patient support groups are helpful (➜ see 'Further reading').

Table 33.3 Complications, prevention, and monitoring in Guillain–Barré syndrome/Miller Fisher syndrome

Complications	Prevention/monitoring
Respiratory failure	Serial vital capacity (sitting and lying)
Lower respiratory tract infection	Examination, chest physiotherapy, antibiotics
Urinary tract infection	Maintaining fluid intake
Malnutrition and dehydration	Use of alternative forms of feeding as required
Contractures	Passive movements, appropriate positioning resting splints; Goniometry
Pressure sores	Appropriate positioning, turning, pressure-relieving mattress and seating
Venous thromboembolism	Prophylactic low-molecular-weight heparin, compression stockings
Autonomic dysfunction	Monitoring of blood pressure, bowels, heart rate; treatment as necessary
Depression	Psychological therapies and antidepressants.
Neuropathic pain	Use of appropriate analgesia (➜ see Chapter 11)

GBS and MFS have been associated with influenza and hepatitis vaccination, although less with newer forms of vaccine. Patients are often concerned about their risk of relapse with vaccination. Currently, there is no evidence that influenza vaccination increases the likelihood of relapse, and, if there is a very low risk, it is likely to be less than the risk of complications from influenza or of recurrent GBS from influenza. Relapses are rare, occurring in about 1–3% of those who have had GBS.

Post-polio syndrome

Acute polio is now rare, having been virtually eradicated in the developed world and is significantly less common in developing countries. However, there are still a large number of people who were affected by the disease, usually in their childhood. Late deterioration after polio can occur and is known as post-polio syndrome. The key points are as follows:

* Post-polio syndrome usually occurs around 30–40 years after the acute illness.
* It is defined as the development of new muscle weakness after a period of stability with evidence of neurogenic change in someone who has had previous polio.
* Other conditions should be excluded.
* Sometimes the resulting disability can be disproportionate to the apparent minor change because of a lack of functional reserve in a person who is already disabled.

Deterioration is usually slowly progressive. It is said that, on average, there is about 1% of loss of muscle strength each year. However, even a modest reduction in muscle strength of, say, 10% can be enough to produce severe further weakness in individuals already disabled after their acute polio.

It can be accompanied by other symptoms such as:
* fatigue
* joint and musculotendinous complex pain
* neurogenic pain from secondary conditions such as nerve compression and disc herniation
* muscle pain and cramps
* neurogenic respiratory failure
* dysphagia
* dysphonia
* cold intolerance.

Aerobic training can improve endurance, and resistance training can improve muscle strength, at least to a limited degree.

Other aspects of rehabilitation focus on methods to assist weak limbs, such as the use of orthoses, mobility aids, wheelchairs, and environmental adaptation.

Charcot–Marie–Tooth disease/hereditary motor and sensory neuropathies

There is an increasing genetic literature on the hereditary motor and sensory neuropathies/CMT, with these terms being used synonymously. There is an overall prevalence of 1 in 2500, many different genetic mutations having been found. The commonest forms, CMT 1 and 2, are pure peripheral neuropathies, but other forms are associated with CNS changes, such as pyramidal tract signs, deafness, and optic atrophy. For a review, see Murphy et al.[5]

Impairments are classically:
- distal and ascending sensory loss
- distal motor weakness, initially involving intrinsic muscles of foot and hand
- foot deformities, most frequently pes cavus
- neurogenic pain.

Due to the progressive nature of the conditions, an important aspect of rehabilitation to minimize the effects of progression and secondary complications, and educating them about the condition and its prognosis. As it is inherited, the patient may well have experience of other family members with the condition.

Rehabilitation interventions centre on the following:
- Maximizing muscle strength and endurance, improving balance, and avoiding falls.
- Appropriate prescription of AFOs and footwear to optimize gait. Custom-made AFOs are often necessary.
- Appropriate prescription of resting hand splints, aiming to reduce the rate of formation of finger contractures.
- Regular chiropody is particularly important for those with sensory loss in the feet and hands.
- Provision of appropriate hand splints and other simple aids to daily living, such as adapted cutlery, pen holders, and so on.
- Prescription of mobility aids, such as walking frames and wheelchairs, and appropriate advice about driving and transport.
- Adaptation of the environment as necessary, such as ramps, lifts, hoists, assistive technology, and so on.
- Screening for respiratory impairment, sleep-disordered breathing, and restless legs syndrome.
- Treating pain.

Due to the slowly progressive nature of the condition, the impact of disability often arises in mid-adult life, with the psychological impact of that on career, family roles, and self-image often being a major problem.

Surgical correction is sometimes helpful. In the LLS, this can involve Achilles tendon lengthening, plantar fasciotomy, tendon transfers (e.g. of tibialis posterior, long toe flexor, and extensor muscles), as well as the possibility of arthrodesis and osteotomies in order to preserve function and prevent complications. Surgery for the UL is less used but may have a role in centres with the necessary experience.

Brachial plexus injuries

Brachial plexus injuries are uncommon but nevertheless around 500 people in the UK suffer permanent disability each year—usually from traction injuries to the plexus. Brachial plexus injuries in childbirth still occur but they are becoming less common as obstetric practice improves. Road traffic accidents account for the great majority, most commonly secondary to motorcycle accidents. The mean age is in the early 20s and the majority are males.

Individuals should be referred as soon as possible to a specialist centre where there is not only a good multidisciplinary rehabilitation team but also where expert surgical advice and treatment is obtainable.

Treatment focuses on a very accurate diagnosis of which parts of the brachial plexus have been damaged. This also involves a careful *functional* UL assessment, often combined with neurophysiological investigation. If avulsion of the spinal nerves is suspected, then surgical exploration should be carried out as soon as possible. There is a clear decline in long-term functional results if surgery is delayed. One series showed full return of function in individuals who were operated on within 3 weeks of the injury. However, the proportion of failed procedures rose to over 60% in those operated on after 6 months. The nerves can be repaired either by grafting or nerve transfers. The optimal timing for surgery to ruptured spinal nerves is 3–6 months post injury.

Specialist splints can be very useful and effectively restore function in individuals who do not make a full recovery after surgery. The following are particularly helpful:
- An elbow lock splint is useful in the absence of active elbow control (C5 and C6 lesions).
- A gauntlet splint is useful when there is major loss of function in the forearm and hand (C7, C8, and T1 lesions).
- The flail arm splint is used when there is irreparable damage to the whole plexus (C5–T1 lesions). The flail arm splint will include an elbow hinge and a wrist platform to which can be attached various devices, such as split hook which is open and closed by a cable and operated from the opposite shoulder. Various other appliances can be attached to the flail arm device, such as attachments to aid ADLs around the house or in the garden. Some individuals can return to work using various splints attachments, such as pliers, sewing devices, and so on.

Neuropathic pain is common and can be difficult to control. Treatment follows the same principles as for any neuropathic pain (➜ see Chapter 11).

In summary, the outlook for people with brachial plexus lesions is good as long as urgent referral is made to a specialist centre and the lesion is surgically explored and repaired as soon as possible. There is often much that can be done for those with residual arm and shoulder weakness.

References

1. Jones LK, Crum BA (2016). Spinal, peripheral nerve, and muscle disorders. In: Wittich CM (ed), *Mayo Clinic Internal Medicine Board Review*, 11 edn, pp. 639–648. Oxford University Press, Oxford.
2. Overell JR (2011). Peripheral neuropathy: pattern recognition for the pragmatist. *Practical Neurology* 11, 62–70.
3. World Health Organization. Fact sheet on diabetes. ℘ http://www.who.int/mediacentre/factsheets/fs312/en/.
4. Wakerley BR, Uncini A, Yuki N, et al. (2014). Guillain Barré and Miller Fisher syndromes—new diagnostic classification. *Nature Reviews Neurology* 10, 537–544.
5. Murphy SM, Laura M, Fawcett K, et al. (2012). Charcot–Marie–Tooth disease: frequency of genetic subtypes and guidelines for genetic testing. *Journal of Neurology, Neurosurgery & Psychiatry* 83, 706–710.

Further reading

Crews RT, Schneider KL, Yalla SV, et al. (2016). Physiological and psychological challenges of increasing physical activity and exercise in patients at risk of diabetic foot ulcers; a critical review. *Diabetes/Metabolism Research Reviews* 32, 791–804.

Gilbert A (ed) (2001). *Brachial Plexus Injuries*. (Federation of European Societies for Surgery of the Hand). Martin Dunitz, London.

Gonzalez H, Olsson T, Borg K (2010). Management of postpolio syndrome. *Lancet Neurology* 9, 634–642.

Kress JP, Hall JB (2014). ICU-acquired weakness and recovery from critical illness. *New England Journal of Medicine* 370, 1626–1635.

Examples of support groups

Brachial plexus injuries

℘ https://www.ubpn.org—there are surprisingly few brachial plexus patient groups, this is the United Brachial Plexus Network based in the US.

℘ https://www.brachialplexuspalsyfoundation.org—a further US-based website.

GBS and MFS

℘ http://www.gaincharity.org.uk/.

℘ http://www.gbsnz.org.nz/guillain_barre_syndrome.

℘ https://www.gbs-cidp.org/canada/.

℘ https://www.gbs.org.uk.

Polio

℘ https://www.britishpolio.org.uk—a large UK charity supporting people with polio and the post-polio syndrome.

CMT

℘ https://www.charcot-marie-tooth.org.

℘ http://cmt.org.uk/.

Muscle disorders

Introduction

There are a wide variety of inherited muscle conditions that result in disability and thus a need for rehabilitation. Table 34.1 shows the estimated prevalence figures for various groups of conditions. Despite missing estimates for some conditions and wide variability of estimated prevalence for others, the combined prevalence of inherited muscle conditions, inflammatory myopathies, and metabolic myopathies is likely to be about 60 per 100,000. In addition, muscle pathology occurs secondary to systemic disease and so will often contribute to disability in patients with other conditions who are seen by rehabilitation professionals.

Muscle function relies on a highly tuned contractile apparatus that depends on a structure, biochemistry, and physiology that is simple in its basic principles but highly complex in the interactions of the many proteins and cellular processes that make that function possible. Defects in any one of the many proteins involved can lead to muscle disease by effects on structure, energy supply, contraction, growth, maintenance, or a combination of these. Fig. 34.1 shows some of the main proteins involved in just one structure involved in muscle function, that of the dystrophin-associated protein complex where most of the proteins illustrated are each known to be associated with at least one type of muscle condition.

Muscle conditions have an impact throughout the lifecycle, from those conditions which manifest at birth and in childhood, such as congenital myotonic dystrophy, congenital myopathies, and Duchenne muscular dystrophy (DMD), to those that predominate in early adult life such as facioscapulohumeral and limb girdle muscular dystrophy, and finally conditions starting in older age such as inclusion body myositis. Rehabilitation can enhance the ability of individuals with a muscle condition to participate in many life areas, such as work, education, family life, and leisure activities.

Table 34.1 Prevalence of different groups of muscle conditions

Conditions	Prevalence per 100,000	Reference
Inherited muscle conditions excluding mitochondrial and metabolic myopathies	37	Single regional muscle centre, Norwood et al. 2009
Muscular dystrophies	19–25	Review, Theadom et al. 2014
Inflammatory myopathies	14	Review, Meyer et al. 2015
Mitochondrial disease (but prevalence of a myopathy phenotype will vary)	9.2	Schaefer et al. 2008

⊖ See 'Further reading' for detailed references.

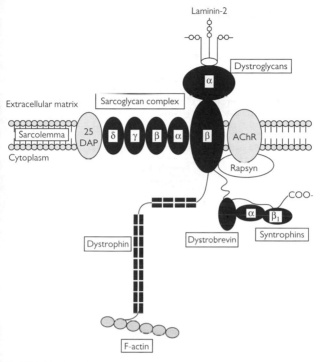

Fig. 34.1 The dystrophin-associated protein complex.

Reproduced with permission from Hilton-Jones D. Muscle diseases in *Brain's Diseases of the Nervous System*, Donaghy M. (Ed.). oxford, UK: Oxford University Press. © 2009 Oxford University Press. Reproduced with permission of Oxford University Press through PLSclear and courtesy of Rosie Fisher. http://oxfordmedicine.com/view/10.1093/med/9780198569381.001.0001/med-9780198569381-chapter-024.

This chapter covers some of the commoner muscle conditions seen by the rehabilitation physician alongside their more frequent impairments. As with many of the conditions described in this book, the general principles of rehabilitation apply and more detailed information given in other chapters remains relevant for specific activity limitations and participation restrictions.

Classification

There is no overall accepted classification for muscle conditions. Table 34.2 illustrates an overview of types of muscle conditions according to whether inherited or acquired and the primary pathological process involved.

Although the rehabilitation physician sees a predominance of the inherited muscle conditions when involved in a specific neuromuscular service, the acquired conditions need to be considered as potential contributors to the complexity of medical problems that rehabilitation physicians will see in other patient groups.

Table 34.2 An outline classification of muscle diseases

Inherited	Muscular dystrophies
	Congenital myopathies
	Myotonic dystrophies
	Channelopathies
	Metabolic myopathies
Acquired	Inflammatory myopathies
	Myasthenic syndromes
	Endocrine induced
	Nutritional deficiency
	Drugs and toxin induced
	Autoimmune
	Paraneoplastic

Impairments

Muscle wasting, weakness, and contractures

Muscle dysfunction understandably leads to weakness. ➔ Chapter 33 gives an overview of the effects of weakness.

Muscle wasting itself has an impact on the patient. Patients can be very aware of the cosmetic impact, especially when it involves the face. It is also a factor in weight loss associated with muscle disease, and the change in proportions of body muscle and fat are important when considering weight changes and nutrition in those with muscle conditions. Pseudohypertrophy occurs in conditions such as DMD and Becker muscular dystrophy, for instance, in the calves, deltoids, and tongue. Those muscles affected are also weak, with pseudohypertrophy being due to replacement of muscle by fat and fibrous tissue, alongside limited muscle fibre hypertrophy.

Contractures often occur, varying in distribution according to condition. They occur as a result of an imbalance in muscle strength across a joint, the effects of gravity once muscles lose antigravity strength, and sometimes may occur due to compensatory mechanisms.

Fatigue

Muscle fatigue limits the extent to which a person with muscle disease can continue an activity and this can have a profound effect on participation—for many activities it is important not only to do them once but to continue to do so throughout the day. Alongside this, those with muscle disease often have high levels of perceived fatigue, which may be due to a combination of physiological muscle fatigue and the effect of many activities being difficult, thus requiring more physical and cognitive effort.

Fatigue is the predominant symptom in many metabolic myopathies, such as McArdle's disease. In such conditions, the ability of the muscle to use energy is impaired resulting in patients often suddenly experiencing muscle weakness and fatigue.

Pain

Myalgia can be a prominent symptom in some muscle conditions, most frequently in Becker muscular dystrophy, facioscapulohumeral muscular dystrophy (FSH), limb girdle muscular dystrophy type 2I, myotonic dystrophy type 2, and metabolic myopathies. It can be associated with several endocrine disorders and nutritional deficiencies (see later sections). Myalgia and muscle fatigue can be associated with rhabdomyolysis and subsequent renal failure. It is therefore important to gain a detailed history of muscle pain, including any history suggestive of myoglobinuria. For a useful review of the assessment and investigation of myalgia see Kyriakides et al.[1]

In addition to myalgia, many people with muscle conditions experience aching associated with the musculotendinous complex that is probably associated with weakness and deterioration in posture. This can be particularly noticeable in the neck and back.

Respiratory impairment
Weakness of respiratory muscles and, in myotonic dystrophy, impaired central control of respiration, leads to type 2 respiratory failure and is the leading cause of death in many muscle conditions. The underlying principles and management are described in ➲ Chapter 17.

Cardiac impairment
Several muscle conditions are associated with cardiac impairment due to pathological involvement of cardiac muscle and the conduction system.

Cardiac conduction disorders can lead to heart block or tachyarrhythmias, including sudden death. It is important to screen by taking a targeted history, and performing ECGs and various forms of heart monitoring, although identifying arrhythmias can be difficult as they may be infrequent and asymptomatic. The severity of the conduction disorder is often not associated with the severity of the skeletal muscle condition. They occur most frequently in the myotonic dystrophies, Emery–Dreifuss muscular dystrophy, limb girdle muscular dystrophy (LGMD) 1B, and desmin myopathies.

Most of the cardiomyopathies are dilated in nature, and treated as any cardiomyopathy would be. They occur in DMD, Becker muscular dystrophy, and many of the limb girdle muscular dystrophies. Use of implantable cardiac defibrillators is becoming more common in line with general heart failure guidelines, although the relative risks of arrhythmia secondary to ischaemic and non-ischaemic cardiomyopathies is uncertain. Specialist cardiology advice, especially with regard to use of implantable defibrillators, is important.

Gastrointestinal impairments
Impairment of smooth and skeletal muscle can lead to several GI problems:
* Dysphagia usually only becomes problematic in those with more advanced muscle disease, although it occurs relatively early in inclusion body myositis. Management is as described in ➲ Chapter 9.
* Delayed gastric emptying has been reported in DMD and myotonic dystrophy and is likely to occur in other muscle conditions.
* Slow intestinal transit time and GI dysmotility probably occur in several muscle conditions. People with myotonic dystrophy often have irritable bowel-like symptoms of diarrhoea, pain, and bloating, sometimes due to bacterial overgrowth.
* Constipation is multifactorial, secondary to immobility, smooth muscle, and skeletal muscle involvement. It can be managed in a similar way to other conditions, by increasing dietary fibre, ensuring an adequate fluid intake, and use of aperients and suppositories.

Extramuscular impairments
Some of the inherited muscle conditions have extramuscular manifestations. The myotonic dystrophies are well-known examples, and the systemic aspects of these conditions will be described in later sections in this chapter. However, it is becoming increasingly recognized that genetic mutations in other conditions can have effects on tissues other than muscle, for instance, in DMD it is recognized that there are changes in the brain and in the renal tubules.

Assessment and diagnosis

Diagnosis is a specialist area and general diagnostic principles are described in this section. It is important for patients to see a myologist for primary diagnosis or if their diagnosis is being re-evaluated. More detailed information regarding neuromuscular disease texts are described in ➜ 'Further reading'.

The pattern of muscle weakness and wasting is important in diagnosis. Most conditions produce symmetrical weakness, but that symmetry may not be exact with some conditions, such as FSH, often being associated with a greater degree of muscle weakness on one side. Apart from the broad distinction between peripheral and proximal patterns of weakness in the early stages of disease, very specific muscle groups are involved in some conditions, for example, wasting and weakness of the long finger flexors in inclusion body myositis (Fig. 34.2).

Creatine kinase (CK) is elevated in some conditions, but not all. The use of MRI in identifying specific patterns of muscle involvement is an expanding trend in evaluation of muscle disease. EMG is rarely of value. Some conditions have specific mutations associated with them, so genetic mutation analysis is important in diagnosis, but other conditions can only be diagnosed by muscle biopsy. There remain individuals in whom a specific genetic mutation cannot be identified.

Various aspects of muscle conditions can be measured in order to assess response to rehabilitation interventions:

- Timed tests, such as the 6-minute walk test.
- Specific impairments, such as respiratory impairment.
- Specific extended ADL scales, such as the performance of UL in DMD.
- Specific QOL using measures, such as the individualized neuromuscular quality of life scale (INQoL).

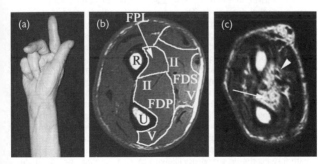

Fig. 34.2 MRI of forearm muscles in inclusion body myositis, showing wasting of flexor digitorum profundus (FDP), flexor digitorum superficialis (FDS), and flexor pollicis longus (FPL).

Reproduced with permission from Takamure M. et al. Finger flexor weakness in inclusion body myositis. *Neurology*, 64(2):389. Copyright © 2005, American Academy of Neurology. https://doi.org/10.1212/01.WNL.0000142980.87159.8C.

Examples of muscle conditions

There are brief descriptions of several muscle conditions, or groups of conditions, in the following sections. They have been chosen as representative of different aspects of muscle conditions and because they are some of the commoner conditions.

Acquired myopathies

In comparison to the many inherited and inflammatory myopathies, acquired myopathies secondary to other conditions receive relatively less attention. However, there is a high probability that anyone involved in rehabilitation will see patients with such secondary disorders. Examples include the following:

Endocrine conditions

Myopathies can occur in:
- hypothyroidism, associated with myalgia and an increase in CK
- hyperthyroidism, associated with proximal weakness
- Cushing syndrome
- hyperparathyroidism
- acromegaly.

Myalgia is associated with:
- hypoparathyroidism
- hypothyroidism
- hypoadrenalism.

Drugs and toxins

Many pharmacological substances are associated with myopathy. Some more frequently encountered in rehabilitation medicine practice include the following:
- *Alcohol*. Most commonly, alcohol causes a slow-onset myopathy, but can cause rhabdomyolysis. The response is dose dependent. It can be compounded by nutritional deficiency associated with alcoholism. A chronic proximal myopathy occurs in 30–70% of heavy drinkers, with type II fibre atrophy and type I fibre hypertrophy. It can be reversed by stopping consumption of alcohol.
- *Antipsychotics* can cause neuroleptic malignant syndrome (NMS). The reaction is partly idiosyncratic, but is more likely if the person is also dehydrated and if the dose of antipsychotic is higher or escalated more quickly. The mechanism is unclear but is associated with a reduction in dopaminergic activation. NMS consists of hyperthermia, rigidity, autonomic instability, and change in mental state. The muscle rigidity can lead to muscle necrosis with increase in CK that can progress to rhabdomyolysis, myoglobinuria, and renal failure. NMS is treated by withdrawing the drug or drugs likely to cause it; cooling; use of muscle relaxants such as benzodiazepines and dantrolene; use of dopamine agonists such as bromocriptine and amantadine; and correcting fluid and electrolyte imbalance. Electroconvulsive therapy has been used successfully when NMS is not responsive to these measures, and can also treat the underlying psychiatric condition.

- *Statins.* There is debate over the terminology of muscle conditions associated with statins, currently the preferred term is SAMS—statin-associated muscle symptoms (SAMS). Broadly, statins can cause a myalgia with or without a rise in CK, a CK rise without myalgia, rhabdomyolysis, and/or a necrotizing myopathy, and more commonly seen with hydrophilic compared to the lipophilic statins. Fortunately, myalgia alone is the commonest complication and is reversible on withdrawing the statin, or changing the type or frequency of statin. Estimates of the frequency of statin-associated myalgia vary between 5% and 30% of those taking statins. A necrotizing myositis is extremely rare but persists when the statin is withdrawn and is an immunological reaction. A common concern is whether it is safe for people with muscle disease to take statins, and current evidence suggests that cautious use and slow introduction at a low dose is safe in the majority of patients, outweighing the risk posed by high cholesterol.
- *Steroids.* Prednisolone and dexamethasone reduce protein synthesis and increase protein catabolism in muscle, leading to atrophy of type II muscle fibres and a predominantly proximal weakness. This can occur acutely, and there is overlap here with critical care myopathy, or the onset can be slow. CK levels are usually normal. Exercise and physical activity possibly ameliorate muscle atrophy secondary to steroids, with trials ongoing.

Electrolyte disturbance
Hypokalaemia, hypomagnesaemia, and hypophosphataemia are all associated with muscle weakness.

Nutritional deficiency
- Vitamin D deficiency. Muscle weakness and falls are associated with reduced levels of vitamin D. There is a positive correlation between vitamin D levels, supplementation, and muscle strength or function.
- Selenium has an antioxidant function in muscle metabolism. Deficiency is associated with muscle weakness and myalgia in areas where intake is low due to selenium poor soil, in conditions associated with starvation such as anorexia nervosa, and in dependency on enteral or parenteral nutrition or malabsorption.
- Thiamine deficiency can cause myalgia.

Systemic disease
Many chronic conditions are associated with muscle atrophy (e.g. renal, hepatic, cardiac or respiratory failure, and cancer) related to increased muscle protein breakdown and a catabolic state. There are various ongoing trials of agents and physical activity that may reduce muscle wasting in these conditions.

Duchenne muscular dystrophy
DMD has a prevalence of 4–5 per 100,000 males. It is due to a mutation of the dystrophin protein on the X chromosome that causes a short non-functional protein to be produced, in contrast to the rarer Becker muscular dystrophy where the dystrophin mutation causes a poorly functioning protein.

DMD becomes apparent in early childhood, usually with a diagnosis at about 5 years of age. Motor milestones are often delayed, and by the age of 5 years the child is usually struggling to run, walk, jump, and climb stairs as easily as his peers. Cognitive function can be affected, especially with regard to verbal immediate memory and language. There is also a higher incidence of autistic spectrum and attention deficit hyperactivity disorders.

Muscle weakness begins proximally, especially with weakness of the hip and knee extensors giving rise to the typical 'Gower's manoeuvre' (Fig. 34.3). Weakness progresses so that, without interventions, the ability to walk is lost between the ages of 10 and 15 years. Death without intervention is at an average age of 17 years. Fortunately, the outlook for DMD is improving due to use of interventions such as NIV, spinal surgery, and steroids. These have improved survival in DMD, so that the mean age of death has increased to the late 20s, with some patients surviving into their 40s.

Young men with DMD are increasingly able to participate in adult life due to equipment such as specialized seating systems, powered wheelchairs, adapted cars, electronic AT, and powered mobile arm supports.

Facioscapulohumeral muscular dystrophy

FSH is one of the commoner muscular dystrophies of adult life. Prevalence is usually quoted as being about 5 per 100,000, although a recent Dutch study gave an estimate of 12 per 100,000.[2] It is an autosomal dominant condition, with a deletion in the D4Z4 repeat sequence on chromosome 4q. Symptoms most frequently begin around 20 years of age, but can start in childhood or later in adult life. The first muscles affected are those of the face, shoulder girdle, and foot dorsiflexors, with gradual progression to other muscles over time. Approximately 20% of people with FSH need to use a wheelchair after 50 years of age. The lumbar lordosis becomes exaggerated relatively early in the course of the condition. Respiratory involvement occurs in about 10%. The severity of facial weakness leads to reduced eye closure, so corneal irritation and keratitis can occur, with eye drops being useful in symptom management and reduction of secondary inflammation.

There are two important extramuscular manifestations:
• Sensorineural hearing loss, commoner when onset is in childhood, so it is important to screen for hearing loss in children with FSH.
• Retinal vascular disease, rare but commoner in those with larger deletions, so it is recommended that those with deletions of 10–20 kB are referred for specialist ophthalmological examination.

Important interventions:
• AFOs can control the degree of foot drop and improve gait, although there are the practical limitations of difficulties associated with comfort and cosmesis outweighing efficacy, as found in other conditions.
• Scapular fixation can be used to improve the ability to elevate the upper limbs. It is done while there is still normal strength in deltoid to 45° of abduction.
• There is some evidence for the safety and efficacy of aerobic and strengthening exercise in FSH, with benefits shown for muscle strength, VO_2 max, walking, and fatigue.
• Fatigue can be a problem and has been shown to benefit from both CBT and aerobic exercise approaches.

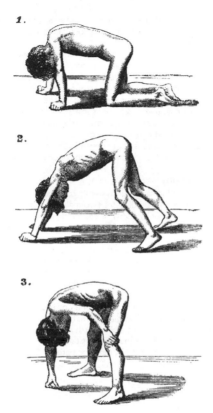

Fig. 34.3 Gower's manoeuvre showing a method of getting off the floor adopted by boys with DMD.

Reproduced from W. R. Gowers. *Pseudo-hypertrophic Muscular Paralysis: A Clinical Lecture*. London, UK: J. & A. Churchill. 1879.

Idiopathic inflammatory myopathies

These include the following:

• Sporadic inclusion body myositis (IBM). This is a condition of older adult life, with approximately 80% of patients being older than 60 years at presentation. Weakness is found first in the long finger flexors and quadriceps, with dysphagia occurring relatively early. It can be associated with autoimmune conditions but behaves more as a neurodegenerative condition. There is a poor response to immunosuppressants, and there is no evidence that they make a difference to the course of the

condition. There is evidence that aerobic and strengthening exercise is
safe, tolerated, and can lead to mild improvements in aerobic capacity
and muscle strength.
• Dermatomyositis, juvenile dermatomyositis, and polymyositis. These
conditions present with limb girdle and anterior neck flexor muscle
weakness, fever, and myalgia. In dermatomyositis there are additional
dermatological features of an erythematous rash over the face,
neck, and upper chest, heliotropic periorbital oedema, and a raised
erythematous rash over the extensor surfaces of joints (Gottron's
papules). Muscle weakness can progress early to cause dysphagia and
dysarthria. Table 34.3 shows some of the complications and associations
of inflammatory myositis. As with other muscle conditions, benefit has
been shown from aerobic and strengthening exercise programmes.

Myotonic dystrophy

The myotonic dystrophies are multisystemic conditions, affecting many organs as well as causing muscle disease. Two main types are recognized:
• Type 1 myotonic dystrophy (DM1) is caused by a CTG trinucleotide
repeat on chromosome 19. It is the commonest muscular dystrophy
of adult life. Prevalence varies between countries, being about 9–13/
100,000 in most countries. It is rarer in non-Caucasians and commoner
in specific populations where there has been a founder effect, such as
in Quebec, Canada. There are subtypes of congenital, childhood-onset,
adult-onset, and minimal myotonic dystrophy.
• Type 2 myotonic dystrophy (DM2) is due to a tetranucleotide repeat
expansion of the zinc-finger protein 9 gene on chromosome 3. It is
less common, and possibly less diagnosed, than DM1, with prevalence
being highest in countries with a high north European component to the
population, for example, Finland has an estimated prevalence of about
10/100,000 compared to the UK (approximately 0.2/100,000) and Italy
(approximately 1/100,000).

Table 34.3 Conditions associated with the three commonest
inflammatory myopathies.

Association	Juvenile dermatomyositis	Dermatomyositis	Polymyositis
Malignancy		√	√
Interstitial lung disease		√	√
GI vasculopathy	√		
Myalgia	√		√
Rhabdomyolysis	√	√	√
Calcinosis	√		
Lipodystrophy	√		
Cardiac disease	√	√	√

Non-skeletal muscle features of DM1 include:
- early-onset cataracts
- frontal pattern balding
- reduced androgen and follicle-stimulating hormone levels, increased luteinizing hormone levels
- pseudohypoparathyroidism with poor sensitivity of parathyroid hormone receptor (PTH) receptors and increased levels of PTH
- increased incidence of diabetes mellitus type 2 and impaired glucose tolerance
- cardiac rhythm and conduction disorders
- cognitive changes, with impairment of executive functioning, social functioning, and increased levels of apathy
- excessive daytime sleepiness
- learning disability in all with congenital DM1 and some with childhood-onset DM1
- dysphagia
- slow GI transit, with increased rates of constipation and bacterial overgrowth
- increased incidence of gallbladder disease
- abnormal response to specific anaesthetics
- sensitivity to opiates
- prolonged labour and increased incidence of postpartum haemorrhage due to uterine smooth muscle dysfunction
- increased incidence of various cancers, although not sufficiently high for screening to be of use.

There is considerable variation between individuals in the development of these features.

Skeletal muscle impairments include myotonia, weakness, and poor fatigue resistance of muscles. Facial, cervical, finger flexor, and ankle dorsiflexor muscles are the first to be affected, with gradual progression to other muscle groups. Respiratory muscles, especially the diaphragm, can be affected relatively early, causing type 2 respiratory failure. DM2 differs by the distribution of muscle weakness, being more proximal than distal with muscle stiffness, more prominent myotonia, and myalgia. There is not a congenital form of the condition and anaesthetic complications have not been reported. The other features found in DM1 can occur.

Given the variety of problems that a person with myotonic dystrophy can experience, there is considerable scope for a rehabilitative approach to maximize participation. In addition to screening for and minimizing potential complications, aerobic and strengthening exercise has been shown to be beneficial. The dysexecutive problems and apathy that are common in myotonic dystrophy mean that any rehabilitation programme needs to accommodate and adapt for them when considering work, education, relationships, and other aspects of participation.

Rehabilitation management

Although there are important differences between these muscle conditions, paying attention to the following aspects can assist in rehabilitation management. The rehabilitation medicine physician can play a vital role in recognition and coordination of the different areas of management to optimize activity and participation:

- Respiratory management (for details, ⟴ see Chapter 17):
  - Cough augmentation, using breath stacking, a lung volume recruitment bag, or cough assist device.
  - NIV.
  - Respiratory emergency management plans.
  - Influenza and pneumococcal vaccination.
- Bone health: currently the risks and benefits of long-term bisphosphonates are uncertain, but it is logical to at least ensure normal vitamin D levels. Enabling a person to stand will also assist in maintaining bone health.
- Nutrition: following the principles of good nutrition, maintaining a BMI in the normal range, and use of modified diet and enteral nutrition as necessary when swallowing is affected.
- Bowel management: to avoid constipation and pseudo-obstruction.
- Cardiac management: screening those at risk of arrhythmia, conduction block, and cardiomyopathy. Pharmacological management of cardiac impairments is the same as for any other cause of these.
- Good posture, seating, and contracture management.
- Use of electronic AT.
- Exercise: research has shown that exercise can be tolerated without harm if prescribed appropriately and can have some positive benefits. Various modalities of exercise have been studied, for instance, endurance and strengthening gym-based exercises, yoga, Qi-gong, and Pilates. The details of an exercise prescription will vary according to individuals and muscle condition but general principles are as follows:
  - Using exercise that the person themselves is interested in and will be able to maintain.
  - The person should be advised to look out for signs of over-exercising. Muscle pain the following day is an indicator they have done too much. Greater caution needs to be taken in conditions that carry a risk of rhabdomyolysis but exercise is still possible.
  - Using a variety of prescribed exercises, alone or within a group programme, including strengthening, endurance, and flexibility.
  - Considering exercise for basic fitness as well as to achieve specific personal goals (e.g. related to pain or a particular activity).
  - Recognizing incidental exercise as a valid supplementary approach to a prescribed exercise programme.
  - Making allowance for the lower muscle strength and greater fatigue, and the slower rate of improvement in these when devising an exercise prescription.

- Information and peer support. As with many conditions, the optimal format and rate at which people acquire information about their condition is very individual. It is therefore important to ascertain what information a person needs and how they prefer to have that information. Enquiry about information needs should be revisited periodically, as they may change over time. Patient support groups can provide such education and are available for most conditions, examples of some of these are given in ➲ 'Further reading'.
- Transition from paediatric to adult care. Those diagnosed in childhood will require transition to adult care. Use of a transition service can ensure that this happens as smoothly as possible and can help to address the extra needs a young person has at that time.
- Role of family. As many muscle conditions are inherited, family members often have prior knowledge of the condition, and some may also be affected. Genetic counselling is important in these circumstances, along with a sensitivity to the needs of family members playing a caring role. Support groups are often invaluable sources of support.

References

1. Kyriakides T, Angelini C, Schaefer J, et al. (2013). EFNS review on the role of muscle biopsy in the investigation of myalgia. *European Journal of Neurology* 20, 997–1005.
2. Deenen JC, Arnts H, van der Maarel SM, et al. (2014). Population-based incidence and prevalence of facioscapulohumeral dystrophy. *Neurology* 83, 1056–1059.

Further reading

Bushby K, Finkel R, Birnkrant DJ, et al. (2010). Diagnosis and management of Duchenne muscular dystrophy, part 1: diagnosis, and pharmacological and psychosocial management. *Lancet Neurology* 9, 77–93.

Bushby K, Finkel R, Birnkrant DJ, et al. (2010). Diagnosis and management of Duchenne muscular dystrophy, part 2: implementation of multidisciplinary care. *Lancet Neurology* 9, 177–189.

Hilton-Jones D, Turner MR (2014). *Oxford Textbook of Neuromuscular Disorders*. Oxford University Press, Oxford.

Meyer A, Meyer N, Schaeffer M, et al. (2010). Incidence and prevalence of inflammatory myopathies: a systematic review. *Rheumatology* 54, 50–63.

Norwood FL, Harling C, Chinnery PF, et al. (2009). Prevalence of genetic muscle disease in Northern England: in-depth analysis of a muscle clinic population. *Brain* 132, 3175–3186.

Rizos CV, Elisaf MS (2017). Statin myopathy: navigating the maze. *Current Medical Research and Opinion* 33, 327–329.

Schaefer AM, McFarland R, Blakely EL, et al. (2008). Prevalence of mitochondrial DNA disease in adults. *Annals of Neurology*, 63, 35–39.

Theadom, A, Rodrigues M, Roxburgh R, et al. (2014). Prevalence of muscular dystrophies: a systematic literature review. *Neuroepidemiology* 43, 259–268.

Useful websites

⅍ http://www.enmc.org/home/—the European Neuromuscular Centre website, with summaries of workshops concerning neuromuscular conditions.

⅍ http://www.musculardystrophyuk.org/—the Muscular Dystrophy UK website.

⅍ http://www.myotonicdystrophysupportgroup.org/—the Myotonic dystrophy support group website, an example of one of many support groups for specific types of muscle condition.

⅍ http://neuromuscular.wustl.edu/—the Neuromuscular Disease Centre at Washington University (St. Louis, MO, US) giving synopses of different neuromuscular conditions.

Common musculoskeletal conditions

Global burden of musculoskeletal conditions

The Global Burden of Disease study identified musculoskeletal (MSK) conditions as the largest single cause of years lived with disability, and the second largest cause of disability-adjusted life years in developed countries.[1] These include back pain, osteoarthritis (OA), inflammatory arthritis, chronic pain, and other overuse-related conditions. MSK conditions affect more than 10 million people in the UK and cost society around £5.7 billion per year. Over 9 million working days are lost in a year due to MSK conditions, second only to mental ill health. Co-morbid anxiety and depression are common in chronic MSK pain and around one-quarter of patients have major depressive symptoms. Chronicity of the condition is associated with poorer outcome for the individual and the society.

MSK medicine and rehabilitation services worldwide are heterogeneous in nature in terms of patient pathway and involvement of various healthcare professionals. The service can be led by consultants in different medical specialties: in primary care by GPs with a special interest in MSK disorders and in secondary care by rheumatologists, orthopaedic surgeons, neurosurgeons, pain specialists, rehabilitation, and MSK physicians. Allied health professionals such as physiotherapists and extended scope practitioners now have a far greater role in managing MSK conditions in some countries such as the UK.

Screening for serious pathology/'flags'

Clinicians use colour 'flags' to highlight risk factors in MSK conditions and to identify potential barriers to rehabilitation[2]:

- *Red flags*: indicate serious pathology which often requires action for urgent surgical opinion. For example, bowel or bladder incontinence in back pain.
- *Yellow flags*: indicate psychosocial factors that influence chronicity and response to treatment. For example, fear avoidance behaviour in spinal pain.
- *Blue flags*: indicate modifiable work perceptions.
- *Black flags*: denote work conditions that could inhibit progress with recovery, for example, a desk at the wrong height or a requirement to do repetitive or heavy lifting.
- *Orange flags*: indicate drug abuse or abnormal psychological processes.

Principles of patient education and promotion of self-management

Effective patient education is likely to depend as much on the method of delivery as the content. It is both helpful and constructive to dispel any misconceptions which may act as a barrier to recovery. The clinician needs to give credible explanations to provide the patient with confidence to carry out rehabilitation and to return to normal activities as soon as reasonably practicable.

The American College of Sports Medicine's exercise prescription guidelines (8th edition) recommend that no medical consultation is required prior to exercise for healthy adults.[3] Screening prior to exercise is advised in:

- women aged 55 and older, men aged 45 and older
- those patients with more than two cardiovascular disease risk factors
- patients with signs or symptoms of coronary heart disease
- patients with known cardiac, pulmonary, or metabolic disease.

Exercise prescription must be tailored to level of readiness for change. Individuals progress through four key stages: pre-contemplation, contemplation, action, and maintenance prior to developing a habit.

Osteoarthritis

OA is the commonest form of arthritis and is the main cause of locomotor disability worldwide.

Aetiopathogenesis

OA results from an imbalance in catabolic and anabolic processes leading to progressive cartilage damage. The reparative process leads to replacement of hyaline by fibrocartilage, subchondral bone damage and marginal osteophyte formation.

Risk factors for OA

- Age—OA is uncommon in those less than 45 years of age but is seen in 80% of those older than 55 years.
- Sex—females are more likely than men in the age group over 50 years.
- Occupation—for example, farmers are associated with hip OA.
- Genetic—inherited component to hand, knee, and hip OA.
- Lifestyle—for example, obesity.
- Hormonal factors—oestrogen deficiency after menopause.

Diagnosis of OA

- The diagnosis of OA is based on clinical and radiological findings—laboratory tests are normal.
- Physical examination reveals joint effusion, joint line tenderness, crepitus, restricted range of movement, and pain and stiffness on activity.
- Plain X-rays show joint space narrowing, osteophytes, subchondral cysts, and subchondral sclerosis (Fig. 35.1).
- Often too much importance is given to radiographic change and a poor correlation exists between structural changes and symptoms.
- Analysis of synovial fluid can also be useful.

Clinical features of OA

OA commonly affects the hips, knees, distal interphalangeal joints (DIPs), thumb joint (first carpometacarpal joint), lower cervical spine, and first metatarsophalangeal joint. Specific finding in the hand include bony enlargement of proximal interphalangeal joints (Bouchard's nodes) and the distal interphalangeal joints (Heberden's nodes). Clinical features the patient may experience include:

- pain on activity
- post activity stiffness
- joint swelling
- reduced joint function
- bony enlargement
- joint instability
- joint effusion
- gait abnormalities
- Heberden's nodes on DIPs
- Bouchard's nodes
- crepitus
- restricted joint movement
- muscle weakness and wasting.

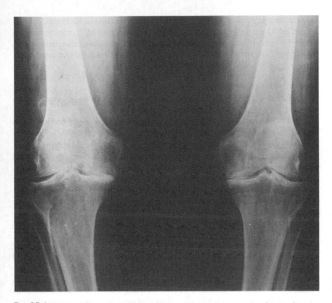

Fig. 35.1 Bilateral knee osteoarthritis showing joint space narrowing, bony sclerosis, and osteophytes.

Reproduced with permission from Brion P.H. and Kalunian K.C. Osteoarthritis in *Oxford Textbook of Medicine*, Warrell D.A. et al. (Eds.). Oxford, UK: Oxford University Press. © 2010 Oxford University Press. Reproduced with permission of Oxford University Press through PLSclear. http://oxfordmedicine.com/view/10.1093/med/9780199204854.001.1/med-9780199204854-chapter-1909.

Secondary causes of OA

- Mechanical—obesity, trauma, and previous joint surgery.
- Neuropathic disorder—diabetes mellitus.
- Inflammatory arthritis—rheumatoid arthritis (RA), gout, and septic arthritis.
- Anatomical abnormalities—bone dysplasia.
- Metabolic/endocrine—haemochromatosis, acromegaly, and hyperparathyroidism.
- Developmental—hypermobility, congenital dislocation of the hip, Perthes disease, and epiphyseal dysplasias.

Management of OA

The aims of treatment include educating the patient so self-management strategies can be adopted, pain management, and maintaining function. The misconception that OA is due to ageing often leads to patients to believe that little can be done when in fact, there are many coping strategies that the patient can engage in. A patient's mood is an important factor in determining how successfully symptoms are managed and should be assessed along with sleep during the assessment process and treatment advocated if necessary. Consequently it is important to involve the patient in all aspects of care management so that they can become an active participant in their care.

Drug management

Paracetamol is the drug of choice and the patient may need educating on the benefits of taking paracetamol at regular intervals to achieve maximum effect. Topical non-steroidal drugs or capsaicin can be useful for hand and knee OA. If oral non-steroidal drugs are required they should be used for a short time span and at a low dose during a flare of the symptoms. Non-steroidal drugs are not recommended for use in elderly patients. Some studies have demonstrated improvement with the use of the health supplement glucosamine and chondroitin salts but evidence is inconclusive. Joint aspiration and injection with corticosteroid can be used for symptomatic relief. Intra-articular injection of hyaluronic acid has become popular, but any effect is likely to be small.

Exercise

The most helpful advice to give a patient with OA is to carry out regular exercise. Many patients are fearful that exercise will increase their pain and lead to the affected joint 'wearing out'. It is important to reassure the patient that this is not the case and in fact a reduction in activity will lead to an escalation of their symptoms. The type of exercise that is required includes strengthening exercises for specific joints as well as advice on aerobic exercise to improve stamina and fatigue. Exercise can also help with weight reduction, joint proprioception, and psychological status. Versus Arthritis produces a range of educational booklets that provide advice on exercise.[4]

Reducing of biomechanical stress

- Weight reduction can reduce pain and improve stamina and general levels of fitness.
- Insoles and the use of shoes with deep cushioning—such as trainers— can redistribute stress and reduce impact loading.
- The use of walking sticks and other mobility aids need to be considered to improve function.
- Increased muscle balance (length/strength) around affected joints will support biomechanical alignment.

Surgery

- Surgery should be considered for patients who have failed conservative management, those with uncontrolled pain, especially at night, and considerable limitation in function.
- Surgical options are joint lavage, menisectomy (knee), synovectomy, realignment, partial joint replacement, and total joint replacement. Hip and knee replacements have been proven to greatly improve a person's QOL.
- Surgery has also become more common on shoulder, elbow, and thumb joints.

Inflammatory arthritis: rheumatoid arthritis

RA is the most common inflammatory arthritis, which primarily causes syno-vitis that leads to cartilage destruction and bone erosions. The condition has potential to impact physical, psychological, and social function. Many patients find it difficult to remain in work and leisure activities are often curtailed. Early diagnosis and treatment is required to try and minimize dis-ability and morbidity. Patients can experience a combination of acute pain, which often occurs when there is a 'flare' of disease activity as well as daily (chronic) pain affecting the muscles and the joints. The frequency of the pain can result in fatigue, low mood, and impinge on functional activities.

Incidence of RA

Population studies suggest an incidence of 3.4 per 10,000 in women and 1.4 per 10,000 in men. Although RA affects all ages, the commonest time of onset in women is in the third to fifth decades while in men the incidence increases over the age of 45 years.

Cause of RA

The cause is unknown but there is a genetic predisposition that may be triggered by infective, hormonal, or environmental factors. First-degree re-latives are twice as likely to develop RA than the general population and approximately 50% of patients will carry the antigen HLA DR4. Cigarette smoking has been shown to be associated with development of RA.

Diagnosis of RA

Diagnosis is arrived at through a combination of clinical and laboratory tests. Onset is insidious with inflammation, pain, and stiffness present in synovial joints. The small joints (metacarpophalangeal, proximal interphalangeal, wrist, and metatarsophalangeal joints) are commonly affected with sym-metrical changes (Fig. 35.2). Laboratory tests and radiographs are used to support the clinical impression of RA and exclude other differential diagnosis. The American College of Rheumatology and European League against Rheumatism 2010 criteria for the classification of RA are shown in Fig. 35.3.

Clinical features of RA

RA has both articular and extra-articular features as listed:
- Polyarticular swelling
- Early morning stiffness
- Joint pain
- Nodules
- Fatigue
- Myalgia
- Weight loss
- Muscle wasting
- Renal—glomerulonephritis and amyloidosis
- Ocular—episcleritis, scleritis, Sjögren's syndrome, and keratoconjunctivitis sicca

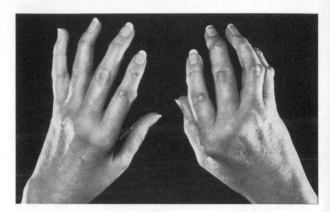

Fig. 35.2 Hands of a person suffering from rheumatoid arthritis. Features include symmetrical soft tissue swelling of second and third metacarpophalangeal (MCP) joints, early swan-neck deformity of left ring finger, ulnar deviation of MCP joints, wasting of small muscles of hand, and small rheumatoid nodules.

Reproduced with permission from Maini R.N. Rheumatoid arthritis in Oxford Textbook of Medicine, Warrell D.A. et al. oxofrd, UK: Oxford University Press. © 2010 Oxford University Press.

Reproduced with permission of Oxford University Press through PLSclear.
http://oxfordmedicine.com/view/10.1093/med/9780199204854.001.1/
med-9780199204854-chapter-1905.

- Cardiac—pericarditis, myocarditis, and valve abnormalities
- Pulmonary—pleural effusions, interstitial disease, and nodules
- Neurological—peripheral neuropathy
- Vascular—vasculitis, rashes
- Skin—rash, ulcers, and vascular lesions
- Spinal cord—cord compression
- Haematological—anaemia and Felty syndrome.

Management of RA

The aim of treatment is to optimize physical, psychological, and social function and to prevent structural damage and deformity. To achieve this, a multidisciplinary approach is required.

Drug therapy

The aims of drug therapy are to provide symptom relief and suppress the activity of the condition. First-line therapy consisting of analgesia and NSAIDs are used to reduce pain and stiffness. Second-line therapy including disease-modifying antirheumatic drugs (DMARDs) and cytotoxic and biological therapy is used when the disease is active. It is important to commence DMARDs as soon as diagnosis is confirmed to minimize structural damage and preserve function. The different DMARDs include:

- traditional small-molecule DMARDs—hydroxychloroquine, sulfasalazine, gold injections, methotrexate, leflunomide, azathioprine, and penicillamine

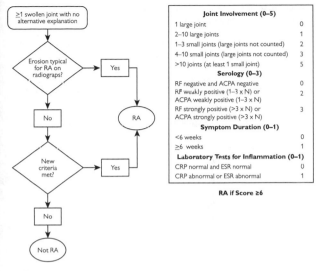

Fig. 35.3 Classification criteria for rheumatoid arthritis (RA).
Note on abbreviations: RF: Rheumatoid Factor; ACPA: Anti-Citrullinated Peptide.

Reproduced with permission from Michet C.J. Rheumatoid Arthritis and Spondyloarthropathies. In *Mayo Clinic Internal Medicine Board Review* (11 ed.), edited by Christopher M. Wittich. © 2016 Oxford University Press. Reproduced with permission of Oxford University Press through PLSclear. Adapted with permission from Gaujoux-Viala C et al. Recommendations of the French Society for Rheumatology for managing rheumatoid arthritis. *Joint Bone Spine*, 81(4):287–297. Copyright © 2014 Société française de rhumatologie. Published by Elsevier Masson SAS. Adapted with permission from Aletaha D et al. Rheumatoid arthritis classification criteria: an American College of Rheumatology/European League Against Rheumatism collaborative initiative. *Ann Rheum Dis*, 69(9):1580–1588. Erratum in: *Ann Rheum Dis*, 69(10):1892. Copyright © 2010 by the American College of Rheumatology. Published by John Wiley and Sons.

- biological DMARDs such as adalimumab, etanercept, infliximab, and rituximab.
- emerging small-molecule DMARDSs.

For a flare of disease activity, intramuscular or intravenous steroid can be administered.

Education and management

It is important that a patient learns to self-manage the daily symptoms of the condition. Education can be provided in individual or group format and often involves many members of the MDT including the following:

- Specialist nurse—to provide information about the condition, monitor drug therapy, provide psychological support, and advise on symptom management (e.g. fatigue and sleep disturbance). ➔ See 'Fibromyalgia' for advice regarding sleep.

- Physiotherapist—in the acute phase, the focus is upon reduction of pain and inflammation with hot/cold modalities (heat is useful for muscular pain and ice packs can reduce the swelling of inflamed joints), transcutaneous electrical nerve stimulation (TENS) (pain gating), and hydrotherapy. In the rehabilitation phase, joint protection and function are the focus with therapeutic exercise to address muscle weakness, range of movement, and pain management; assistive equipment (gait aids); and patient education. Immersion in warm wax baths can help hand pain and stiffness.
- Occupational therapist—joint protection, use of aids, splints to reduce the pain of a swollen joint, hand function, and work and leisure assessment
- Podiatry—foot care and provision of orthoses and insoles to improve posture and function.

Surgery

The aim of surgery is to restore function and/or provide pain relief. Surgery is most effective when the systemic aspect of the condition is under control. The commonest surgery is hip and knee replacement. Replacement of other joints, including shoulder and elbow, is also increasing. Urgent surgery is required for septic arthritis, tendon rupture, and spinal cord decompression. Due to the potential vulnerability of the cervical spine, a preoperative spinal X-ray is required and a cervical collar may be required during surgery to remind theatre staff of the potential problems at the neck. Carpel tunnel syndrome occurs more often in patients with RA and if the symptoms are troublesome, a decompression of the carpel nerve can be carried out.

Factors associated with poor prognosis

- High titre of rheumatoid factor.
- Many active joints at onset.
- High level of disability at onset.
- Presence of extra-articular manifestations.
- Early evidence of radiological erosions.
- Low socioeconomic status.

Evaluating the outcome of RA

There are many tools and markers that can be used to assess the progress of RA. These include the following:

- The disease activity score (DAS)—this is a composite score which includes the number of swollen and tender joints, ESR, and patient global assessment using a visual analogue scale.
- Pain can be assessed using a visual analogue scale, a questionnaire such as the McGill questionnaire, or by palpating the patient's joints for tenderness—the Ritchie articular index.
- Blood markers—such as the ESR and CRP—to indicate a reduction in inflammation.
- Documenting the duration of early-morning stiffness—the higher the duration, the more active the condition will tend to be.

- Measuring functional ability using the Health Assessment Questionnaire which records the patient's physical ability to carry out eight aspects of daily living including dressing and personal hygiene.
- The Arthritis Impact Measurement (AIM) scales focuses on the physical, psychological, and social impact of the condition.
- The Hospital Anxiety and Depression Scale assesses the psychological impact of the condition.

Inflammatory arthritis: spondyloarthropathies

Aetiopathogenesis

The spondyloarthropathies are a group of inflammatory rheumatic diseases affecting the spine, sacroiliac joints, peripheral joints, and entheses. Conditions involved in this group are shown in Table 35.1.

Causes

- HLA B27 is a genetic risk factor.
- Different types of spondyloarthropathies can be found in members of the same family.
- In reactive arthritis, infection is the major cause with the condition triggered by gastroenteritis or urethritis.

Investigations

- Haematology—indicators of inflammation and acute phase response (e.g. ESR and full blood count).
- Immunology—HLA B27 positive in: greater than 90% of ankylosis spondylitis, greater than 80% of reactive arthritis, 75% of enteropathic spondylitis, and 50% of psoriatic spondylitis.
- Absence of rheumatoid factor.
- ESR, CRP may be raised.
- Microbiology—urethral swabs.
- Joint aspiration.
- Radiological investigations.

Clinical features

See Table 35.1.

Treatments for spondyloarthropathies

- *Drug therapy*—to relieve symptoms, analgesia, NSAIDs, antibiotics for reactive arthritis, intramuscular or intra-articular corticosteroid injections. To suppress disease activity, disease-modifying drugs and biological agents.
- *Physiotherapy*—all patients require daily exercises to maintain function, posture, and spinal movement. Ideally this should be done with the support of a physiotherapist. Hydrotherapy is a good medium to improve muscle strength and range of movement. Ultrasound can help with enthesitis and TENS assists some patients in pain management.
- *Surgery*—the most common intervention is hip arthroplasty especially for ankylosing spondylitis patients. Knee and shoulder replacements can also be required.

Table 35.1 Clinical features of spondyloarthropathies

Spondyloarthropathy	Features
Ankylosing spondylitis	Low back and buttock pain
	Peripheral arthritis
	Iritis
	Enthesopathy
	Reduced chest expansion
Reactive arthritis	Urethritis/gastroenteritis
	Lower limb arthritis
	Triad of arthritis, conjunctivitis, and urethritis
	Enthesopathy
	Inflammatory spinal pain
	Keratoderma blennorrhagica
	Amyloidosis
Psoriatic arthritis	Psoriasis
	Monoarthritis or dactylitis ('sausage toe')
	Inflammatory spinal pain
	Enthesopathy
	Nail changes
	Amyloidosis
	Arthritis in several joints
Enteropathic arthritis	Bowel disease
	Lower limb peripheral arthritis
	Spinal pain
	Enthesopathy
	Tendinopathy
SAPHO syndrome	Synovitis
	Acne
	Pustulosis palmaris et plantaris
	Hyperostosis
	Osteitis

Fibromyalgia

Definition

A condition characterized by widespread MSK pain, non-restorative sleep, fatigue, and a host of other physical and psychological associations (Fig. 35.4).

Incidence

Fibromyalgia occurs in 0.5% of men and 3.4% of women. The onset in women usually occurs between 25–45 years. Fibromyalgia is the third commonest reason to be referred to a rheumatologist. Work absenteeism is high among those in work and disability payments are received by one-third of fibromyalgia patients.

Cause

No single pathophysiological causative mechanism has been identified and it would appear that fibromyalgia is a multifactorial syndrome. There is strong familial aggregation reported in fibromyalgia. Fibromyalgia can be associated with other MSK conditions such as rheumatoid arthritis where it is referred to as 'secondary fibromyalgia'.

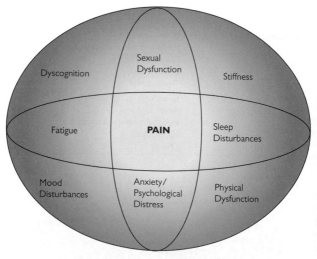

Fig. 35.4 Fibromyalgia domains.

Reproduced with permission from Smith H.S. et al. Fibromyalgia in *Pain Medicine: An Interdisciplinary Case-Based Approach*, Hayek S.M. et al. (Eds.). © 2015 Oxford University Press. Reproduced with permission of Oxford University Press through PLSclear. http://oxfordmedicine.com/view/10.1093/med/9780199931484.001.0001/med-9780199931484-chapter-26.

Possible factors involved in development of fibromyalgia include:
- abnormal pain processing (increased wind-up or central sensitization and reduction of descending analgesic activity)
- genetic predisposition to pain sensitivity
- neurohormonal dysfunction
- neuroendocrine disturbances
- neurotransmitter regulation dysfunction
- allergy, infection, toxicity, and nutritional deficiency
- physical trauma—road accidents and whiplash
- emotional trauma.

Diagnosis

In clinical practice, the diagnosis is made on the basis of the clinical history and examination. The modified American College of Rheumatology criteria for fibromyalgia can be used for clinical and research purposes (Box 35.1).

Box 35.1 The American College of Rheumatology 2010 modified criteria for fibromyalgia

A patient satisfies diagnostic criteria for fibromyalgia if the following three conditions are met:
- Either (A) or (B) is met:
  - (A) Widespread pain index (WPI) ≥7 and a Symptom Severity (SS) scale score of ≥5.
  - (B) A WPI of 3–6 and an SS scale ≥9.
- Symptoms have been present at a similar level for at least 6 months; and,
- The patient does not have a disorder that would otherwise explain the pain.

Widespread pain index

Note the number of areas in which the patient has had pain over the last week. Score 0–19 possible points (areas of pain in past week); areas include left/right for each: shoulder girdle, upper/lower arm, hip/buttock/ trochanter, upper/lower leg, jaw, chest, abdomen, upper/lower back, neck.

Modified Symptom Severity (SS) Scale

SS scale score = sum of the three symptoms + sum of three items

Three symptoms: for each symptom score: 0 = none; 1 = slight, mild, or intermittent; 2 = moderate, considerable; 3 = severe, life disturbing:
- Fatigue
- Waking unrefreshed
- Cognitive symptoms.

Three items: present = 1; absent = 0 for each of following:
- Headaches during previous 6 months
- Pain or cramps in lower abdomen during previous 6 months
- Depression symptoms during previous 6 months.

Clinical features from the history

- Widespread MSK pain.
- Pain is a constant feature.
- Tired all the time.
- Joint stiffness.
- Non-restorative sleep.
- Difficulty carrying out normal activities.
- Physical associations could include irritable bowel, irritable bladder, temperature changes, paraesthesia, perception of swelling, migraine, muscle spasm, and dizziness.
- Psychological associations: panic attacks, anxiety, depression, irritability, memory lapses, word mix ups, and reduced concentration.

Examination

The main finding is the presence of symmetrical tender/painful sites around the body. In patients without fibromyalgia these sites are uncomfortable to firm pressure but in patients with fibromyalgia the same pressure causes the patient to cry out and withdraw the area being examined.

Investigations

Limited investigations are required to exclude other causes for the symptoms. Polymyalgia rheumatica, spondyloarthropathy, and hypothyroidism can also give rise to similar symptoms. Investigations include:

- full blood count
- inflammatory markers (e.g. ESR and CRP)
- biochemical profile—serum calcium, alkaline phosphatase, CK, and blood sugar
- thyroid function tests.

It is important to make a diagnosis of fibromyalgia after the clinical history and examination and explain to the patient that the blood tests are simply to ensure there is no underlying condition. Radiological investigations are not required.

Management

- Reassurance that there is no sinister underlying pathology and other possible rheumatological conditions have been ruled out.
- Coping strategies such as CBT or Acceptance and Commitment Therapy (ACT).
- Graded exercise and pacing strategies.
- Relaxation techniques, yoga, and meditation
- Neuropathic medications such as pregabalin or amitriptyline can be tried to improve pain sensitization, sleep, and anxiety symptoms.
- SSRIs such as fluoxetine or sertraline or newer serotonin and noradrenaline reuptake inhibitors such as duloxetine or milnacipran can be used for low mood and anxiety symptoms.
- Chronic opioid use is inappropriate in the treatment of fibromyalgia.[5]
- Some clinicians offer trigger point injections to tender spots but the evidence is inconclusive.
- Other strategies in chronic pain management (➔ see Chapter 11).

Chronic fatigue syndrome

Definition

Chronic fatigue syndrome (CFS), also known as myalgic encephalopathy (ME), post-viral fatigue syndrome (PVFS), or chronic fatigue immune dysfunction syndrome (CFIDS) is characterized by chronic mental and physical fatigue, myalgia, arthralgia, unrefreshing sleep, dizziness, breathlessness, gastric upset, headache, and cognitive problems such as poor memory and concentration. There are fluctuations in the condition with recovery and relapse. Some patients believe that the illness is purely 'medical' and being active will harm them.

Prevalence

It is estimated that 0.5% of the population have CFS. There seems to be higher incidence in age groups 10–20 and 30–40 years. It is reported more commonly in females (two to three times more common than males).

Cause

The aetiology is not entirely understood but associations with genetics, infection (Epstein–Barr virus, Q fever), immune dysfunction, sleep problems, neuroendocrine and neurotransmitter abnormalities, personality, and chronic stress have been identified.

Diagnosis

Diagnosis is based on clinical history (Box 35.2).

Box 35.2 The international consensus definition of chronic fatigue syndrome

1. Complaint of fatigue:
   - of new onset
   - not relieved by rest
   - duration of at least 6 months.
2. At least four of the following additional symptoms:
   - Subjective memory impairment
   - Sore throat
   - Tender lymph nodes
   - Muscle pain and joint pain
   - Headache
   - Unrefreshing sleep
   - Post-exertional malaise lasting more than 24 hours.
3. Impairment of functioning.
4. Other conditions that might explain fatigue excluded.

Differential diagnosis

- General—occult malignancy, autoimmune disease, endocrine disease, cardiac/respiratory/renal failure
- GI—malabsorption including coeliac disease
- Neurological—MS, myasthenia gravis, Parkinson's disease, early dementia, cerebrovascular disease
- Infectious disease—chronic active hepatitis (B or C), Lyme borreliosis, HIV, tuberculosis
- Respiratory disease—nocturnal asthma, obstructive sleep apnoea
- Chronic toxicity—alcohol, solvents, heavy metals, irradiation
- Psychiatric—major depressive disorder, dysthymia, anxiety and panic disorder, somatoform disorder.

Some patients who satisfy criteria for CFS also fulfil criteria for psychiatric conditions such as depression, anxiety, neurasthenia, and somatoform disorders and it might be difficult to differentiate CFS from these conditions. If such dilemma arises, it might be better to use both to describe the condition, for example, CFS/depression.

Management

CFS has a prolonged course of illness that can last several years if not permanently. Patients who have strong views on 'medical illness' seem not to do well in the long term. None of the medications seem to have strong evidence that merit consideration. Graded exercise and activity has been shown to help improve function. Psychological approaches (such as CBT) have convincing evidence of efficacy.

References

1. Global Burden of Disease Study 2013 Collaborators (2015). Global, regional, and national incidence, prevalence, and years lived with disability for 301 acute and chronic diseases and injuries in 188 countries, 1990-2013: a systematic analysis for the Global Burden of Disease Study 2013. *Lancet* 386, 743–800.
2. Main CJ, Watson PJ, Clough AE, et al. (2015). Psychological aspects of musculoskeletal pain. In: Hutson M, Ward A (eds), *Oxford Textbook of Musculoskeletal Medicine*, 2nd edn, pp. 186–199. Oxford University Press, Oxford.
3. The American College of Sports Medicine (2009). *Guidelines for Exercise Testing and Prescription*, 8th edn. Lippincott Williams and Wilkins, Hagerstown, MD.
4. Versus Arthritis. Exercises to manage pain. ℘ https://www.versusarthritis.org/about-arthritis/managing-symptoms/exercise/exercises-to-manage-pain/.
5. Painter JT, Crofford LJ (2013). Chronic opioid use in fibromyalgia syndrome: a clinical review. *J Clinical Rheumatology* 19, 72–77.

Further reading

Hakin A, Clunie G, Hakim A (2006). *The Oxford Handbook of Rheumatology*, 2nd edn. Oxford University Press, Oxford.
Main C, Spanswick C (2000). *Pain Management: An Interdisciplinary Approach*. Churchill Livingstone, Edinburgh.
Sharpe M, Wessely S (2012). Chronic fatigue syndrome. In: Gelder M, Andreasen N, Lopez-Ibor J, et al. (eds), *New Oxford Textbook of Psychiatry*, 2nd edn, pp. 1035–1042. Oxford University Press, Oxford.
Snaith M (2004). *ABC of Rheumatology*, 3rd edn. BMJ Books, London.

Useful websites

Arthritis and Musculoskeletal Alliance: ℘ http://www.arma.uk.net.
British Pain Society: ℘ http://www.britishpainsociety.org/people-with-pain/—links and information for People with Pain.
British Society for Rheumatology: ℘ http://www.rheumatology.org.uk.
CFS/ ME Association: ℘ http://www.meassociation.org.uk.
Fibromyalgia Association UK: ℘ http://www.fmauk.org.

Musculoskeletal problems of upper and lower limbs

Common upper limb conditions

The shoulder (glenohumeral) joint is a complex joint which achieves a high degree of mobility at the expense of stability. The shoulder girdle includes the bones that attach the arm to the chest (clavicle and scapula) and comprises three joints (sternoclavicular, acromioclavicular, and scapulothoracic) (Fig. 36.1). The glenohumeral joint is stabilized by static (capsule and ligaments) and dynamic stabilizers (rotator cuff muscles). The muscles involved in shoulder movement are listed in Table 36.1. The rotator cuff comprises of four muscles: subscapularis, supraspinatus, infraspinatus, and teres minor.

Chronic conditions of the shoulder girdle are usually multifactorial and the whole functional chain needs to be considered while making a diagnosis. Any condition affecting muscular strength or function may alter the biomechanics of component joints or the rotator cuff muscles and cause pain. Degenerative changes in the neck (C5 nerve compression), brachial plexus dysfunction, trapezius muscle spasm, and diaphragmatic and pericardial conditions may all result in referred shoulder pain, but these will not be considered in detail here.

Research has identified that common shoulder pathologies have a key feature: loss of translational control and both the static and dynamic positioning of the scapula play an important role in any shoulder pathology.

As a general principle, a shoulder must keep moving to maintain function and a fall may produce soft tissue damage and extreme pain, such that the patient stops moving the limb. The restriction of movement can very quickly lead to a true frozen shoulder, that is, an adhesive capsulitis.

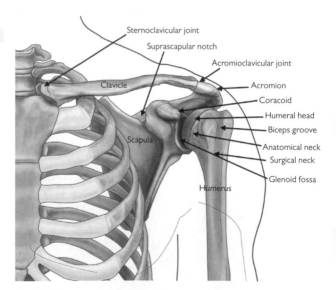

Fig. 36.1 Bones and joints of the shoulder.
Reproduced courtesy of Funk L. ShoulderDoc, Wilmslow, UK. www.shoulderdoc.co.uk.

Table 36.1 Muscles involved in shoulder movement

Muscles	Ele	Dep	Pro	Flx	Ext	Int rot	Ext rot	Abd	Add
Supraspinatus								+	
Deltoid				(+)	(+)	(+)	(+)	+	
Pectoralis major		+		+		+			+
Subscapularis						+			
Latissimus dorsi		+			+	+			+
Teres major					+	+			+
Teres minor							+		
Infraspinatus							+		
Trapezius	+								
Serratus anterior		(+)	+						
Pectoralis minor			+						

Abd, abduction; Add, adduction; Dep, depression; Ele, elevation; Ext, extension; Ext rot, external rotation; Flx, flexion; Int rot, internal rotation; Pro, protraction.

Adhesive capsulitis of the shoulder

Adhesive capsulitis or frozen shoulder is a condition characterized by painful restriction in shoulder range of movements. It is generally seen in individuals between 40 and 60 years of age and is two to four times more common in women than men. The aetiology is generally idiopathic but there is a slightly increased prevalence in diabetes, cardiac disease, and stroke. Secondary frozen shoulder is seen in immobilization/disuse after surgery, trauma, or neurological weakness. The underlying aetiopathological process is not fully understood but is characterized by capsular shrinkage and fibroblastic proliferation with increased collagen and nodular band formation.

Shoulder X-rays do not reveal any abnormality. Shoulder joint arthrography or arthroscopy can reveal reduction in shoulder volume. The standard three stages of adhesive capsulitis are:
- 'freezing'—characterized by pain and progressive reduction in the range of movement of shoulder
- 'frozen'—when pain reduces but reduction in range of movements remains
- 'thawing'—when there is a gradual improvement in the range of movement of shoulder.

Latest thinking is to classify it into two stages: 'pain predominant' or 'stiffness predominant'.

Management

Pain predominant
- Explain the timescale (will spontaneously resolve in 18–24 months, although often range of movement may not be recovered without physiotherapy).
- Advise on avoidance of aggravating activities (e.g. overhead activities or stretching).
- Can use oral analgesia (e.g. NSAIDs).
- Offer an early intra-articular glenohumeral corticosteroid injection for pain relief.
- Avoid vigorous stretching/exercise in the early/painful phase of frozen shoulder as it will exacerbate the pain.
- Gentle graded manual therapy—passive mobilization, mobilization with movement, and gentle pendular swinging exercises.

Stiffness predominant
- Graded range of movement therapy.
- Local 'heat' via hot pack or wheat bag prior to exercise.
- Grade 'B' mobilization (end-of-range stretches into the 'plastic' range of connective tissue) under care and direction of a physiotherapist.
- Advice on posture/positioning/prophylactic advice and home exercise programme.

Some patients who fail with conservative measures may be offered alternative interventional procedures: guided glenohumeral joint distension with normal saline, manipulation under anaesthesia, or arthroscopic capsular release.

Glenohumeral joint arthritis

Articular cartilage is avascular, alymphatic, and aneural. It forms a friction-free, shock-absorbing surface that enables joints to have a smooth, pain-free movement. Arthrosis/arthritis refers to progressive loss of articular cartilage. In the shoulder it is commonly idiopathic but can also result from trauma or poor function of the rotator cuff. Idiopathic arthritis is poorly understood but is characterized by changes in fluid and biomechanical structural of the cartilage. The highly innervated and vascular subchondral bone becomes more exposed to joint forces as the cartilage thickness reduces causing significant pain. Stiffness and crepitus occur due to loss of joint lubrication. The body's response to increased forces on the subchondral bone is to increase bone production in the form of osteophytes.

Management

- Control pain and maintain movement.
- Regular oral/topical analgesia.
- ROM and muscle strengthening exercises.
- Joint injections with either corticosteroids or hyaluronic acid can be considered.
- Joint replacement (arthroplasty) is considered in severe arthritis with considerable functional limitations.

Acromioclavicular joint arthritis

Osteoarthritis of this joint is common in people over 40 years of age. There is joint tenderness and pain on stressing flexion and abduction of the arm between 60° and 90°. Radiographs or diagnostic ultrasound show loss of joint space and possibly osteophytes, which may cause an impingement syndrome by reducing the space underneath the joint for the supraspinatus tendon to glide during abduction of arm. Management is similar to any joint OA with conservative management and arthroscopic shaving of the under-surface in advanced cases.

Rotator cuff disease

Rotator cuff lesions are relatively common and often asymptomatic. Subacromial impingement accounts for 44–65% of all shoulder complaints and is the second most common MSK condition after back pain. Impingement encompasses pain, which is likely to be generated by any pathology of the contents of the subacromial space (rotator cuff and subacromial bursa). The other rotator cuff pathologies are calcific tendinopathy and cuff tears. The three mechanisms that are believed to lead to rotator cuff problems are as follows:

1. *Intrinsic*—age-related tendinopathy (tendon degeneration). As a non-inflammatory process it results in decreased integrity and function of the tendon. It may be influenced by tendon vascularity, systemic disease, or repetitive injury.
2. *Biomechanical* abnormalities involving both the rotator cuff and scapula as a result of either poor posture, response to pain, or tendon damages. Often results in increased pressure within the subacromial space due to abnormal shoulder kinematics.
3. *Extrinsic* mechanical impingement, for example, osteophytes from the acromioclavicular joint or enthesophyte of the coracoacromial ligament; causing increased subacromial pressure generating an inflammatory process within the bursa and resultant significant pain.

Assessment

Arc of pain (i.e. pain-free, then an 'arc' of pain, and again a pain-free ROM) on active abduction indicates an impingement. Generally there is an abnormality of the structure passing under the acromion process (supraspinatus, infraspinatus, or subacromial bursa). Severe rotator cuff or shoulder muscle lesions are easy to diagnose by a resisted static test of the muscle:

- Supraspinatus tendinopathy—resisted abduction.
- Infraspinatus tendinopathy—resisted external rotation of the shoulder with the elbow flexed to 90°.
- Subscapularis tendinopathy—resisted internal rotation of the shoulder with the elbow flexed to 90°.
- Biceps tendinopathy—resisted elbow/shoulder flexion.

X-ray can be used to assess arthritis or calcific deposits in the tendon. Ultrasonography can diagnose cuff degeneration or tears and has the advantage of being a dynamic assessment. MRI can diagnose cuff problems and/or intra-articular labral problems but are most useful if forgery is being contemplated.

Management

- The majority of cases respond to exercise therapy to correct the biomechanical problems that cause impingement.
- There is no convincing evidence for use of oral analgesia (paracetamol, NSAIDs, or codeine) or topical medications. However, steroid injections can provide a pain-free window to enable the rehabilitative exercises. Ultrasound-guided barbotage of calcific deposits is being done by some clinicians for calcific tendinopathy.
- The value of arthroscopic surgical decompression for impingement syndrome is being debated and evidence is inconclusive. Cuff repair is recommended for cuff tears in younger individuals with higher function. Surgical removal of calcific deposits is done in calcific tendinopathy not responding to conservative measures.

Tennis elbow/lateral epicondylalgia and golfer's elbow/medial epicondylalgia

These two elbow conditions are usually seen in people over the age of 40 years, and are thought to be part of an UL overuse syndrome resulting from excessive tension on the common forearm extensor and flexor muscles respectively, which in turn results in localized tenderness and pain on gripping and twisting the hand (Box 36.1). Both syndromes often impair hand function, particularly in lifting weights. Self-reported symptoms may be associated with pain referred from the neck or be neurodynamic in origin.

Management includes identifying and correcting the cause. Resting from aggravating activities while maintaining function and strengthening of the whole UL is helpful.

There is no particular treatment that has been shown to be superior to another. An epicondylitis clasp worn reasonably tightly around the upper forearm just below the common extensor or common flexor origin is thought to protect the common muscular origin by transmitting forces away from the enthesis (where the tendon attaches to bone). Localized taping techniques can have similar benefit. This can usefully allow people to continue to work. If these measures are insufficient, dry needling or local hydrocortisone injection may diminish and treat symptoms. Hydrocortisone alone should be used in preference to fluorinated corticosteroids, as the latter may cause subcutaneous fat atrophy and local disfigurement. Autologous blood or platelet rich plasma injections in the treatment of lateral epicondyle tendinopathy is a new approach increasing in popularity.

Box 36.1 Definitions of tennis elbow and golfer's elbow

Tennis elbow
- Tender lateral humeral epicondyle.
- Epicondylar pain on resisting wrist or finger extension supporting arm (straight elbow).
- Forced pronation of the forearm with the elbow straight also produces pain.

Golfer's elbow
- Tender medial humeral epicondyle.
- Epicondylar pain on resisting wrist or finger flexion supporting arm (straight elbow).
- Pain on resisted supination less reliable.
- Sensory symptoms do not typically occur.

De Quervain's tenosynovitis/ intersection syndrome

There is pain and tenderness on the radial aspect of the wrist due to inflammation of abductor pollicis longus and extensor pollicis brevis tendon sheaths. The condition is referred to as De Quervain's tenosynovitis if symptoms are localized to the tendon sheath distally at the wrist and known as intersection syndrome if located at the musculotendinous intersection area proximally (that also involves the second dorsal compartment extensor wrist muscles).

Occupational activity is often responsible and a positive Finkelstein's test is indicative. This is carried out by flexion and opposition of the thumb into the palm of the hand and held down by the fingers. The wrist is then subjected to an ulnar deviation force, thus stretching the affected tendons and reproducing pain.

Management includes physiotherapy utilizing graded transverse friction massage and/or local ultrasound therapy. Alternatively, an injection of local anaesthetic with corticosteroid into the tendon sheath of the two affected muscles (in De Quervain's syndrome) can be done. Although physical intervention can be successful, addressing the (occupational) cause is important and protecting the wrist in a resting wrist splint may occasionally be helpful in the short term.

Dupuytren's contracture

Dupuytren's contracture is a progressive fibroproliferative disorder. A hand deformity is characterized by visible and palpable hard lumps of connective tissue in the palmar fascia, most commonly affecting the ring and little finger. As the tissue tightens, the fingers are pulled towards the palm and there is a resultant shortening of the fingers due to contracture. The cause is unknown but is known to have a genetic predisposition, is more common in patients who also have diabetes mellitus, and has a male:female ratio of more than 4:1. If the contracture is not causing any functional difficulty, treatment may not be needed.

Those patients with metacarpophalangeal (MCP) joint contractures of 30° or less with no proximal interphalangeal joint contractures can be treated with corticosteroid injection, needle aponeurotomy, or percutaneous fasciotomy. Early cases can also be treated with *Clostridium histolyticum* collagenase injections as an outpatient procedure.

Surgery (needle fasciotomy, open fasciotomy/fasciectomy) is recommended when function is impaired or a severe and disabling deformity is present. Patients with MCP joint contractures of 30° or more can be considered for this option.

Carpal tunnel syndrome

Carpal tunnel syndrome (CTS) is the most common entrapment neuropathy in the general population, with an adult prevalence rate of 3–6%. CTS results from entrapment of the median nerve as it passes through the carpal tunnel under the flexor retinaculum at the wrist. It is usually idiopathic but is also seen secondary to some systemic conditions (Box 36.2). Obesity and pregnancy can be risk factors for CTS. It is more common in women and can be bilateral in 50% of cases.

The diagnosis is made by examination and suggested by a positive *Tinel's sign* where percussion of the nerve at the wrist produces pain and paraesthesiae in the median nerve territory. A similar result may also be achieved by sustained full flexion or extension of the wrist (*Phalen's sign*). The sensitivity of these tests is in the range of 30–50%. Nerve conduction studies and EMG provide more accurate results, identify the site of median nerve compression, and rule out the differentials such as cervical radiculopathy and other proximal compression syndromes. In some cases, there is double-crush syndrome with compression of an UL nerve at more than one site.

Mild carpal tunnel syndrome

There is pain and paraesthesiae occurring in the territory of the median nerve (i.e. the radial aspect of the palmar surface of the hand and of the lateral 3½ fingers). Symptoms are often nocturnal pain, which may cause patients to wake up and may gain relief by shaking the hand or hanging the hand out of bed). Management involves using a resting wrist splint to prevent excessive extension and flexion. Local steroid injections under the retinaculum around the nerve are indicated if splinting alone does not resolve symptoms.

More severe carpal tunnel syndrome

There is motor involvement with weakness and atrophy of abductor pollicis brevis and opponens pollicis muscles. Management is surgical decompression of the carpal tunnel (particularly where active denervation is present) by open or endoscopic methods. The procedure generally has a favourable outcome with recurrence rate of around 10%.

Box 36.2 Causes of carpal tunnel syndrome

- Fluid retention—pregnancy or oral contraceptive (commonest association).
- Osteoarthritis or rheumatoid arthritis of the wrist.
- Colles and scaphoid bone fractures.
- Direct trauma.
- Hypothyroidism.
- Acromegaly.
- Amyloidosis.
- Mucopolysaccharidosis
- Myelomatosis.

Work-related upper limb disorders

Work related upper limb disorder (WRULD) is an umbrella term for conditions thought to have caused in the workplace (see Box 36.3 for a definition). This is also referred to as repetitive strain injury (RSI), overuse syndrome, and cumulative trauma disorder (CTD).

Type 1 WRULD refers to demonstrable pathomorphology. There are numerous disorders in this category, the nine commonest being:

- rotator cuff tendinopathy
- biceps tendinopathy
- shoulder capsulitis
- lateral epicondylalgia
- medial epicondylalgia
- De Quervain's tenosynovitis
- tenosynovitis of wrist
- CTS.

Type II WRULD refers to persistent pain and dysaesthesia in the UL. This is also referred to as neuropathic arm pain (NAP). The discomfort/pain initially is experienced peripherally, often in the hands (extensor surface) and then extends diffusely to the shoulder, neck and upper back. The pain has a burning 'toothache' quality, sometimes accompanied by subjective sensation of swelling, numbness, hypersensitivity, or hyperalgesia. It is more common in women than men and generally seen in repetitive stereotyped activities of the hands and digits, such as typing in an administrative job. In longstanding cases, sleep is disturbed and psychological symptoms develop such as depression, headache, chronic fatigue, and frustration.

The typical patient is a young or middle-aged person with a long history of fibromyalgia, prolonged morning stiffness, chronic sleep disturbance, and easy fatigue and poor exercise tolerance. The individual may have other unrelated tender points and there is often subjective swelling of the hands along with paraesthesia (pins and needles in a limb, over and above a nerve root territory). On examination, a degree of self-reported impairment of function is present. Pain may be present on moving the neck, but often the range of movement is normal. Neurological examination is essentially normal but with pain-induced weakness on muscle power testing.

Box 36.3 Definition of WRULD

A number of well-recognized MSK conditions of the workplace which are associated with acute, cumulative, and chronic 'injuries' and illnesses of soft tissue caused by mechanical stress, strain, sprain and vibration, inflammation, or irritation.

Management

- Identification of cause.
- Treatment of the specific UL disorder (that might include physical agents, exercise therapy, manipulation, steroid injection, or surgery).
- Modification of aggravating factors.
- Ergonomic assessments and adaptations—better design of tools, equipment, and work layout.
- Maintain active range of movement.
- Advice on pacing activity and prevention of chronicity.
- Address psychological risk factors (low mood, somatizing tendency, job dissatisfaction, negative perceptions about work environment).
- Rehabilitation programme to support with phased return to work.
- Medications can be used for neuropathic symptoms and sleep. Low-dose amitriptyline is preferred by many clinicians.

Common musculoskeletal problems of the lower limb

The hip joint is a synovial ball and socket joint between the femoral head and acetabular socket, deepened by the cartilaginous labrum. The hip is much more stable and has less range of movement when compared to the shoulder joint. The muscles involved in hip movements and their innervation are summarized in Table 36.2.

Table 36.2 Muscles involved in hip movement

Muscles	Flx	Ext	Int rot	Ext rot	Abd	Add
Gluteus maximus		+		+		
Gluteus medius	(+)		+		+	
Gluteus minimus			(+)	(+)	+	
Lateral rotators[a]				+		
Tensor fascia lata	+		+		+	
Iliopsoas	+			(+)		
Sartorius	+			+		
Rectus femoris	+					
Semitendinosus/ semimembranosus		+	+			
Biceps femoris		+		(+)		
Adductors	(+)					+
Gracilis						+

Abd, abduction; Add, adduction; Ext, extension; Ext rot, external rotation; Flx, flexion; Int rot, internal rotation.

[a] Lateral rotators include piriformis, quadratus femoris, obturator internus/externus and the gemelli.

The ones with (+) show that parts of the muscle/s can assist in that movement.

Osteoarthritis

The most commonly affected joints are the hip, knee, ankle, subtalar, and first toe. Hip arthritis is a common cause of hip pain, disability, and reduced QOL. The pain is often felt in the groin radiating to the anterior thigh, but can also be felt in the knee on occasion. Referred pain from the spine must be carefully excluded in suspected cases of hip arthritis. Knee arthritis can affect either the medial tibiofemoral compartment, the lateral tibiofemoral compartment, the patellofemoral compartment, or all three compartments.

Management

Optimal management of patients with OA of the knee or hip requires a combination of non-pharmacological and pharmacological modalities following feedback from the Osteoarthritis Research International members on draft guidelines:

- Non-pharmacological modalities:
  - Education and self-management
  - Weight reduction
  - Low-impact aerobics, muscle strengthening, and water-based exercises
  - Regular telephone contact/monitoring
  - Referral to a physiotherapist
  - Walking aids/joint supports
  - Cushioned insoles and footwear adaptations
  - Thermal modalities, TENS, and acupuncture.
- Pharmacological modalities:
  - Acetaminophen, oral NSAIDs, and opioid medications
  - Topical NSAID gel and capsaicin
  - Intra-articular injections of local anaesthetic agent, corticosteroids or hyaluronates. This can be done under fluoroscopic or ultrasound guidance, particularly for the hip joint.
- Surgical interventions:
  - Arthroscopic debridement surgery (although current literature is not supportive).
  - Joint arthroplasty (either partial or total) is the gold standard treatment that substantially improves pain and function in severe arthritis.

Greater trochanter pain syndrome

This is a relatively new term used to describe pain and tenderness in the region of the greater trochanter and the juxtaposed soft tissues of lateral buttock and proximal thigh. This syndrome is the LL equivalent of shoulder impingement syndrome.

• Gluteal medius/minimus dysfunction/tendinopathy/tear
• Trochanteric bursitis
• Iliotibial band friction syndrome (snapping hip)
• Radiculopathy from spinal compression.

Conservative management includes activity modification to avoid exacerbating movements, ice, physical agents, and analgesic medications. Eccentric strengthening exercises of the gluteal muscles is the mainstay treatment for gluteal tendinopathy. Stretching of tight structures such as the iliotibial band and tensor fascia lata and core and pelvic stability exercises should be addressed. Leg length discrepancy of more than 1.5 cm needs to be adjusted with orthoses or insoles. Foot overpronation poses a risk and should be corrected where present. Steroid injections, dry needling, extracorporeal shock wave therapy, or prolotherapy can be useful in resistant cases. Surgery is rarely used for gluteal tendon repair and iliotibial band lengthening.

Tendinopathy: patellar tendon/Achilles tendon/tibialis posterior tendon

Patients present with pain localized to the tendon and is seen in those involved in repetitive movements of the joint by the tendon. The term 'tendinopathy' replaces the old term 'tendinitis' when it was believed there was an element of inflammation of the tendon. It is now established that tendinopathy is an overuse injury in which the tendon develops collagen disarray, increased hydrophilic ground substance, increased poor quality blood vessels (neovascularization), and lacks an inflammatory process as previously believed.

The biomechanical changes that lead to unequal distribution of forces along the links of the kinetic chain need to be addressed in rehabilitation exercises. Eccentric strengthening exercises have the best available evidence in these conditions. Other procedures such as dry needling, steroid injections, high volume distension, sclerosing therapy, autologous blood, and platelet-rich plasma injections have been used in selective cases with ongoing trials investigating their efficacy.

Plantar fasciopathy

This is similar to tendinopathy and is one of the most common causes of heel pain. It is believed to result from chronic overload either from lifestyle or exercise. The term plantar fasciitis is being phased out as the pathology is of a degenerative nature rather than inflammation.

The classic signs and symptoms are severe pain in the morning and pain after rest that improves with movement but is aggravated by long periods of weight bearing. Palpation identifies tenderness over the medial calcaneal tubercle and often self-reported discomfort on passive flexion of the big toe. Ultrasonography shows thickness of the plantar fascia.

Treatment includes modification of aggravating activity, use of a supportive insole/heel pad; stretching of plantar fascia, gastrocnemius, and soleus; self-massage with a frozen bottle or golf ball; strengthening exercises of intrinsic foot muscles; taping; steroid injection and dry needling in selective cases; extracorporeal shock wave therapy; and surgery (plantar fasciectomy) in resistant cases.

Morton's neuroma

This is a common cause of metatarsalgia and refers to swelling along the course of the interdigital nerve between the metatarsal bones in the foot. There is pain in between the toes accompanied by neuropathic symptoms in the toes innervated by the nerve. Examination reveals a palpable click with squeezing the metatarsal heads. Treatment consists of using shoes with a wide toe box, a plantar metatarsal pad to spread the load over the combined metatarsals, and intrinsic foot muscle strengthening exercises. Injection of steroid and local anaesthetic is undertaken when not responding to these conservative measures. Surgery (excision of the nerve) is reserved for resistant cases.

Further reading

Bruckner P, Khan K (2012). *Clinical Sports Medicine*, 4th edn. McGraw-Hill, Sydney.

Cochrane T, Davey S (2005). Randomised controlled trial of the cost effectiveness of water- based therapy for lower limb osteoarthritis. *Health Technology Assessment* 9, 1–14

Conaghan PG, Dickson J, Grant RL (2008). Care and management of osteoarthritis in adults: summary of NICE guidance. *BMJ* 336, 502–503.

Global Burden of Disease Study 2013 Collaborators (2015). Global, regional, and national incidence, prevalence, and years lived with disability for 301 acute and chronic diseases and injuries in 188 countries, 1990–2013: a systematic analysis for the Global Burden of Disease Study 2013. Lancet 386, 743–800.

Hutson M, Ward A (eds) (2015). *Oxford Textbook of Musculoskeletal Medicine*, 2nd edn. Oxford University Press, Oxford.

MacAuley D (2013). *Oxford Handbook of Sport and Exercise Medicine*. Oxford University Press, Oxford.

Main CJ, Watson PJ, Clough AE, et al. (2015). Psychological aspects of musculoskeletal pain. In: Hutson M, Ward A (eds), Oxford Textbook of Musculoskeletal Medicine, 2nd edn, pp. 186–199. Oxford University Press, Oxford.

Silman AJ, Newman J (1996). A review of diagnostic criteria for work related upper limb disorders (WRULD). ℘ www.hse.gov.uk/research/misc/silman.pdf.

The American College of Sports Medicine (2009). *Guidelines for Exercise Testing and Prescription*, 8th edn. Lippincott Williams and Wilkins, Hagerstown, MD.

Useful websites

℘ http://www.hse.gov.uk/pubns/indg438.pdf—the Assessment of Repetitive Tasks (ART) tool.

℘ http://www.hse.gov.uk/msd/uld/art/resources.htm—a task rotation worksheet.

Further reading

Spinal problems

Introduction

Low back and neck pain are extremely common symptoms in modern societies. The pain may result from abnormalities occurring within the trunk
muscles, the vertebrae, the intervertebral discs, the facet joints, the ligaments, and from the spinal canal and the nerve roots themselves. Pain may
also be referred from distant sites—such as the abdomen—and in some
cases may be functional or psychogenic in nature. As discussed in ➔
Chapter 11, pain can be described as acute or chronic; pain present for
more than 3 months is considered as chronic.

Low back pain

The lifetime prevalence of low back pain has been reported as high as 84%. At a given time, about 40% of the population has had low back pain in the past 6 months. It is the leading cause of work absenteeism and has huge financial implications. Modern societies spend more on management of back pain than any of the following conditions: coronary heart disease, stroke, diabetes, mental health problems, dementia, and peripheral vascular disease. For example, in 2000, the NHS in the UK spent one-fifth of its entire budget on direct and indirect costs related to management of back pain. These costs are, however, reducing given the increased emphasis on non-surgical and non-interventional management in the condition.

History

A careful history must be elicited to rule out the 'red flags' that need further work-up such as imaging and referral to a specialist. These are listed in Box 37.1. The presence of 'yellow flags' (➔ see Chapter 11) must be explored as well.

Physical examination includes observation of the overall posture, spinal range of movement, and gait; palpation of spine; neurological and musculoskeletal examination; and special tests of neural tension (highlighted in ➔ Chapter 5) (Box 37.2).[1] Investigations should be considered in appropriate cases (Fig. 37.1).[2]

Box 37.1 Red flags in back pain

- Age less than 18 years or greater than 55 years.
- Recent significant trauma.
- Progressive pain at night.
- Fever and/or systemic illness.
- Weight loss.
- Systemic steroids/immunosuppression.
- Marked morning stiffness with raised inflammatory markers.
- Iritis, skin rashes, colitis, and urethral discharge.
- Loss of anal sphincter tone or faecal incontinence.
- Saddle anaesthesia.
- Widespread progressive motor weakness or gait disturbance.

Box 37.2 Differential diagnosis of low back pain

1. Regional mechanical low back pain (90%):
   * Non-specific mechanical low back pain (sprain, strain, lumbago, etc.)
   * Degenerative changes in discs and/or facet joints
   * Osteoporotic compression fractures
   * Traumatic fractures
   * Deformity (severe scoliosis, kyphosis)
   * Symptomatic spondylolisthesis
2. Mechanical low back pain with neurogenic leg pain (7–10%):
   * Intervertebral disc herniation
   * Spinal stenosis (± spondylolisthesis)
3. Non-mechanical spine disorders (1%):
   * Neoplasia (metastases, lymphoid tumours, spinal cord tumours, etc.)
   * Infection (bacterial or tuberculous spondylodiscitis, epidural abscess)
   * Seronegative spondyloarthritides (ankylosing spondylitis, psoriatic arthritis, reactive arthritis, Reiter syndrome, inflammatory bowel disease)
4. Visceral disease (1–2%):
   * Pelvic (prostatitis, endometriosis, pelvic inflammatory disease)
   * Renal (nephrolithiasis, pyelonephritis, renal papillary necrosis)
   * Aortic aneurysm
   * Gastrointestinal (pancreatitis, cholecystitis, colon carcinoma, peptic ulcer disease)
5. Miscellaneous:
   * Paget's disease
   * Parathyroid disease
   * Haemoglobinopathies

Adapted with permission from Lurie J.D. What diagnostic tests are useful for low back pain? *Best Pract Res Clin Rheumatol*, 19 (4): 557–75. Copyright © 2005 Elsevier Ltd. All rights reserved. https://doi.org/10.1016/j.berh.2005.03.004.

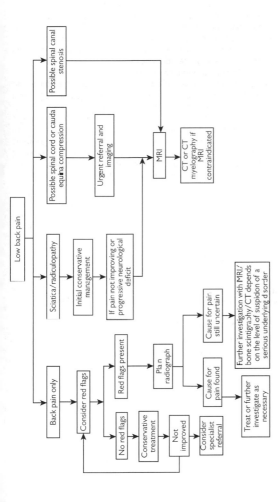

Fig. 37.1 Algorithm for the investigation of patients with low back pain.

Mechanical low back pain

This is also referred to as non-specific low back pain, back strain, or spinal degenerative pain. The cause can be multifactorial including abnormal posture, deconditioning of core muscles, degenerative changes in lumbar spinal segment (lumbar spondylosis), or psychological factors. The potential anatomical pain generators in the back are the innervated structures summarized in Box 37.3. In addition, some patients have negative beliefs about pain and develop movement avoidance behaviours.

Treatment is primarily around reassurance that there is no serious pathology and encouraging movement and back exercises. Flexibility and strengthening exercises have been shown to improve posture, segmental stability, and restore normal pattern of muscle activity in the kinetic chain.[3] Exercise is recommended in the acute phase of a pain episode to prevent deconditioning and reduce the chances of recurrence. Aerobic fitness exercises, aquatic exercises, Pilates, and yoga are beneficial. An ergonomic assessment to encourage and maintain correct posture in the working environment is useful. There is a role for medications, group classes, and multidisciplinary programmes in chronic low back pain as detailed in ➲ Chapter 11.

Box 37.3 Pain generators of back

Innervated structures
- Bone: vertebral body
- Joint: zygapophyseal/facets
- Disc: external annulus
- Ligaments: anterior longitudinal ligament, posterior longitudinal ligament, and interspinous
- Muscles: anterior (psoas, quadratus lumborum) and posterior (latissimus dorsi and paraspinal)
- Fascia: thoracolumbar fascia

Non-innervated structures
- Disc: internal annulus and nucleus pulposus
- Ligaments: ligamentum flavum

Sciatica/lumbosacral radiculopathy

The most common cause for radicular pain in the leg is compression of the nerve in the vertebral segment (disc prolapse or spinal stenosis). The segments L4–L5 and L5–S1 are commonly affected with compression of L5 or S1 nerve roots. Which nerve root is compressed depends on the type of disc prolapse: a central disc compresses the transiting root (e.g. the L4–L5 disc compressing the L5 nerve root) and a lateral foraminal disc compresses the exiting nerve root (the L4–L5 disc compressing the L4 nerve root) (Fig. 37.2). A large central disc has the potential of compressing all the traversing nerve roots in the thecal sac causing an acute cauda equina syndrome that is a surgical emergency, with decompressive surgery recommended within 48 hours of presentation.

More than 90% of disc prolapse pain regresses spontaneously and hence a conservative approach is favoured. Relative rest is indicated in the first 1–3 days. Thereafter, the activity levels need to be increased along with supervised exercise therapy and/or an active rehabilitation programme. Anti-inflammatory medications can be used in the acute stage but have no benefit in the long-term management of radicular pain. Oral steroids in

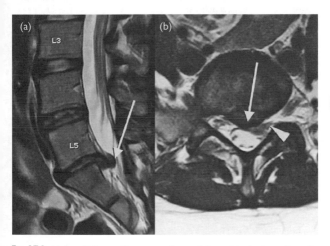

Fig. 37.2 (a) A sagittal magnetic resonance image of the vertebral column shows the herniated L5/S1 disc (arrow) protruding posteriorly into the vertebral canal, where it impinges on the nerve roots of the first sacral nerve. (b) An axial magnetic resonance image at the level of the L5/S1 disc shows a herniated nucleus pulposus (arrow) in the vertebral canal where it impinges on a spinal nerve (arrow head).

acute disc prolapse lack substantial evidence of efficacy, even though they are used in many countries. Lumbar epidural steroid injections (particularly targeted transforaminal injections at affected level) can be used as an adjunct in management of neuropathic pain. Surgery (microdiscectomy) is indicated in carefully selected cases when conservative management has been tried for 6–8 weeks or there is progression of neurological deficits. The patient needs to be counselled that the objective of the surgical approach is to minimize leg pain; relief of back pain is difficult to predict and cannot be guaranteed. The patient is likely to have persistent chronic low back pain due to the degenerative nature of the prolapsed intervertebral disc.

Chronic disc and facet joint degeneration can lead to degenerative spinal canal stenosis either at central or foraminal level. The classical presentation is of neurogenic claudication that comes on after walking and is relieved by forward flexion of the spine (e.g. leaning forward on a shopping trolley). The stenosis can be graded as mild (>75% of normal anteroposterior canal dimension), moderate (50–74%), or severe (<50%). The management is mainly conservative with pain control and improving function by flexion-based lumbar stabilization exercises. Surgical decompression (a laminectomy to create more space in the lumbar canal) is indicated in severe symptoms not responding to conservative measures and those with progressive neurological deficits.

Differential diagnoses for radicular-type pain should be considered including vascular claudication (walking aggravated pain that is relieved only by stopping rather than bending forward), sacroiliac joint problems, pyriformis syndrome, and peripheral polyneuropathy.

Spondylolysis/spondylolisthesis

Spondylolysis is a defect of the pars interarticularis in the vertebral segment which can be developmental, traumatic, or a combination of both. It is a known cause of back pain in adolescents with repetitive hyperextension injuries, such as in gymnasts. The degenerative defects are commonly seen in the L5–S1 level and can be unilateral or bilateral. When bilateral, it can cause slippage of one vertebra over another (spondylolisthesis). Oblique X-ray views of the lumbar spine reveal the 'break in neck of the scottie dog' appearance. Bone scan, single-photon emission CT (SPECT) scan, and CT scan are more sensitive than plain X-ray films. Conservative management with a core muscle stability rehabilitation programme and avoidance of activities that worsen the pain is mostly successful in alleviating symptoms.

Spondylolisthesis can present in various forms. The isthmic type is characterized by the pars defect as described previously. Other types are congenital (dysplasia of facet joints), degenerative (instability due to facet joint degeneration), or traumatic. The common complaint is back pain associated with radicular pain in cases with nerve compression due to the slippage. The Meyerding grading system describes five grades in the lateral plain film (grade 1 <25% slip; grade 2, 25–49%; grade 3, 50–74%; grade 4, 75–99%; and grade 5, 100% or more slip).[4] Spontaneous progression of the slip is rare in adults, hence the mainstay treatment is conservative and includes a back strengthening and stabilization rehabilitation programme. Surgery is only indicated in resistant cases with significant progression of slippage and neurological deficit; or in young patients who have not achieved skeletal maturity and have more than 50% (grade 3 or higher) of slip.

Spinal infection

Spinal infections are commonly diagnosed late as the presentation is not straightforward. Unfortunately, these infections have the potential to cause paralysis if not diagnosed early and appropriately managed. The incidence of osteomyelitis, discitis, and epidural infections is increasing with the growing number of immunocompromised patients (those on immunosuppressive agents, diabetics, IV drug users, tuberculosis, haemodialysis, and infected IV lines and in critically ill patients). The classical symptoms of fever and signs of raised white cell count and inflammatory markers (ESR and CRP) may not be present in many cases (estimated to be around 50% of cases) and hence diagnosis is challenging. X-rays might be normal in early stages and more sensitive modalities such as MRI should be used to rule out spinal infection, particularly in immunocompromised patients. Once diagnosed, prompt treatment with appropriate antibiotics for 4–6 weeks and surgical evacuation (with or without fusion) in select cases can reduce mortality and long-term disability

Neck pain

The prevalence of neck pain in the general population ranges from 10% to 18%. Cervical axial pain is defined as pain localized to the midline extending from the inferior occiput to the superior interscapular region. Cervical radicular pain is pain radiating to the shoulder girdle and distal upper limb. Understanding the pattern of pain helps in diagnosis and treatment.

Cervical spondylosis/disc prolapse

Degenerative changes in the cervical intervertebral disc, facet joints (zygapophyseal), uncovertebral joints, and ligamentous hypertrophy is referred to as cervical spondylosis. These changes can cause axial neck pain or radicular pain (when there is compression to exiting nerve root) or myelopathy (when there is compression to spinal cord). A thorough examination is needed to establish the dermatomal and myotomal pattern of peripheral neurological deficit and UMN signs of spinal cord involvement (Hoffman sign, Babinski's plantar response, LL weakness pattern, gait disturbances, bowel and bladder involvement).

Plain radiographs have limited utility in assisting management. A CT scan is ideal for osseous details and a MRI scan in those with radiculopathy or myelopathy. Nerve conduction studies are used in cases to establish the site of nerve compression or double-crush phenomenon, where a proximal compression makes the nerve susceptible to a compression injury distal in its course.

Cervical spondylosis with axial cervical pain needs a non-operative rehabilitation approach. Maintaining the ROM and strengthening the spinal muscles helps reduce the pain. Posture education and ergonomic assessment is useful. Short duration use of a soft collar can only be advocated in acute episodes of pain and muscle spasm (along with analgesic medications). There is a role of guided steroid injections or radiofrequency ablation of nerve roots in select cases with clearly identified facet joint pain generation.

Cervical radiculopathy (either due to disc prolapse or spondylosis) generally settles with a conservative approach and only a minority (10–15%) will eventually need any surgical intervention. A soft collar acts as a kinaesthetic reminder of the proper neck position in the acute phase and can reduce extreme painful movements. Anti-inflammatory medications and neuropathic agents such as amitriptyline, gabapentin, and pregabalin can be used for pain relief in acute and chronic stages. Selective nerve root blocks are used for diagnostic and therapeutic purpose but are not as popular as lumbar nerve root blocks due to the possible rare adverse event of spinal cord ischaemia. Surgical interventions (e.g. foraminotomy or discectomy and fusion) is recommended for those with a progressive neurological deficit or progression to myelopathy.

Cervical myelopathy can occur when there is more than 30% reduction in the cross-sectional area of the spinal canal. The cause culprit might be the disc and/or the vertebral body or posterior elements, or a combination of these. Anterior decompression (discectomy or corpectomy) and fusion is carried out when fewer stenotic segments are present. Extensive stenosis across many segments requires both anterior and posterior (laminectomy) decompression and stabilization. There is a limited role for non-operative management in cervical myelopathy unless surgery is contraindicated or the patient refuses to have surgery.

Cervical strain/sprain and whiplash

Cervical strain/sprain accounts for 85% of neck pain from acute, chronic, or repetitive traumatic neck injuries such as road traffic injuries or sporting injuries. The acceleration–deceleration mechanism of the head and neck in such injuries can cause stress injury to the neck muscles (strain) and ligaments (sprain). The commonly affected muscles are the extensor group and the common ligament affected is the anterior longitudinal ligament. There is neck pain associated with range of movement, producing the tendency to guard any movement. There can be associated neck stiffness and headache. Plain radiographs and flexion-extension views are used to rule out any instability. Treatment in the acute phase (2–3 days) involves rest, use of a soft collar, anti-inflammatory medications, and avoidance of aggravating activities. Once the pain is better, rehabilitative exercises and posture to restore spinal biomechanics and cervical muscle strength is recommended to avoid long-term neck stiffness and chronic pain. A short course of tricyclic antidepressants can be used in those with painful muscle spasms and sleep disturbance.

Whiplash-associated disorder is the latest accepted terminology to describe the heterogeneous group of symptoms after rear or side impact in motor vehicle accidents. The symptoms can include pain in the neck, headache, paraesthesias in the arm and hands, dizziness, temporomandibular pain, visual and vestibular symptoms, cognitive symptoms, and emotional/psychological disturbances. The cervical spine is thrown into a S-shaped curve in these impacts and there is evidence of damage to facet joint cartilage and capsule, cervical disc, and anterior and posterior longitudinal ligaments during this non-physiological movement of the cervical spine. Functional brain studies show associated hypoperfusion of brain areas. The popular hypothesis that explains the symptoms is the mismatch in the midbrain between information from damaged cervical structures and other afferents related to visual and vestibular system.[5] Predisposing risk factors for development of whiplash symptoms are a history of previous neck pain, poor coping style, anxiety/stress disorders, depression, catastrophizing, and/or the presence of litigation or secondary gain factors. Management is conservative, involving education and reassurance that 90% of people recover completely within 2–3 months. Active mobilization and strengthening must be encouraged once pain is under control. Around 10% of people have chronic symptoms which require a chronic pain management approach of functional restoration addressing the physical, cognitive, and social aspects of the condition. A soft collar is of little to no use. There is limited evidence on the use of steroids, BoNT injection to paraspinal muscles, and radiofrequency ablation of nerves to facet joints.

Cervicogenic headaches

Nearly one-third of cases of headache are thought to arise from the cervical spine. Various structures have been implicated such as the cervical discs, facets joints, uncovertebral joints, ligaments, muscles, and exiting nerve roots. The hypothesis suggests that pain from these structures and/or the posterior scalp converge on the same second-order intraspinal neurons, resulting in referred pain felt as a headache. These headaches are mostly unilateral, involving the posterior cervical region and radiating towards the vertex. The intensity is typically less than cluster headaches, does not have the other typical features of migraine, and is aggravated by neck movements. Cervical imaging can be useful but can be misleading as cervical degenerative changes are common and present in many asymptomatic individuals. A diagnostic facet joint block can help establish the diagnosis and, if positive, a therapeutic steroid injection or radiofrequency ablation can be useful in select cases.

References

1. Lurie JD (2005). What diagnostic tests are useful for low back pain? *Best Practice & Research Clinical Rheumatology* 19, 557–575.
2. Sibtain N, Cregg R, Purves A (2012). Investigation of patients with back pain. In: Chong S, Cregg R, Souter A (eds), *OPML Back Pain*, pp. 29–46. Oxford University Press.
3. Barr KP, Harrast MA (2011). Low back pain. In: Braddom RL (ed), *Physical Medicine and Rehabilitation*, 4rd edn. WB Saunders, Philadelphia, PA.
4. Wiltse LL, Winter RB (1983). Terminology and measurement of spondylolisthesis. *Journal of Bone and Joint Surgery (American)* 65, 768–772.
5. Vállez García D, Doorduin J, Willemsen AT, et al. (2016). Altered regional cerebral blood flow in chronic whiplash associated disorders. *EBioMedicine* 10, 249–257.

Further reading

Alpini DC, Brugnoni G, Cesarani A (2014). *Whiplash Injuries: Diagnosis and Treatment*, 2nd edn. Springer, Italy
Braddom RL (2011). *Physical Medicine and Rehabilitation*, 4rd edn. WB Saunders, Philadelphia, PA.

Cervicogenic headaches

References

Further reading

Cancer rehabilitation

Background and epidemiology

Cancer has changed from being a condition with a poor prognosis where the emphasis was on treatment aimed at stopping or slowing the cancer to one which frequently is a chronic condition, or at least a condition in which survival may be measured in years rather than months. The natural consequence of this is that rehabilitation has become an important aspect of management, and a vital one if a person is to fully take advantage of successful cancer treatment. The numbers of those who might benefit from rehabilitation are very high: in 2008 there were an estimated 28.8 million people worldwide who had been diagnosed with cancer in the previous 5 years. The numbers of cancer survivors far outweigh those with new diagnoses of cancer at any one time; for example, in 2008 there were estimated to be 17,832,000 cancer survivors in Europe compared with 1,530,000 new diagnoses and 569,000 cancer deaths. Fig. 38.1 shows the prevalence of different types of cancer diagnoses over periods of time up to 5 years post diagnosis.

Cancer rehabilitation is provided sporadically. Recommendations exist that may help to make rehabilitation provision more equitable, for example, the UK NICE guidelines 'Improving supportive and palliative care in cancer patients'[1] and the 'National Standards for Rehabilitation of Adult Cancer Patients for Wales'.[2] In addition, guidelines concerning rehabilitation have been produced for individual types of cancer, such as breast cancer.[3]

Different terminologies are used concerning rehabilitation so it may not be immediately obvious that it is provided: an example is many of the components of cancer survivorship programmes are rehabilitative in nature. The term 'supportive care' often covers rehabilitation, for instance, in publications from the Australian National Cancer Expert Reference Group, such as in 'Optimal Pathway for Patients with Breast Cancer'[4] there are detailed appendices termed 'Supportive Care' that describe aspects of rehabilitation.

In the UK, specialist rehabilitation is more often provided for brain and spinal cord tumours than for other tumour types, possibly because this fits with existing specialist neurological rehabilitation services. In other countries, such as the US, specialist rehabilitation has developed in general cancer care.

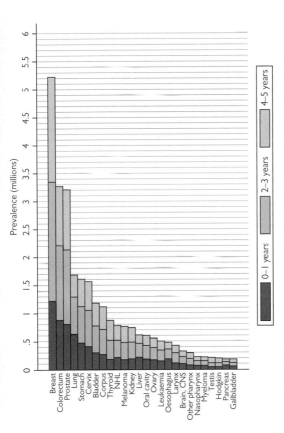

Fig. 38.1 Prevalence of those living with different types of cancer over 0–1-, 2–3-, and 4–5-year periods. CNS, central nervous system; NHL, non-Hodgkin's lymphoma.

Reproduced with permission from Bray, F. et al. Global estimates of cancer prevalence for 27 sites in the adult population in 2008. *Int. J. Cancer*, 132(5): 1133–1145. Copyright © 2012. John Wiley and Sons. doi:10.1002/ijc.2771.

Impairments associated with cancer

Cancer causes many impairments, some that are associated with most forms of cancer, others that are more organ specific. They inevitably have an impact on participation and QOL. There are many possible organ-specific impairments, according to the type of cancer the person has. These are not described here because of the many possible types of cancer.

Generic impairments associated with cancer

The management of many of these impairments is similar to that described in the corresponding chapters in this book. Issues that are more closely related to cancer or not described in other chapters are expanded on in the following sections.

Bladder and bowel impairments

Many GI and renal tract cancers will be associated with bladder and bowel impairment, either due to the cancer itself or treatment for it. Similarly, CNS cancers can cause neurogenic bladder and bowel impairment. Some patients will have ostomies following surgery for cancer affecting the colon, rectum, bladder, uterus, and ovaries.

Breathlessness

Lung cancers cause breathlessness due to structural reasons, but breathlessness may occur in any cancer due to comorbidities and side effects of chemotherapy and radiotherapy. Chemotherapies that cause pulmonary toxicity include:
- bleomycin
- erlotinib, dasatinib, and imatinib
- carmustine
- methotrexate.

Bronchiolitis obliterans can occur as a late effect of bone marrow transplantation.

Cachexia, malnutrition, and obesity

Weight loss and weight gain can be a problem for cancer survivors. Cachexia can occur from the primary effects of the cancer on metabolism, but also from malnutrition related to nausea, depression, medication, and pain while having active treatment. Further muscle wasting can occur due to physical inactivity. Dietary counselling during cancer treatment has been shown in some cancers to improve QOL and diet.

For longer-term survivors, obesity can be an issue, although undernutrition can remain a risk, especially in those with GI cancers. Ongoing input to encourage and advise on how to maintain a healthy weight may therefore be beneficial.

Cardiotoxicity

This can be caused by several types of chemotherapy and by radiotherapy in the region of the chest. Chemotherapies known to cause cardiotoxicity include anthracyclines, cyclophosphamide, taxanes, trastuzumab, and sunitinib. Radiotherapy for lung, breast, and head and neck cancers and directed at the mediastinum for lymphoma can result in cardiotoxicity.

CNS impairment

Brain and spinal injury can occur in cancer patients due to:
- metastases, most frequently breast, lung, prostate, or renal cancers
- primary brain and spinal cord tumours
- radiation myelopathy
- radiation vasculopathy.

The same range of secondary effects can occur as in any other condition affecting the brain or spinal cord, with the complexity of issues involved often leading to such patients requiring inpatient rehabilitation.

Cognitive impairment

Cognition can be affected by brain tumours, surgery, or radiotherapy to the CNS and chemotherapy. Commonly cited cognitive impairments include disorganization, confusion, difficulty concentrating, word-finding difficulties, reduced attention span, memory impairments, fatigue, general 'fogginess', and impaired new learning. The term 'chemo-brain' is often used, but is inaccurate, as these symptoms can occur following a range of treatments including hormone therapy, immunotherapy, radiation therapy, and surgery, in addition to chemotherapy.

Cognitive rehabilitation, combined in some programmes with psychotherapy, has been shown to result in improvement in cognitive function in patients with low-grade brain tumours of various types. Examples of studies of cognitive rehabilitation programmes are given in ➲ 'Further reading'.

Fatigue

Cancer-related fatigue is described by the European Association of Palliative Care as 'A subjective feeling of tiredness, weakness or lack of energy'. Estimates of its prevalence in cancer survivors are from 25% to 33%. Associations with fatigue include:
- medication
- anxiety/depression
- proinflammatory cytokines
- hypothalamic–pituitary–adrenal axis dysregulation
- anaemia
- hypothyroidism
- pain
- co-morbidities
- living alone
- sleep disturbance
- physical deconditioning
- psychological reaction to cancer.

Interventions that reduce fatigue are:
- exercise, but there is uncertainty regarding the optimal type and amount of exercise
- psychotherapeutic interventions based on CBT, mindfulness, or yoga.

Lymphoedema

This occurs secondary to disruption of lymphatic drainage from surgery or radiotherapy, with immobility sometimes being an additional factor. It can lead to pain, decreased function of the limb, and cellulitis. Treatment is based on complete decongestive therapy (CDT) which combines several approaches to reduce the lymphoedema and is more effective if started early. A summary of the initial intensive phase of CDT is shown in Table 38.1.

The intensive phase lasts 10–20 days and is followed by a maintenance phase. The maintenance phase follows similar principles, with the patient and any carer being taught and increasingly involved in the therapy.

Osteoporosis

This can occur secondary to chemotherapy, steroids, premature menopause, immobility, and adopting an indoor lifestyle, and can respond to pharmacological and lifestyle interventions as for other causes of osteoporosis.

Pain

Different estimates suggest 30–90% of cancer survivors experience pain. Table 38.2 shows possible contributors to pain, of which there is often more than one in any individual. The principles of treatment of pain are as described in ⊃ Chapter 11, except for bone pain. An algorithm for treating bone pain is shown in Fig. 38.2.[5]

Sexuality and fertility

There are several ways in which sexuality may be affected:
• Disruption of body image caused by the cancer or treatment for it.
• Chemotherapy affecting libido and sexual function.
• Direct damage to organs or structures involved in sexual activity.
• Depression and anxiety.
• Effects on relationships and roles.

Table 38.1 Intensive phase of complete decongestive therapy.

Activity and goal	Brief description of method
Manual lymph drainage to enhance lymphatic flow and reduce limb volume	Massage for about 60 minutes stretches the skin
Multilayer compression bandaging to provide an even low pressure and a structure that limb muscles can contract against	Several types of bandages, such as foam and elasticated short stretch bandages, are wrapped around the limb following manual lymph drainage
Exercises to promote venous, capillary, and lymphatic flow, and hence drainage	Exercises within the compression garment
Skin care to avoid infection	Skin kept clean and hydrated by cleansing and moisturizing

Table 38.2 Sources of pain in cancer

Pain source	Example
Nerve excision during surgery	Spinal accessory nerve in head and neck cancers contributing to shoulder impairment
Nerve compression or damage	Radiation-induced brachial plexopathy following breast cancer
	Intercostal nerve damage following thoracotomy
Bone	Metastatic prostate cancer
Cytokine and chemokine release	Sensitization of pain receptors in vicinity of tumour or metastasis
Peripheral neuropathy	Secondary to chemotherapy using agents such as cisplatin and vinca alkaloids

The general principles of management are the same as those described in
➲ Chapter 13.

Fertility may be affected, and sperm and ovarian banking are becoming
increasingly available prior to surgery or chemotherapy where this may affect fertility. However, there will be many people who have had treatment
prior to the availability of these methods, particularly survivors of childhood cancer.

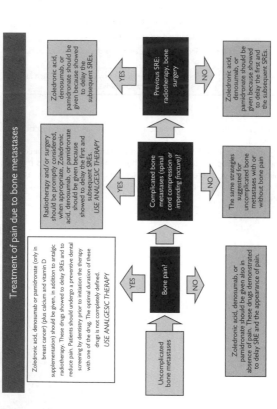

Fig. 38.2 Algorithm describing treatment of bone pain. SREs, skeletal-related events.

Psychological and emotional aspects of rehabilitation following cancer

Cancer causes major disruption to a person's expected life narrative and goals, similar to many other conditions that lead to a need for rehabilitation. Public knowledge of cancer is often greater than for other conditions, which can exacerbate fear to a greater extent than in less well known conditions, but may also result in greater social support and understanding.

The psychological effects of having cancer can range from normal and appropriate distress and worry to a pathological response with depression and/or anxiety. Survivors will have different adjustment styles that will affect rehabilitation overall. Both depression and anxiety occur commonly following cancer and can continue long term. Several studies have shown that the risk is also higher in partners and carers of cancer survivors.

Fear of cancer recurrence is a common source of distress, occurring in 24–70% of cancer survivors. It has been associated with:

- younger age
- having children
- more physical symptoms
- neurotoxicity from treatment
- advanced disease
- higher trait anxiety
- less social support
- low levels of optimism, self-efficacy, and self-esteem
- anxiety and depression
- Pain.[6]

As with many other chronic conditions QOL in cancer survivors has a tendency to return to baseline values. Some of this may be due to patients either continuing to achieve or appropriately adjusting their life goals.

There is evidence that psychological interventions can help following cancer: these can be part of an overall rehabilitation programme (➜ see 'Cancer rehabilitation programmes') or specifically to address the psychological need. CBT, mindfulness, and creative therapies have all been shown to have positive outcomes.

Cancer rehabilitation programmes

As with any rehabilitation programme, those for cancer vary in their content and overall aims, and can be delivered to inpatients or in the community. Programmes contain components that will address some of the impairments listed in previous sections and that will improve aspects of participation such as return to work. Fig. 38.3 demonstrates the areas of intervention that could be included in a rehabilitation programme.

Place of rehabilitation

Those patients with more complex needs may benefit from rehabilitation as an inpatient. There is evidence for both inpatient and community rehabilitation leading to functional improvements both in patients with specific types of cancer and in mixed groups.

Assessment for inpatient rehabilitation follows the principles used for any other patient but the following are important additional factors:

- *Current cancer-related treatment*. The rehabilitation programme should be designed to allow for ongoing chemotherapy and radiotherapy—both logistically and with regard to side effects.
- *Prognosis*. Prognosis will depend on type and stage of cancer and treatments available. In order to plan rehabilitation and negotiate appropriate goals, both the patient and the rehabilitation team need a shared understanding of the patient's prognosis. Goals, and the length of time taken to achieve them, need to be realistic while also allowing the patient a degree of hope.
- *Coordination*. A close ongoing relationship with the treating oncologist is important. In facilities with a higher proportion of cancer patients having inpatient rehabilitation, it is useful for a senior member of the rehabilitation team to join the oncology MDT meetings.

Physical activity

Physical activity programmes using resistance training and cardiopulmonary exercise have been used in many different types of cancer. Cancer survivors have higher risks of obesity, diabetes, secondary cancers, cardiovascular disease, and physical deconditioning all of which are known to be reduced by physical activity in the general population. The current literature suggests that at virtually all points along the cancer trajectory, patients benefit from incremental aerobic exercise, and that exercise intensities as high as 90% of maximal heart rate three times weekly can be safely tolerated.

In cancer, physical activity programmes have been shown to result in improved fatigue, nausea, insomnia, mental health, mobility, well-being, and QOL. Both home-based and group exercise have been shown to be beneficial. Interventions can be directed at complications associated with particular types of surgery, such as shoulder impairment following head and neck cancer surgery, or to improve overall levels of physical activity, function, and fitness.

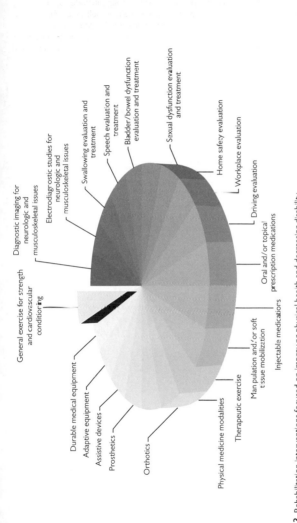

Fig. 38.3 Rehabilitation interventions focused on improving physical health and decreasing disability.

Self-management

Programmes that enable the person to self-manage include aspects giving medical and practical information that will help in self-care and psychological strategies. Programmes can be delivered in different ways, with evidence for group, individual, telephone, and web-based programmes reducing depression and anxiety and improving emotional well-being and self-efficacy.

References

1. National Institute for Health and Care Excellence (NICE) (2004). *Improving Supportive and Palliative Care for Patients with Cancer*. Cancer service guideline [CSG4]. NICE, London. ℜ http://www.nice.org.uk/guidance/csg4.

2. Cancer Services Coordinating Group (2010). *National Standards for Rehabilitation of Adult Cancer Patients for Wales*. ℜ http://www.wales.nhs.uk/sites3/Documents/322/National_Standards_for_Rehabilitation_of_Adult_Cancer_Patients_2010.pdf.

3. Harris S, Schmitz KH, Campbell KL, et al. (2012). Clinical practice guidelines for breast cancer rehabilitation. *Cancer* 118, 2312–2324.

4. National Cancer Expert Reference Group (2016). *Optimal Pathway for Patients with Breast Cancer*. ℜ https://www.cancer.org.au/content/ocp/health/optimal-care-pathway-for-women-with-breast-cancer june-2016.pdf.

5. Ripamonti CI, Santini D, Maranzano E, et al. (2012). Management of cancer pain: ESMO clinical practice guidelines. *Annals of Oncology* 23, vii139–vii154.

6. Mehnert A, Koch U, Sundermann C, et al. (2013). Predictors of fear of recurrence in patients one year after cancer rehabilitation: a prospective study. *Acta Oncologica* 52, 1102–1109.

Further reading

General texts or reviews regarding cancer rehabilitation

Cheville AL (2015). Cancer rehabilitation. In: Cfiu DX (ed), *Braddoms's Textbook of Physical Medicine and Rehabilitation*, 5th edn, pp. 627–652. Saunders/Elsevier, Philadelphia, PA.

Salakari MR, Surakka T, Nurminen R, et al. (2015). Effects of rehabilitation among patients with advanced cancer: a systematic review. *Acta Oncologica* 54, 618–628.

Silver JK, Baima J, Newman R, et al. (2013). Cancer rehabilitation may improve function in survivors and decrease the economic burden of cancer to individuals and society. *Work* 46, 455–472.

Stubblefield MD, Hubbard G, Cheville A, et al. (2013). Current perspectives and emerging issues on cancer rehabilitation. *Cancer* 119, 2170–2178.

Yung RL, Partridge AH (2016). Cancer survivorship and rehabilitation. In: Kerr DJ, Haller DG, van de Velde CJH, et al. (eds), *Oxford Textbook of Oncology*, 3rd edn, pp. 312–326. Oxford University Press, Oxford.

Cognitive rehabilitation

Ownsworth T, Chambers S, Damborg E, et al. (2015). Evaluation of the making sense of brain tumor program: a randomized controlled trial of a home-based psychosocial intervention. *Psycho-Oncology* 24, 540–547.

Pil K, Juhler M, Jakobsen J, et al. (2014). Controlled rehabilitative and supportive care intervention trials in patients with high-grade gliomas and their caregivers: a systematic review. *BMJ Supportive & Palliative Care*, 6, 27–34.

Examples of generic programmes or guidelines

Chasen MR, Feldstain A, Gravelle D, et al. (2013). An interprofessional palliative care oncology rehabilitation program: effects on function and predictors of program completion. *Current Oncology* 20, 301–309.

Harris S, Schmitz KH, Campbell KL, et al. (2012). Clinical Practice Guidelines for Breast Cancer Rehabilitation: Syntheses of Guideline Recommendations and Qualitative Appraisals. *Cancer* 118, 2312–24.

Hauken MA, Holsen I, Fismen E, et al. (2015). Working toward a good life as a cancer survivor: a longitudinal study on positive health outcomes of a rehabilitation program for young adult cancer survivors. *Cancer Nursing* 38, 3–15.

Shahpar S, Mhatre PV, Huang ME (2016). Update on brain tumors: new developments in neuro-oncologic diagnosis and treatment, and impact on rehabilitation strategies. *PM R* 8, 678–689.

Examples of programmes with emphasis on physical activity

Cheville AL, Kollasch J, Vandenberg J, et al. (2013). A home-based exercise program to improve function, fatigue, and sleep quality in patients with stage IV lung and colorectal cancer: a randomized controlled trial. *Journal of Pain and Symptom Management* 45, 811–821

McNeely ML, Parliament MB, Seikaly H, et al. (2008). Effect of exercise on upper extremity pain and dysfunction in head and neck cancer survivors. *Cancer* 113, 1097–10142

Rock CL, Doyle C, Demark-Wahnefried W, et al. (2012). Nutrition and physical activity guidelines for cancer survivors. *CA: A Cancer Journal for Clinicians* 62, 242–274.

Examples of self-management programmes

Gaston-Johansson F, Fall-Dickson JM, Nanda JP, et al. (2013). Long-term effect of the self-management comprehensive coping strategy program on quality of life in patients with breast cancer treated with high-dose chemotherapy. *Psycho-Oncology* 22, 530–539.

Risendal B, Dwyer A, Seidel R, et al. (2014). Adaptation of the chronic disease self-management program for cancer survivors: feasibility, acceptability, and lessons for implementation. *Journal of Cancer Education* 29, 762–771.

Geriatric rehabilitation

Epidemiology and introduction

Between 2015 and 2030, the number of older persons aged 60 years and above will grow by more than 50% to 1.4 billion people worldwide. During this same period, the proportion of old to young people will fall from one to eight to one in six globally. The ageing process is particularly advanced in Europe and North America where survival to age 80 years is norm.

Ageing, however, is strongly associated with co-morbidities, frailty, and disability. The co-morbidity burden is tremendous with at least two-thirds of elderly having three or more chronic diseases. More than a quarter of elderly patients are frail and a similar proportion have ADL difficulties, especially those older than 75 years. The elderly are further characterized by medical *complexity* and 20% or more may have overlapping domains of significant co-morbidity, frailty, and disability.

The MDT approach is particularly important in geriatric rehabilitation due to patient complexity and disability which is often multicausal from a number of diagnoses. This is especially so when addressing the rehabilitation of geriatric syndromes such as falls, delirium and dementia, incontinence, functional decline, and frailty. The rehabilitation physician is well placed to lead and direct the team with his/her skills through a holistic multimodal biopsychosocial approach.

The gold standard clinical tool used to assess this complexity is the Comprehensive Geriatric Assessment (CGA). The use of the CGA is associated with improved outcomes including improving care quality, reduction of readmissions and medical complications, with better functional outcomes and QOL. The CGA is used *together* with the WHO ICF (➲ see Chapter 2) for prognostication, problem-solving, and rehabilitation interventions. For example, the CGA may indicate moderately severe cognitive impairment in a patient. Using the ICF model, this could manifest in activity limitation or participation restriction which is modifiable with environmental, personal, or behavioural interventions.

Physical frailty, sarcopenia, and the consequences of reduced mobility are specific areas that rehabilitation clinicians are well suited to assess and offer interventions for. Falls, and their association with minimal trauma fractures, are characteristic of the elderly and geriatric rehabilitation.

Finally, there is a need to guard against 'ageism', defined as the conscious or subconscious stereotyping or discrimination against someone based on a person's age. Frail older patients should not be excluded from rehabilitation whenever clinically significant outcomes are achievable.

Comprehensive Geriatric Assessment

The CGA is based on the framework that recognizes the cumulative burden of multiple domains operative in an elderly patient (Table 39.1). This is important as clinicians underestimate the extent of disability.

- The CGA involves an interdisciplinary team (team members have skills in domains outside their own expertise) to approach and evaluate the needs of the older person. The results of the CGA are used to guide an overall comprehensive, individualized plan for rehabilitation.
- The CGA is often integrated into specific programmes for the elderly. For example, fall intervention programmes include a home environmental assessment together with the CGA and a geriatric oncology programme will use the CGA to stratify functional recovery, chemotherapy, or surgical interventions in addition to cancer-specific prognostic biomarkers.
- Core domains usually assessed are:
  - ADLs
  - instrumental ADLs (IADLs)
  - cognition
  - emotion and mood
  - co-morbidity
  - polypharmacy.
- Depending on specific programmes or individualized needs, other common domains assessed include:
  - mobility and falls
  - social support
  - nutritional status.
- A common critique of the CGA is that it is time-consuming. Composite screening measures have been developed for use in various healthcare settings, such as the Vulnerable Elders Survey-13 (VES-13) to determine which seniors may benefit from more detailed assessment. This is an area that requires further research before more widespread adoption.
- There is also varying expertise required in administering various scales within each domain. Geriatric programmes and units often stratify scales into simpler ones with high sensitivity which can be administered by junior clinicians to determine which domains require more comprehensive assessment.

Table 39.1 Comprehensive Geriatric Assessment with domains measured. Examples of screening and more detailed assessment tools given in each domain and listed in WHO-ICF standardized order

Domain	Screening tool example	More detailed assessment tool example
Cognition	Abbreviated Mental Test (AMT)	Mini-Mental State Examination (MMSE)
Mood	Patient Health Questionnaire-2 Screening Instrument (PHQ-2)	Geriatric Depression Scale (GDS)
Co-morbidity	Simple Count of diseases ICD Code Count	Charlson Comorbidity Index (CCI)
Medications	Direct count of potentially inappropriate medication use in older adults with Beers' Criteria with subsequent medication review	Measurement incorporated into systems designed to evaluate polypharmacy. A well-known system is the STOPP-START
Nutrition	Height, weight, BMI Mini Nutritional Assessment Tool (MNA)	Dietician assessment with: Calculations on energy expenditure Measurement of body fat through skinfold calipers
Daily basic ADLs	Katz Index	Functional Independence Measure (FIM) Barthel Index
Instrumental ADLs (IADLs)	Direct questioning: 'Do you do shopping, housework or manage money yourself?'	The Lawton IADL Scale
Social support	Family tree diagram Direct questioning: 'Do you live alone?' 'Do you have a caregiver?'	Zarit Caregiver Burden Inventory Community Integration Questionnaires
Physical function/ mobility	Grip strength Gait speed Timed Up and Go Functional Reach Test	Cardiopulmonary exercise testing Muscle mass analysis: DXA scan Body impedance analysis

STOPP: Screening tool of older people's prescriptions and START: screening tool to alert to right treatment.

Practical assessment and investigation pointers for geriatric rehabilitation

When assessing patients for geriatric rehabilitation programmes, a comprehensive history and physical examination is essential to avoid missing diagnoses or impairments that may impact rehabilitation. Specific points include the following:

* Allow time to establish good rapport, which often requires initial informal conversations revolving around latest news, social activities, or other family members (particularly grandchildren!). This facilitates more open sharing and discussions and often allows invaluable insights into social support dynamics.
* Screening the sensory systems for impairments, particularly visual, hearing, vestibular, and the integrity of the peripheral nervous system for loss of sensation and proprioception. Cataracts and sensorineural hearing loss are prevalent in the elderly and can impact significantly on the ability to participate in rehabilitation. Peripheral neuropathy with loss of pain sensation or position sense may require targeted rehabilitation strategies to minimize falls.
* Assessment for postural hypotension. Check blood pressures in both arms, with a systolic blood pressure drop of 20 mmHg or more being significant. Consequences include falls, stroke, and cardiovascular complications if not treated.
* Three widely used simple physical tests are conducted in geriatric assessment and rehabilitation units. They are strongly associated with underlying physiological processes including frailty and sarcopenia. They predict a wide range of outcomes from falls, ADL and IADL status, readmissions, discharge to nursing homes, and mortality.
  * *Walking speed* (WS). Its importance in geriatric rehabilitation has led it to be designated a *vital sign*. It is an independent predictor of mortality in this population. Subjects walk at their comfortable speed and are timed over a fixed distance usually 5 or 10 metres. Normal WS ranges from 1.2 to 1.4 metres/second. A threshold of 0.8 metres/second or less often indicates an elder 'at risk', necessitating further assessment. A meaningful improvement would be a gain of 0.05 metres/second from initial measurements.
  * *Grip strength* (GS). GS is significantly associated with overall health, strength, and muscle mass. Subjects perform maximum voluntary GS contractions with a grip dynamometer. Averages of two or three values from each hand are taken and scores are normalized against the BMI. Norms stratified by age, sex, and race are widely available for reference.
  * *Timed Up and Go (TUG) test*. The TUG is an excellent composite screen of physical performance. Like WS and GS, the TUG associates strongly with functional outcomes and frailty. The patient is timed rising from a chair, walking 3 metres, turning around, walking back to the same chair, and sitting down. Generally timings of longer than 30 seconds are associated with disability in the elderly and norms are available for common geriatric conditions including PD, OA, and recurrent fall cohorts.

- Simple, inexpensive, rapid diagnostic tests with high yield should be performed in the elderly presenting with disability to the rehabilitation inpatient unit or outpatient clinics. These include:
  - complete blood count
  - electrolytes, blood urea nitrogen (BUN), glucose, and creatinine
  - vitamin D, calcium, and phosphate levels
  - vitamin B12 and folate levels
  - thyroid function tests
  - chest X-ray and ECG.

Medications in the elderly

More than two-thirds of people above 65 are on regular medication and up to one-quarter may have adverse drug reactions in ambulatory care. Medication selection and dosing is challenging in the elderly, with limited evidence to guide choices. Management is guided by prior experience, clinical guidelines, and minimizing polypharmacy. In addition, rational decisions to commence drugs include considerations of future life expectancy and a respect for the patients' care goals.

Non-pharmacological approaches are often effective and can be tried first. These include nutritional guidance, exercise advice, and weight reduction. When prescription is necessary, all drugs should have a documented response to therapy to determine effectiveness and continuation.

Periodic drug reviews are essential. Medication reconciliation is a deliberate process where current and prior medication lists are compared and summative decisions made on the most optimal list. Herbal, complementary, and over-the-counter medication use are common and patients need to be specifically told to bring these during consults. Consideration for safer alternatives, dose simplification, and reduction to the minimum effective dose should be actively performed. The Beers Criteria and START-STOPP are two well-known and practical guides in appropriate prescribing for the elderly.

In the elderly, an adverse drug reaction or interaction requires consideration as a differential in any new impairment. The *prescribing cascade* occurs when an adverse drug reaction is diagnosed as a new impairment or medical condition and additional drugs are then prescribed to address these. An example in the rehabilitation setting is the prescription of new medications for Parkinsonism when the manifested impairments are actually extrapyramidal side effects of antipsychotic drugs for agitation control in brain injury.

Clinicians need not withhold important drugs just to avoid polypharmacy and fear of side effects. However, 'start low and go slow' is an important maxim for prescriptions as the elderly have altered sensitivity to higher doses. Conversely, avoid suboptimal prescription of beneficial drugs as well. Under-treatment for systolic hypertension results in a significant risk of major cardiovascular events. Older women with untreated osteoporosis have a four times increased risk of developing a fragility fracture compared to those with normal bone mineral density. Older patients suffer from chronic pain more commonly than younger people because of multiple co-morbidities. Inadequate management of pain may result in delirium in the elderly. NSAIDs should be used with particular care due to adverse effects on the cardiovascular, GI, and renal systems and potentially covered with a gastroprotective agent. Opioids are preferred second-line therapy after acetaminophen and options include codeine for mild pain and morphine and fentanyl for moderate to severe pain. A common issue is that older patients are suboptimally treated because of the reluctance to prescribe opioid analgesics and even if given, doses are often inadequate.

Finally, compliance is a common issue in geriatric patients. Patients or caregivers require education on the use of drugs and informed about adverse events. Financial considerations have also emerged as an important reason why prescriptions may be written but not filled. Further measures to improve compliance include simplifying drug packaging, increasing label size, using liquid or suspension formulations where tablets are hard to swallow, utilizing pill boxes, and avoiding the need for divided doses.

Frailty and sarcopenia

Frailty and sarcopenia are core concepts in geriatric rehabilitation. The cornerstones of interventions are well-prescribed nutrition and therapeutic exercise which are familiar to rehabilitation clinicians.

Frailty

Frailty is defined as a geriatric syndrome of increased vulnerability due to diminished physiological reserve. Close to half of people older than 85 years are frail and even higher proportions are in the pre-frail categories.

Important points:

- The term *increased vulnerability* is key and denotes an 'at-risk' cohort. This concept is illustrated by the frailty (or disability) cascade (Fig. 39.1).
- Frailty is associated and often precedes the development of the geriatric syndromes, particularly falls, and cognitive, physical, and functional decline.
- There is also a significantly higher risk of worse outcomes after surgery, postoperative complications, readmissions, nursing home admissions, general morbidity, and mortality.
- The underlying basic science processes are explained by the concept of system redundancy. There is reserve built into organ systems to withstand stressors. However, due to cumulative intrinsic (physiological changes with ageing) or extrinsic (e.g. poor nutrition or lack of exercise) factors, a health threshold is crossed. This then manifests clinically and can rapidly lead to permanent disability and eventual institutionalization.
- The well-known phenotype model has five indicators of frailty:
  - Weight loss of at least 4.5 kg or 5% per year
  - Self-reported exhaustion of (3–4 days per week or most of the time) on the Center for Epidemiological Studies depression scale.
  - Low energy expenditure of less than 383 kcal/week (men) or less than 270 kcal/week (women).
  - Slow WS.
  - Weak GS.

A diagnosis of 'frailty' requires three or more indicators, while 'pre-frail' elderly people fulfil one or two criteria.

- The other well-known model is the cumulative deficit paradigm and the frailty index. More than 90 variables of symptoms, signs, laboratory values, co-morbidities, and disabilities are collected and frailty is ascertained when crossing a predefined cumulative threshold.
- The two best established interventions for frailty are exercise and adequate nutrition after a comprehensive assessment. In healthy individuals, exercise delays the onset of frailty. In frail elderly people, exercise slows the progression of frailty. A short summary of exercise in the elderly follows.
- Important nutritional interventions:
  - Protein and protein-energy undernutrition. This is common and under-recognized. Acute illness and chronic co-morbidities induce inflammatory responses and hormonal changes creating a state of muscle catabolism and lipolysis. Altered swallowing ability and appetite loss causes further malnutrition.

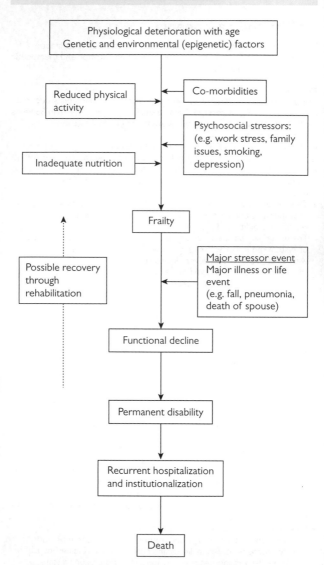

Fig. 39.1 Development of frailty and the frailty cascade.

- Quick estimates for daily energy requirements are 25–30 kcal/kg to maintain weight, increasing to 35–45 kcal/kg in acutely ill or stressful conditions. Guidelines also recommend a protein intake for elderly adults of 1.0–1.25 g/kg/day rising to 1.5 g/kg/day in acutely ill patients. Supplementation is often required and referral to the team dietician is appropriate for complex cases or when patients are not able to take food orally.
- Micronutrient insufficiently, specifically calcium and vitamin D. The recommended calcium daily allowance is 1200 mg/day in older people over 70 years. Vitamin D deficiency is common in frail patients and supplementation reduces falls and hip fractures, and improves muscle function and mortality. A level of less than 30 ng/mL is a threshold for repletion with ergocalciferol (vitamin D_2, e.g. 50,000 IU weekly) or cholecalciferol (vitamin D_3, e.g. 2000 IU daily).

Sarcopenia

Sarcopenia is defined as the age-associated loss of muscle mass which may also manifest as a loss in muscle strength or performance. As in frailty, it is associated with geriatric syndromes and has similar rehabilitation outcomes. It is commonly studied in parallel with frailty, as the underlying physiological basis of both conditions overlap. Sarcopenia can precede physical frailty or frailty can give rise to sarcopenia. The common end points of both conditions are mobility impairments and disability.

- With ageing, body weight increases till about 60 years, after which it stabilizes and begins to decline.
- Weight changes are attributed to increased fat mass, with intra-abdominal (visceral) fat increasing relatively more than peripheral fat. There is accompanied by a progressive loss in muscle mass proportionately greater peripherally in the limbs compared to centrally in the trunk.
- The diagnosis of sarcopenia requires confirmation of low muscle mass. This is measured classically by dual energy X-ray absorptiometry (DXA). Lately, bioimpedance analysis (BIA) instruments offer a portable alternative.
- Most international criteria also require demonstration of low muscle strength usually through GS tests or low physical performance either with WS or the TUG test.
- The ability to increase muscle mass is impaired in the elderly, but it is still possible to do so. The elderly require greater amounts of protein post exercise to stimulate muscle growth compared with younger adults. Muscle growth can be stimulated by an improved diet and resistance training but with lesser gains than in younger adults.
- The mainstays of treatment are similar to frailty including the need to perform a comprehensive and nutritional assessment as well as exercise interventions. The use of pharmacological treatments such as testosterone or growth hormones is experimental.

Physical activity and exercise in older adults

Physical activity (PA) includes any movement that increases energy expenditure above baseline. Exercise is planned, structured, and repetitive PA with the goal of improving fitness and health. Ageing is associated with diminished PA from physical, cognitive, and social reasons such as increasing sedentary behaviour. With advancing age, physical reductions in aerobic capacity, muscle strength, and performance occur even in the absence of co-morbidities.

The benefits of PA and exercise in the elderly are numerous, and include the following:
* Increases average life expectancy.
* Improves cardiovascular fitness, muscle and bone mass, and strength.
* Reduces the risk of developing chronic disease common in the elderly such as ischaemic heart disease, stroke, type 2 diabetes, depression, and anxiety.
* Mitigates or even improves the functional status in already developed disease including OA and osteoporosis.
* Effective in the geriatric syndromes including cognitive impairment, falls, and frailty.
* Improves a broad range of psychological systems and is a major lifestyle factor for successful ageing.
* Significant benefits across the geriatric continuum from healthy to frail elderly and in patients with established chronic disease or those requiring palliative care. *Pre-habilitation* is a rehabilitation concept important in older adults and refers to PA or exercise prior to developing disease, disability or preceding major surgery or medical intervention (e.g. chemotherapy).

Exercise is so important that the term 'Exercise is Medicine' has been coined and is a global initiative. It emphasizes the therapeutic value of exercise at the same level as any medication intervention.

Current guidelines on activity for older adults are the same as all adults with some specific recommendations. These are as follows:
* Total of 150 minutes/week of moderate-intensity activities or 30 minutes/day in intervals of about 10 minutes each, *or* 75 minutes/week of high-intensity activities *or* a combination of both. This correlates to an average energy expenditure of about 1000 kcal/wk.
  * Examples of moderate-intensity exercises include brisk walking, swimming, or cycling. The latter are useful to reduce biomechanical stress in the lower limbs in elderly people with limited tolerance to walking.
* Resistance training on 2–3 days/week at moderate intensity. Apart from progressive resistance exercise using free or machine weights, stair climbing is a useful exercise for geriatric patients or healthy older people when weights are not readily available.
* Balance training should be incorporated as this improves performance of usual ADL activities. Balance exercises include static exercises

(reducing base of support by tandem or one-legged stance), dynamic exercises (e.g. stretching out to touch an object or tandem walking), and sensory substitution exercises (e.g. standing with eyes closed or walks with uneven surfaces).
- Incorporate flexibility and ROM exercises in the exercise programme with prolonged sustained stretches of major muscle groups.
- Multimodal exercises are often appealing and improve motivation through use of the group setting. The use of weighted vests for walking in the community and the practice of yoga are examples.
  - Another established modality in geriatric rehabilitation in many parts of the world is Tai-chi. Tai-chi originated as a martial art in ancient China but has spread throughout the world with robust evidence of health benefits. Tai-chi improves balance, flexibility, and strength, in addition to psychological health improvements through meditative techniques and its thought philosophy. Tai-chi is often performed in groups which adds to its appeal.
- Exercise stratification and PA limitations may be needed in elderly patients especially with the higher prevalence of cardiopulmonary disease (➔ see Chapters 16 and 17) and chronic musculoskeletal conditions (➔ see Chapters 35 and 36).
- Understanding difficulties with initiating exercise in sedentary elderly people is important. Any PA is better than none, and participation in any amount of activity has health benefits. Thus, if the exercise thresholds above are not reached, they should still be as physically active as their capacities and co-morbidities allow. Even low-intensity activities of walking, gardening, and shopping in the community are beneficial.
- The use of technology such as pedometers and wearables that measure steps, heart rate, and activity approximations are increasingly popular. Preliminary studies indicate that they improve activity through biofeedback and are promising tools to encourage exercise in the elderly in the future.

Hip fracture rehabilitation example

Hip fracture is the diagnosis that epitomizes geriatric rehabilitation.

Comprehensive management not only rehabilitates the hip fracture, but also addresses the geriatric syndromes of falls, frailty, and functional decline. A brief example follows.

A 75-year-old old woman was referred for a rehabilitation consult after a fall at home complicated by a left intertrochanteric hip fracture. She had a sliding hip screw fixation and is currently in her third postoperative day. The orthopaedic surgeon had indicated 'weight-bearing as tolerated' in the operative notes.

She was assessed comprehensively through a CGA and the WHO ICF framework (listed by standardized ICF order) with a focus on addressing falls:

- Cognition: 23 out of 30 in the MMSE (mild cognitive impairment). She feels she is more forgetful recently.
- Mood: 6 out of 15 on the Geriatric Depression Scale (mild depression). Admits to feeling bored, fatigued, and sad that her children do not visit her any more at home.
- Co-morbidities: hypertension, diabetes mellitus, ischaemic heart disease, CHF, and chronic kidney disease. She recently developed vision problems.
- Medications: atenolol, hydrochlorothiazide, nifedipine, enalapril. metformin, glipizide, furosemide, and aspirin.
- ADLs: prior to fracture, independent in all ADLs including dressing and toileting.
- IADLs: independent prior to fracture including food preparation, housekeeping, and laundry. However, takes a much longer time to complete tasks over the past few months. Requires a walking cane when she takes public transportation and does shopping.
- Mobility: no specific exercises but walks for about half an hour on most weekdays. History of a fall about 6 months ago which she attributed to tripping over an old rug.
- Social and personal: lives with 78-year-old husband who is active in the community. Her children live in another city. Enjoys social gatherings with a group of friends but this is becoming less frequent.
- Environment: lives in one-storey house which is over 50 years old. Admits to being a 'hoarder' and her rooms are cluttered with sentimental belongings collected through her lifetime.

Salient points in clinical examination:

- Thin woman (BMI = 17) who is alert, responsive, but appears dehydrated. Her supine blood pressure is 105/60 mmHg which falls to 85/50 mmHg when she stands up. Resting pulse rate is 50 beats/minute.
- She is in some pain (pain score 3/10) in the left hip but is manageable and tolerating therapy.
- Diminished lower limb strength generally with the hip extensors, knee flexors, and extensors all graded 4/5. Has glove-and-stocking distribution of peripheral neuropathy in the lower limbs.
- Systemic examination revealed bilateral cataracts and reduced hearing. She has poor dentition with tooth caries. Evaluation of the cardiovascular, respiratory, abdominal, and neurological system is otherwise normal.
- Relevant laboratory tests: haemoglobin 10 g/dL (normochromic, normocytic), creatinine 130 μmol/L, vitamin D 20 ng/mL (low); calcium, albumin, vitamin B_{12}, folate and thyroid function tests are normal

- Currently requires moderate assistance in lower body dressing, transfers, toileting and requires minimal assistance with a walker to cover 5 metres. She also has poor GS compared to age and BMI norms.

The rehabilitation plans would include the following:
- Medications: furosemide and nifedipine were removed due to dehydration and postural hypotension. Metformin was stopped due to risk of lactic acidosis with renal impairment in the elderly.
- DVT prophylaxis with low-molecular-weight heparin was continued with a plan to continue for at least 10 days postoperatively.
- Vitamin D supplementation with ergocalciferol 50,000 IU was commenced once weekly and a scheduled recheck of levels planned in 2 months.
- Subcutaneous denosumab was started for osteoporosis as bisphosphonates were relatively contraindicated in her as she had renal impairment. A bone mineral density DXA scan was ordered to chart baseline values for follow-up later.
- Supplementation with a high-caloric milk drink with breakfast and a protein supplement was prescribed. Referral to a dietician was also done for detailed nutritional assessment and more eating choices in view of her co-morbidities. Dental assessment was performed to evaluate for mechanical impairments to swallowing.
- Physical and occupational therapy interventions for therapeutic, mobility, and functional exercises, including:
  - TENS for hip pain
  - isometric exercises for the hip muscle groups with gentle resistive exercises for the rest of the muscle groups
  - using assistive devices including long-handle reachers and walking aids
  - foot care and education as well as customized footwear with antislip soles were prescribed due to the risk of falls from peripheral neuropathy
  - education and training in fall prevention strategies.

Prior to discharge, reasonable measures would be as follows:
- Physician and pharmacist review for medication conflicts, patient education, and compliance.
- Promote activity with clear, reasonable prescriptions for continuing PA and exercise in the community. It helps to state exactly what is required, for example, 20 minutes of brisk walking a day, five times a week rather than vague phrases like 'Exercise as much as you can'.
- Caregiver training for the husband to be provided. Also, if the patient still required ADL assistance, a referral to home-based care or continued home rehabilitation is appropriate.
- An occupational therapy home assessment for recommendations to reduce falls risk due to the cluttering at home and facilitation of mobility. This could include non-slip flooring, grab bars, rails, and raised toilet seats.
- A detailed continuity of care plan is provided to the GP incorporating assessments and interventions thus far. Indication of monitoring necessary for cognitive and mood impairment for possible dementia or depression. Referrals also made for outpatient assessments of vision, hearing, and dentition with the relevant specialties.
- Liaison between hospital social work and community services including support groups to reduce risk of loneliness and depression. This can be tailored to her hobbies and personality if peer group support is available.

Further reading

American College of Sports Medicine, Chodzko-Zajko WJ, Proctor DN, et al. (2009). American College of Sports Medicine position stand. Exercise and physical activity for older adults. *Medicine & Science in Sports & Exercise* 41, 1510–1530.

Clegg A, Young J, Iliffe S, et al. (2013). Frailty in elderly people. *Lancet* 381, 752–62.

Morley JE (2016). Frailty and sarcopenia: the new geriatric giants. *Revista de Investigación Clínica* 68, 59–67.

Phillips EM, Bodenheimer CF, Roig RL, et al. (2004). Geriatric rehabilitation. 4. Physical medicine and rehabilitation interventions for common age-related disorders and geriatric syndromes. *Archives of Physical Medicine and Rehabilitation* 85, S18–S22

Scottish Intercollegiate Network (SIGN). *Management of Hip Fracture in Older People.* ℘ http://www.sign.ac.uk/guidelines/fulltext/111/.

United Nations, Department of Economic and Social Affairs, Population Division (2015). World Population Ageing 2015—Highlights (ST/ESA/SER.A/368). ℘ https://www.un.org/en/development/desa/population/publications/pdf/ageing/WPA2015_Highlights.pdf.

Wells JL, Seabrook JA, Stolee P, et al. (2003). State of the art in geriatric rehabilitation. Part I: review of frailty and comprehensive geriatric assessment. *Archives of Physical Medicine and Rehabilitation* 84, 890–897.

Burns rehabilitation

Introduction

A burn injury is an unexpected and dramatic event in a person's life, with a strong likelihood of persistent physical and psychological impacts. Overall, the incidence of burns is relatively low; however, it is higher in developing countries, in lower socioeconomic and disadvantaged groups, in children under 2 years of age, and in the workplace. Immediately post burn, first aid focuses on survival of the individual and the prevention of additional burn damage (e.g. by pouring copious amounts of cold water on thermal burns).

How well a person copes following a burn injury depends on multiple factors including those relating to the burns themselves (e.g. area, depth, and type), secondary issues relating to treatment (e.g. efficacy of pain management and multiple operations), associated long-term implications (e.g. contractures, cosmesis, and psychology), along with personality, family, and societal influences. As with all rehabilitation, the goal is to maximize quality of life by minimizing adverse outcomes, maximizing adaptation, and encouraging positive psychological coping mechanisms.

People with significant burns will have been hospitalized, and it is this group who have the highest rehabilitation needs. Of all the various factors that go towards determining the personal impact of burns, the basic predictors of outcome following a burn injury (i.e. burn type, surface area, and depth) will be addressed first.

Types/mechanism of burns

Three primary types of burns are recognized: thermal, chemical, and electrical. Other burn modalities include friction burns (i.e. where skin is lost due to abrasion from a hard surface) and burns from ionizing radiation. The primary burn types include the following:

- *Thermal burns* are caused by the application of sources of heat or cold to body tissues. Heat burns can be radiative (e.g. standing near a large fire or high-power radio transmitter) or from direct contact (e.g. steam, hot liquids, or hot objects). Cold burns occur from exposure to temperatures that are sufficiently cold to prevent tissue warming through blood flow (e.g. frostbite) through to contact with temperatures which freeze tissue. Around 80% of burns are related to thermal causes.
- *Chemical burns* occur from exposure to chemicals in liquid, gas, or solid form. Chemicals continue to cause damage as long as they are in contact with body tissues. For this reason, chemical burns require close examination to ensure all sources of chemical have been removed. In addition, some chemicals can be absorbed through the skin and produce systemic toxicity (e.g. cement).
- *Electrical burns* occur from exposure to an electrical source. Low-voltage electrical burns produce superficial injury whereas high-voltage burns can produce extensive dermal and subdermal damage. Electrical burns have an entry and exit point from the body and produce deep damage between these points, particularly along the more conductive tissues such as muscle and nerve. These 'electrical passage burns' may cause greater internal injuries than suggested by the extent of the external burn. The severity of damage depends on the amount of energy the person is exposed to (i.e. voltage, current, and time) and the pathway the current takes through the body.

Estimation of burn area

The total area of burns is a vital determinant of medical acuity, having a strong correlation with both morbidity and mortality. A number of approaches have been established to help in determining the total surface area of the burn. For smaller burns, the 'hand method' is simple and effective. Here, burn estimation is completed by considering the palmar surface of the patient's hand and fingers as 1% of their total body surface. The number of 'hands' of burn over the body is estimated and a total percentage calculated from this. In adults with larger burns, the 'Wallace rule of nines' is a relatively simple process for ready estimation. This rule divides the body into areas approximating multiples of 9% of the body (Fig. 40.1):

Body region	% surface area	
Head	9%	
Chest	18%	
Back	18%	
Arm	Right 9%	Left 9%
Leg	Right 18%	Left 18%
Perineum	1%	

In children (whose body proportions differ from adults) it is more accurate to use a Lund and Browder chart (Fig. 40.1). These charts estimate the percentage of surface area burned with reference to changes in children's body shape and size in 5-year increments during their development through to adulthood.

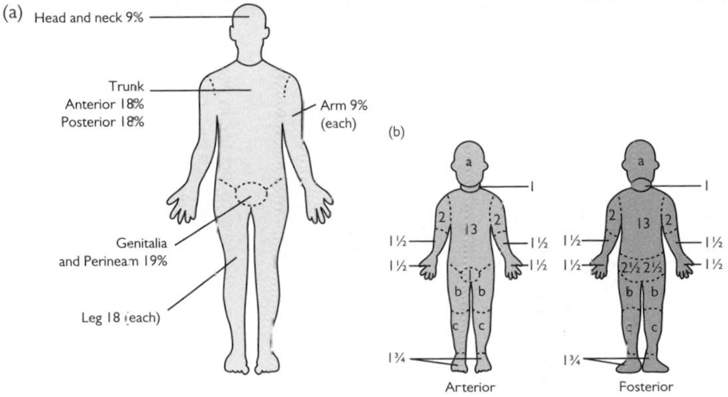
(a)
Head and neck 9%
Trunk
Anterior 18%
Posterior 18%
Arm 9%
(each)
Genitalia
and Perineum 19%
Leg 18 (each)
(b)
a
1
2
13
2
1½
1½
1½
1½
b b
c c
1¾
Anterior
a
1
2
13
2
1½
1½
1½
1½
2½ 2½
b b
c c
1¾
Posterior

Relative percentage of body surface area (% BSA) affected by growth

	Age				
Body Part	0 yr	1 yr	5 yr	10 yr	15 yr
a = ½ of head	9½	8½	6½	5½	4½
b = ½ of 1 thigh	2¾	3½	4	4¼	2¼
c = ½ of 1 lower leg	2½	2½	2%	3	3¼

Fig. 40.1 (a) The Wallace rule of nines. (b) The Lund and Browder chart.

Reproduced from Crouch R. et al. (Eds.). Skin emergencies in *Oxford Handbook of Emergency Nursing* (2 ed.). Oxford, UK: Oxford University Press. © 2010, Oxford University Press. Reproduced with permission of Oxford University Press through PLSclear. http://oxfordmedicine.com/view/10.1093/med/9780199688869.001.0001/med-9780199688869-chapter-12?rskey=MOS5Ib&result=1.

Classification of burn thickness

It can be challenging in the immediate post-burn period to accurately determine the thickness of burns. The classification of burn depth is usually undertaken with reference to the anatomical structures of the skin (Fig. 40.2). Distinction between classes of burns is important as it is a major determinant of the likely success of spontaneous healing, and helps to predict the need for surgical management and other interventions. A standard grading scale of burn thickness is as follows:

- *First-degree burns* are superficial, only involving the epidermis. They are usually painful and heal over a number of days with minimal or no scarring.
- *Second-degree burns* involve the epidermis and the dermis, they can be divided into superficial and deep partial thickness burns:
  - Superficial partial thickness burns involve the superficial dermis. They appear red and often blister, with the skin colour blanching to touch. These burns are painful but re-epithelialize over 1–2 weeks from underlying intact epidermis, hair follicles, and sweat glands. While scarring is minimal, the healed skin may lack normal pigmentation.
  - Deep partial thickness burns incorporate damage of the deep dermis. They do not blanch to pressure and the person may or may not retain pain to pinprick testing. These burns may heal over 2–5 weeks from intact cells around the bases of hair follicles and sweat glands, but often with severe scarring.
- Full-thickness burns involve complete loss of all dermal structures. *Third-degree burns* involve loss of all structures above the subcutaneous fat. *Fourth-degree burns* involve burn damage through subcutaneous fat to underlying tissues such as muscle or bone. If managed non-surgically, these burns can only heal from viable skin at the wound edges and over prolonged timeframes.

While burns at either end of the scale may be easy to identify, in practice it can be difficult to determine the dividing line between classes, particularly around the margins of a burn. Debridement and serial observations of a burn over time may help to demarcate boundaries in this case.

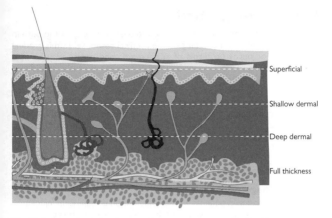

Fig. 40.2 Burns depth classification relative to structures within the skin.

Reproduced with permission from Norman A. T. et al. Pain in the patient with burns. *Continuing Education in Anaesthesia Critical Care & Pain*, 4 (2): 57–61. Copyright © 2004 British Journal of Anaesthesia. Published by Elsevier Ltd. All rights reserved. https://doi.org/10.1093/bjaceaccp/mkh016.

Burns management

These factors in combination determine the overall severity of the burn in terms of survival and the extent of the medical response. In this grading scheme, minor burns (in terms of surface area and depth) may be able to be managed on an outpatient basis. Major burns are usually considered those with an inhalational component, resulting from chemical or high-voltage sources, cover more than 20% surface area, or are associated with trauma. These burns require intensive care management and a specialized multidisciplinary burns team. Burns of an intermediate severity usually still require inpatient management but not necessarily the attention of a dedicated burns unit. Burn severity is also influenced by any coincident internal injuries, either associated with the circumstances of the burn (e.g. motor vehicle accident) or the type of burn (e.g. myocardial and other organ involvement in electrical burns).

Acute management

- *Airway management*: patients with any suggestion of inhalation injuries require urgent airway management, before laryngeal oedema can complicate airway access or exacerbate deoxygenation. Bronchoscopy helps determine if there is any evidence of damage to the bronchial tree. Oxygen levels may also be impaired by the effects of smoke inhalation and carboxyhaemoglobin, although metabolic acidosis is more common in the latter case.
- *Fluid resuscitation*: large burns produce fluid shift from the intravascular space to body tissues along with fluid loss through burnt areas. This can produce significant hypovolaemia with a particular risk for renal failure, among other organ damage. Catabolism and protein loss can produce significant hypoalbuminaemia that may require replacement to maintain oncotic pressure within the vascular tree.
- *Pain management*: pain is the most frequent complaint following burn injury, particularly in first- and superficial second-degree burns. For minor pain, cooling and non-opioid simple analgesics may be effective. More severe pain may require short- or long-acting opioids, such as oxycodone through to parenteral narcotics. Providing adequate pain relief timed around dressing changes or surgical procedures is also important. Effective pain relief is vital in both the early and late phases of burns management as data shows that the incidence of PTSD is lowest where early and effective pain relief has been provided.
- *Wound management*: infection control is particularly important in burns. Non-intact skin, coupled with leakage of body fluids and a potentially compromised immune system, form ideal conditions for bacterial growth.
- *Debridement*: wound cleaning and assessment helps to determine whether a conservative or surgical approach will be necessary. The decision to debride a burn is based around infection risk, scar formation, depth of burn, and the sensitivity of the site. Debridement may be completed mechanically (through washing) or surgically in the operating theatre. In minor burns, recent data suggest that blisters greater than the size of the patient's little fingernail should be debrided to facilitate

full assessment of burn depth and improve patient recovery. Deep dermal and full-thickness burns require excision with skin grafting to heal the wounds in a timely fashion.

- *Surgical wound management*: burnt tissues lack normal elasticity and quickly become oedematous. Swelling and rigidity in circumferential full-thickness burns can compromise tissue blood flow, potentially leading to additional tissue damage. To avoid this, escharotomies or fasciotomies may be required. Escharotomies involve an incision through the burn tissue but not through the fascia. Incisions are made along the medial or mid-lateral aspect of a limb or though creation of a 'chest plate' on a chest with circumferential burns. Where a compartment syndrome is evident or threatened, a fasciotomy may be required to relieve pressure in deeper tissue compartments.
- *Wound dressings*: standard approaches to wound management involve the use of moist wound healing, topical antimicrobial agents (such as silver sulphadiazine (SSD) cream), minimizing oedema through limb elevation, and maintaining adequate nutrition and hydration. Obtaining good control of systemic diseases such as diabetes and avoiding smoking are also advantageous to wound healing. Dressing changes are often painful procedures, the effect of which can be minimized with preprocedural analgesia.

Approaches to wound closure

Grafting

The main role of grafting is to ensure early wound coverage. A number of approaches are available, with options determined by the context of the burn. 'Autografting', or grafting from the patient to themselves, is the optimal approach. It is important to educate the patient about graft donor site pain prior to any procedure. Donor site pain may be worse than that at the wound site due to exposure of intact sensory nerve endings. If the patient's own skin cannot be used as a donor, skin banks are available. This is termed an 'allograft', utilizing skin from deceased donors. While this will cover the wound, 'graft rejection' due to immunological incompatibility will occur after 1–3 weeks.

Split skin grafts

Split skin grafts (SSGs) consist of the first two layers of the skin (the epidermis and part of the dermis) taken from an unburned area to cover a skin defect elsewhere. Common donor sites are the back, buttocks, forearm, upper arm, and abdominal wall. The technique leaves sufficient dermis in the donor site to allow skin regeneration. SSGs are held in place by sutures or staples, with dressings applied over the top. SSGs can be meshed to increase the wound coverage; however, this gives a poorer cosmetic result. Meshing is therefore avoided around the face, neck, and hands. SSGs are more likely to contract over time than full-thickness grafts.

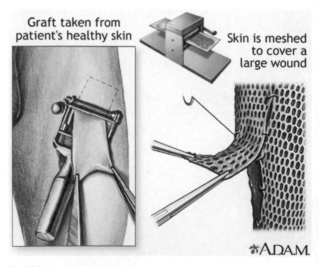

Fig. 40.3 Skin grafts.
Reproduced from https://medlineplus.gov/ency/imagepages/19083.htm.

Full thickness grafts

These involve removing the skin, muscle, and blood supply from the graft donor site to apply to the wound site. Full-thickness grafts are often smaller in size than SSGs, as the graft site requires primary closure as skin cannot regenerate over the site. Full-thickness grafts provide a much better long-term cosmesis and are often used on exposed areas of skin such as the face and the neck.

Spray-on skin

This is a promising new approach. The common theme of the different commercial systems is to take skin from intact areas and separate and grow large numbers of stem cells *in vitro* before spraying them over the debrided burn surface. While the approach has promise, the technique has a limited literature base and has not been widely adopted to date.

Post-acute management/rehabilitation

The duration of post-acute burns management is dependent on the patient's unique situation and can therefore be extremely variable between individuals. Rehabilitation should commence early while noting that the intensity tends to increase as the need for surgical intervention decreases. Burn dressings often need to be continued in the longer term and may adversely impact rehabilitation. The dominant factors influencing the duration of the rehabilitation phase are influenced by the extent/depth of burns, the number of joints with overlying scar tissue, the presence of heterotopic ossification, tissue loss (particularly of the digits), and so on. Durations of 1–2 years (or longer) are not uncommon for adults with severe burns. The rehabilitation needs for children with burns often extend through their entire growth phase.

In general, many of the rehabilitation approaches required for burns management are consistent with general rehabilitation goals, for example, preventing avoidable deconditioning and other predictable complications (e.g. DVT, hypostatic pneumonia, balancing nutritional needs, and so on). These issues are addressed throughout this handbook. However, there are also rehabilitation areas that are more burns specific. These include the following:

- Pain management; chronic pain persisting for more than 12 months post event is common in people with severe burns. Many repetitive procedures, including dressing changes and physical therapy, can be extremely painful and become aversive experiences. Breakthrough or pre-procedure analgesia is encouraged in these circumstances. Neuropathic pain is also a common problem as nerve function recovers. Types of neuropathic pain can include pruritus, hyperalgesia (increased response to a painful stimulus), and allodynia (a painful response to a non-painful stimulus). Approaches to chronic pain management are discussed in detail in ➲ Chapter 11.
- Scar management can be a protracted process. Scar tissue is relatively inelastic and contracts as it matures. Contracture management has two main components—therapy based and garment based. Therapy aims to maintain muscle length through active and passive range of movement exercises and/or providing prolonged low-load stretch from splinting (➲ see Chapter 21). Hand therapy is vital for patients with burns to their fingers. Other contracture management techniques include compressive garments such as masks and suits. These garments are thought to promote wound healing and encourage the flattening of scars through the more organized laying down of collagen fibres in the scar tissue. Silicone gel dressings and facial masks are often used with the aim to improve scar cosmesis. Patients with major burns may have lost sufficient sweat glands to make temperature homeostasis difficult in hot climates.
- Reconstructive surgery is often required in both the short and long term. This may include surgery to release contractures of skin or musculotendinous units where conservative approaches have proved

inadequate in maintaining range of movement. Contracture release surgery is particularly important in children, whose scars may not allow muscles to lengthen as they grow. Surgery is often necessary to maximize the cosmetic result of facial and neck burns.
- Psychological rehabilitation takes on a number of aspects. Consideration of social and psychological adjustment following burns is important, and support for issues such as anxiety, depression, and PTSD are vital. Patient/family education may allay some of the fears regarding the future and provide opportunities to maximize quality of life after a burn injury. Formal psychological counselling may be an advantage for many people post injury.
- Functional rehabilitation; re-establishing the person's involvement and independence in activities such as those of daily living should be commenced as soon as practicable. The aim is to get back to work/school/community as quickly as possible to normalize their experiences as much as possible.
- Vocational retraining needs to be considered, taking into account the person's strengths and abilities. Grafted and donor skin often lack adequate natural sun protection and education regarding sun care should be provided.

Further reading

Agency for Clinical Innovation (2014). *Burn Patient Management: Summary of Evidence*, 4th edn. ℘ http://www.aci.health.nsw.gov.au/__data/assets/pdf_file/0016/250009/Clinical_Practice_ Guidelines_Summary_of_Evidence_ACI_Statewide_Burn_Injury_Service.pdf.

British Burn Association (2001). *National Burn Care Review*. ℘ http://www.britishburnassociation.org/ downloads/NBCR2001.pdf.

Latenser BA (2009). Critical care of the burn patient: the first 48 hours. *Critical Care Medicine* 37, 2619–2626.

Hettiaratchy S, Papini R (2004). Initial management of a major burn: I—overview. *BMJ* 328, 1555–1557.

Amputee rehabilitation

Introduction

Amputee rehabilitation involves the multidisciplinary assessment of all amputees and the resultant advice and therapy delivered. It is essential that treatment is delivered in a patient-centred manner and timely fashion. Amputee rehabilitation includes patients over a wide spectrum of ages—from a baby born with an upper or lower limb (LL) deformity or deficiency to an elderly patient with vascular disease and multiple medical comorbidities. It is a challenging and greatly rewarding subspecialty of rehabilitation medicine. Please note that whilst the term "amputee" is still currently used in rehabilitation medicine, when terminology advances in this area of practice, the term "person with an amputation" may replace the term "amputee."

Amputee rehabilitation is no longer concerned with only patients who are suitable for limb fitting. It is inclusive of all amputees and the specialist amputee MDT should be able to provide valuable advice and therapy to all amputees.[1] It is now recognized that there should be a dedicated care pathway for all amputees beginning ideally in the pre-amputation phase and extending during the acute phase post amputation and up until and including the assessment by the MDT at the prosthetic and amputee rehabilitation centre.[2] It is vital that there is excellent communication between the surgeons, rehabilitation staff, and the community services if patients with amputations are to realize all of their potential.

Epidemiology

Demographics of amputations undertaken in the UK can be found in the National Amputee Statistical Database up until 2007 and since 2010 from data collated by the United National Institute for Prosthetics and Orthotics Development Group (UNIPOD). In the UK, there were around 5900 referrals to the prosthetic and amputee rehabilitation centres in 2011–2012 of which around 30 were congenital deformities.[3] Upper limb (UL) amputations make up around 10% of all referrals. The Amputee Coalition of America estimates that there are 185,000 new lower extremity amputations each year within the United States. It is estimated that there are more than 1 million amputations globally each year.

The most common level for LL amputation is transtibial and this is followed closely by transfemoral amputation. Knee disarticulation is becoming more accepted and is the third most common level of amputation. The transradial level for UL amputations is the most frequent level, followed by absent digits and the transhumeral level.

Peripheral vascular disease is the major cause of LL amputation in the UK and is due to arteriosclerosis. Risk factors for this include hypertension, diabetes mellitus, obesity, hyperlipidaemia, and smoking. Diabetes mellitus causing end-organ obliterative arterial disease, microangiopathy, and resultant neuropathy is frequently the cause of an amputation. Trauma and congenital deficiency are the next most frequent causes of amputation, followed by infections and neoplasia. Neurological disease, for example, spina bifida, is an uncommon cause of amputation.

The major causes of UL amputation or deficiency are trauma, congenital abnormality, neoplasia, and peripheral vascular disease with or without diabetes mellitus. There is a gender bias with more males having an UL amputation; this is due to the most common cause being trauma.

Pre-amputation consultation

Whenever possible, any patients who are likely to need a LL or UL amputation should be referred to the physician in rehabilitation at the prosthetic and amputee rehabilitation centre. An appointment can then be scheduled for the patient to meet the physician and the amputee rehabilitation team. Level of amputation, the rehabilitation process, phantom limb sensation, and pain can be discussed. Realistic expectations of mobility and life as an amputee should be clearly presented. The need for home equipment and a self-propelling wheelchair for LL amputees can also be highlighted. It is also usually beneficial for the patient to meet an established amputee patient and discuss 'life as an amputee'.

The nature of amputations of vascular and traumatic origin often means that there may not be time for the amputee to attend the rehabilitation centre, it is therefore important that the physician in rehabilitation medicine affords time to visit the vascular and orthopaedic wards to meet patients pre- and postoperatively. Written information is useful for patients and relatives. Discussion prior to amputation about the need for changes to the home including ramps and rails can reduce patient anxiety and allow planning. It is recognized that physiotherapy should be encouraged preoperatively as this can reduce muscular strength, deconditioning, and allows patients to start on their rehabilitation even before the amputation has occurred.[4]

The rehabilitation physician should liaise promptly with referring surgeons and the GP and advise on the best level for amputation and highlight any social issues, confounding medical problems, or contralateral limb limitations. It is important that preoperative pain control should be adequate and may include preoperative epidural anaesthesia.[5] Involvement of an amputee coordinator to plan admissions and facilitate a patient's journey from the pre-amputation phase to discharge and on to community services could improve patient experience.[2]

Levels of limb amputation

Upper limb

- Forequarter
- Shoulder disarticulation
- Transhumeral
- Elbow disarticulation
- Transradial
- Wrist disarticulation
- Partial hand (various types)
- Digits.

Lower limb

- Hemipelvectomy.
- Hip disarticulation.
- Transfemoral.
- Knee disarticulation.
- Transtibial.
- Ankle disarticulation:
  - Symes—disarticulation of tibia from calcaneum.
  - Boyd—as per Symes but with the addition of fusion of the calcaneum to the tibia.
- Partial foot:
  - Chopart—removes the forefoot and midfoot, saving talus and calcaneum.
  - Bona Jager—transtarsal amputation between navicular and cuneiforms leaving the proximal cuboid.
  - Lisfranc—disarticulation of mid-foot between tarsal and metatarsal.
- Transmetatarsal.
- Ray.
- Digit.

Level of amputation

When considering the best level for limb amputation, be mindful of the following:

- In general, a transtibial amputation rather than a more proximal one should usually always be the first choice for LL amputees with peripheral vascular disease.[6] Preservation of a functioning knee is a priority.
- Where a more proximal amputation is clinically indicated: a knee disarticulation is a quicker, less complicated operation than a transfemoral amputation. It does not require muscle rebalancing and results in less blood loss. It could be suitable for prosthetic users and also those who will be wheelchair reliant. The resulting full length of femur allows pressure distribution in sitting for non-prosthetic users and affords a long lever arm and a socket with lower trims for prosthetic users. There is a cosmetic sacrifice with having a knee disarticulation as the prosthetic knee will sit proud of the contralateral side, there will also be a shortened shin section. These issues should be explained to patients who will likely be prosthetic users.

- A hip flexion deformity of greater than 30°, in a patient who is likely to mobilize with a prosthesis but is not able to have a transtibial amputation, may mean that a knee disarticulation should be avoided and a transfemoral amputation performed. This is due to difficulty with attaining alignment and positioning prosthetic foot.
- For patients with peripheral vascular LL disease, a transtibial amputation is usually the best choice rather than a Lisfranc or Chopart amputation due to difficulty with wound healing.
- A severe fixed knee flexion deformity of greater than 45–50°, if considered longstanding, would usually mean that a knee disarticulation or transfemoral amputation is indicated if walking mobility is the goal.
- The Chopart level of amputation, for a patient who has a patent arterial supply, can allow indoor mobility without a prosthesis. This allows less fuss with donning a prosthesis, especially at night if moving to the toilet. If there are contralateral LL issues, weakness, or arthritis it is helpful to the patient to have full leg length on the amputated side and sensory feedback from the heel area.
- For UL amputees, long transradial or transhumeral stumps can have a negative impact on function and cosmesis. A long transradial stump for a prosthetic user will mean any added components will add length and place the prosthetic hand further away from the body. A long transhumeral stump may mean that to keep arm proportions, side steels are needed instead of a prosthetic elbow. This will result in reduced prosthetic elbow position options and poorer cosmesis.

Perioperative care

Preoperative care

It is recommended that amputations are only carried out by surgeons experienced in the procedure and that amputations are carried out within 48 hours of a decision having been made to amputate. Early referral to an anaesthetist for pre-assessment is prudent given the multiple co-morbidities many patients will have. Optimized perioperative analgesia reduces chronic phantom limb pain intensity, prevalence, and frequency.[5]

Intraoperative care

The optimum length of tibia should be 8 cm per metre of patient height. A tibia as short as 7 cm can be accommodated within a socket by an experienced prosthetist. A rigid thigh length postoperative dressing (plaster of Paris or pneumatic) for transtibial amputations is recommended. There is evidence of better control of oedema and a shorter period to prosthetic rehabilitation if a rigid dressing is applied. Other variables previously assumed to be advantages of rigid cast dressings, such as fewer falls, shorter hospitalizations, reduced mortality, or less prosthetic failures, did not show a significant difference in small comparative studies.[7]

For transfemoral amputations a myodesis is preferred rather than a myoplasty. Myodesis refers to the anchoring of muscle or tendon to bone using sutures that are passed through small holes drilled in the femur bone. Myoplasty is the attachment of the flexor to the extensor (antagonist) muscles at the end of the transfemoral stump. This can lead to prominence of distal end of the femur due to muscle atrophy and laxity.

Immediate postoperative care

When a patient is medically stable, early physiotherapy and occupational therapy input, ideally on day one, is beneficial. Weekly ward rounds by a physician in rehabilitation with the MDT can be a means of promptly deciding what rehabilitation environment is needed for each patient. This allows patients to build on their confidence and strength. Some patients do not like the remaining leg to be called a stump and the term residuum could be used. Adequate pain control is needed to allow participation in therapy and transfer practice. Neuropathic medication may be needed for phantom pain. Involvement from the pain team may also be needed. Patients with diabetes mellitus should have review by the diabetic outreach team to advise on blood sugar control and medication. Any rigid postoperative dressings should be checked regularly to avoid skin blistering. LL amputees with peripheral vascular disease and diabetes mellitus are high-risk patients for ulceration developing on the contralateral limb. They should have regular podiatry care post amputation every 2 months.[8] Referral to the community podiatry team by the hospital podiatrist post amputation is an important means for information flow and helps to ensure amputees are followed up for contralateral foot care once they have returned to the community.

Postoperative rehabilitation: 2–6 weeks

Some patients with amputations will be able to return home quickly and avail of community therapy input once or twice per week. Many others, however, are fatigued postoperatively and need daily therapy in order to improve in strength and ability to transfer from bed to chair and so on. An amputee ward is ideal for this as nurses and other staff are experienced in the care of amputees. Care of the elderly wards are also very good environments to avail of therapy. Regaining sitting balance, learning pivot transfers or sliding transfers, and sit to stand practice (especially important for transfemoral amputees) are all very important goals for patients. This period of rehabilitation is most important for non-prosthetic users as it is an opportunity to teach independence with transfers or minimal assistance, which can reduce the need of hoists and the care package for the same. Bilateral transfemoral and bilateral transtibial amputees can be taught forwards–backwards transfers or sliding transfers that can facilitate getting into a car etc.

Referral to the prosthetic and amputee rehabilitation centre

It is recommended that all amputees are referred for multidisciplinary assessment regardless of the likelihood of using a prosthesis. Integrated working of the team during the appointment will result in gleaning of important information, recording of muscle strengths and joint movements, and identification of cognitive issues. Many patients have peripheral vascular disease and diabetes mellitus. Fig. 41.1 highlights the areas that should be enquired about when assessing these patients. The patient's aims should be enquired of and freely discussed. At the first appointment it is important that the physician and therapists undertake a global assessment of the patient.

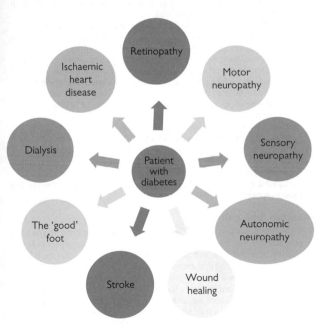

Fig. 41.1 Conditions and problems to consider when assessing a patient who has had an amputation and also has diabetes mellitus.

Postoperative problems

- Delay in wound healing is worrying for the patient. Experience of the amputee team in treating wounds can be an excellent adjunct and an encouragement for the patient. Early mobilizing with a non-healed stump is possible with a pneumatic post amputation mobility aid, femurette, or prosthesis. Close wound monitoring is important.[9]
- Cognitive problems make rehabilitation with or without a prosthesis more difficult. Poor carryover of information and skills between sessions can slow or halt progress. However, especially for transtibial amputees, walking may still be possible. If the patient has a carer or resides in a nursing home then the donning of a prosthesis may be overseen by the carer. Cognitive tools, for example, the Montreal Cognitive Assessment (MoCA), can be applied by the occupational therapist and the results of these can guide the team. Providing written instructions to patients with cognitive problems can be beneficial.
- Severity of respiratory and cardiac disease should be considered. Optimizing cardiac medication and respiratory medication should always be done and may require referral onto or advice from a specialist.
- Identification of joint flexion contractures is very important. Focused exercise therapy to reduce the joint flexion is essential and may be pursued before fabrication of a prosthesis. A knee joint flexion contracture of 40° can be accommodated in a transtibial prosthesis. The prosthetic alignment need not be fully corrected as mobilizing may encourage the prosthetic heel to contact the ground. The prosthetic drawbacks should be explained to the patient before a decision is made to move forward with fabrication of a prosthesis—heavier prosthesis, difficulty accommodating in a normal width trouser, and short step length.
- Commencement or increasing of medication for nociceptive and neuropathic pain is vital to allow the patient to participate in therapy and home exercises.

Phantom limb pain

This was first described by Charles Bell in the 1800s but reported as early as the 1500s by Ambroise Pare. The prevalence of phantom pain in amputees varies between 50% and 70%. Phantom pain is more common in patients who have suffered pre-amputation pain. It is very important to clarify with patients if they are experiencing phantom sensations, or phantom pain, or both. In general, treatment is focused for patients with phantom pain. Those who have phantom sensations can usually accept and grow accustomed to these and do not need any focused treatment.

No treatment can completely eliminate phantom pain and over 70 treatment options are available. Pharmacological treatment includes tricyclic antidepressants—amitriptyline, duloxetine, and anticonvulsants—pregabalin, gabapentin, and local anaesthetics. Tramadol and topical lidocaine patch are also options. TENS machine and liners which incorporate electromagnetic shielding can produce beneficial effects. Mirror box therapy, psychological techniques, and eye movement desensitization reprocessing (EMDR) are also reported to be useful.

Secondary prevention of morbidity and mortality

Symptomatic peripheral vascular disease carries a 30% risk of death within 5 years and almost 50% within 10 years, primarily due to myocardial infarction (60%) or stroke (12%). Risk factor modification unfortunately has not been shown to prevent progression of peripheral vascular disease or loss of limbs; however, an aggressive approach to modifying risk factors in order to reduce the risk of fatal and non-fatal myocardial infarction and stroke is worthwhile. Patients are advised to stop smoking and maintain BMI within normal range, hyperlipidaemia and hypertension should be treated, and diabetic control should be as good as is possible and safe (avoidance of hypoglycaemic episodes).

Return to function

At 6 weeks post amputation and at assessment with the MDT it may be evident that a patient has still further goals to achieve in relation to wheelchair mobility, transfers, and self-care. Daily input of physiotherapy and occupational therapy will likely be needed to achieve success moving from hoisting transfers to a more active type of transfer, for example, with or without a sliding board. Extended ADLs should be explored— getting back to driving, work, and so on.

Lower limb prosthetic rehabilitation

The decision to make a prosthesis should be multidisciplinary and have the patient at the centre of the discussion. The rehabilitation physician should prescribe the prosthesis based on agreement with the team and the most suitable components given. Patients who are deemed suitable to use a prosthesis will require adequate time to learn how to don and doff a prosthesis, adjust socks to afford the correct fit, regain balance and practice walking, and working within the home and beyond.

A LL prosthesis is made up of a socket, a shin tube, a prosthetic foot (Fig. 41.2), and for transfemoral amputees, a knee unit in addition (Fig. 41.3). A socket is usually, for a new patient, made out of polypropylene plastic which can be easily heated out and Pelite™ as the inner liner. Once a more definitive stump volume has been reached, glass reinforced plastic can be used or even silicone for UL sockets.

Transtibial prosthesis

The transtibial amputation is the amputation of choice for the dysvascular amputee. This level avails of the preserved knee joint and provides the patient with a comfortable prosthesis that is easy to don and doff, a highly functional prosthesis, and a cosmetically acceptable limb replacement. Walking with a transtibial prosthesis requires a lower level of energy expenditure, around 40% above baseline as compared with the transfemoral amputation which requires around 80%.

Suspension of the prosthesis

For a primary patient, suspension of the prosthesis may be supracondylar, sleeve, or cuff. At 12–18 months post amputation, when the stump has stabilized in volume, a shuttle lock suspension can be chosen or a liner system with valve and sleeve.

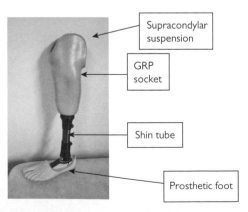

Supracondylar suspension

GRP socket

Shin tube

Prosthetic foot

Fig. 41.2 A transtibial prosthesis. GRP, glass reinforced plastic.

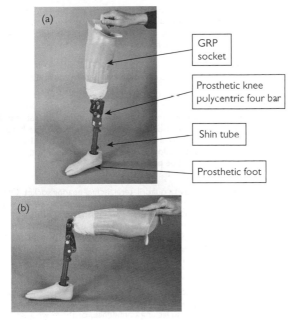

Fig. 41.3 A prosthesis, at fitting stage and without cosmetic cover for a transfemoral amputee. Note the socket, shin tube, polycentric four-bar knee, and prosthetic foot. GRP, glass reinforced plastic.

Weight bearing

A patellar tendon-bearing type prosthesis allows weight acceptance over the inferior patella tendon, the tibial flares, and posteriorly, avoiding pressure at the end of the stump which may be tender in the first few months post surgery.

A total surface-bearing type socket can be used once the stump volume has reduced, stabilized, and the stump wound has healed

Prosthetic feet

Prosthetic feet can be classified into five conceptual groups based on their biomechanical performance.[10] The single-axis ankle–foot due to its set up reaches foot flat most quickly and can increase knee stability. The solid ankle, cushion heel (SACH) is lightweight, simple, and durable. The multi-axial ankle foot can allow some accommodation to uneven surfaces and this may improve the socket comfort. The flexible keel foot has a flexible fore foot which tightens due to plantar straps, this can provide a smooth roll over. The dynamic response foot has a carbon fibre spring-like keel. The keel deflects under loading and releases some energy at late stance. There are many choices of dynamic response feet. Some prosthetic feet have in addition shock absorbers, hydraulic units *in situ*, some even with a microprocessor control allowing better compliance on rough ground. Powered ankle–foot units are also available but are comparatively heavy.

Transfemoral prosthesis

This type of prosthesis is heavier than a transtibial prosthesis and is technically more difficult to walk with.

Suspension of the prosthesis

Primary patients will usually require a Silesian belt (thin, low-set leather belt), a total elasticated support belt, or a rigid pelvic band. The latter is especially good for patients who have a short stump or who have hip weakness. After 12–18 months, a suction socket, shuttle lock, liner with seal, or lanyard type suspension might be preferred.

Weight bearing

Most primary patients will have a quadrilateral, ischial-bearing socket. Other choices at a later date when stump volume has stabilized can be an ischial containment socket: this is where the ischium, trochanteric head, and the symphysis pubis are contained within the socket as the Icelandic, Swedish, New York (ISNY) flexible type sockets. The ISNY concept uses flexible thermoplastic vacuum-formed sockets supported in a rigid (or semi-rigid) fenestrated frame or socket retainer.

Prosthetic knees

A prosthetic knee can be categorized into two major types, locked or unlocked.

For elderly patients or those lacking confidence, or those who walk on rough terrain or who are weak/deconditioned, a semi-automatic locking knee (SAKL) is safest.

Unlocked knees can be single axis or polycentric four bar or six bar in set up.

The single-axis knees as the name suggests have one point of rotation. The polycentric knees on the other hand provide a changing centre of rotation. This is advantageous for patients with proportionally long stumps and also allows better clearance of the ground as the shank inherently shortens during flexion. The polycentric knees are inherently stable at heel strike and less stable at toe off allowing for easier initiation of the swing phase. There are now lightweight polycentric knees which are available for children also.

The correct alignment of a prosthesis is vital, especially for transfemoral amputees using a free prosthetic knee.

Some prosthetic knees also offer weight-activated stance control up to a fixed degree of flexion beyond which the prosthetic knee will flex, this type of knee is extremely stable when used correctly.

Manufacturers of single-axis and polycentric prosthetic knees can offer friction control or pneumatic swing phase control or hydraulic swing phase control. Pneumatic and hydraulic units consist of cylinders with pistons which contain air or fluid respectively. Pneumatic units are lighter, less expensive, and simpler than the hydraulic units. In general, a patient who is able to walk at a variety of speeds would be best suited to use a hydraulic type knee unit.

Microprocessor-controlled prosthetic knees are also available. They feature sensors, a microprocessor, software, a resistance system, and a battery. The internal computer monitors each phase of the gait cycle and the continuous monitoring allows the processor to make adjustments in resistance allowing walking down stairs leg over leg and greater variability in walking speed. The increased cost of these types of knees should be measured against the reduced number of falls, better gait symmetry, and more controlled sitting and standing.

Not all prosthetic knees allow the same amount of knee flexion. Therefore care must be taken to discuss with the patient their goals for activity and any particular hobbies. Increased prosthetic knee flexion may be very important for amputees who wish to kneel down and so on. The patient's weight and the weight limit of the knee unit are also important to consider. Therefore, all aspects of a prosthetic knee and the lifestyle, goals, and ability of the patient should be considered to ensure that the correct choice of prosthetic knee is made for each patient.

Torque absorbers and rotation devices can be useful for specific activities. All additional components will, however, add weight to the overall prosthesis and this should be considered and discussed with the patient.

Knee disarticulation prosthesis

A knee disarticulation amputation is becoming a more frequent level of amputation. There are a greater variety of highly functioning prosthetic knee units also becoming available for this level of amputation than before therefore making it the preferred level of amputation as compared to a transfemoral level.[11] There is a cosmetic sacrifice at this level of amputation as the end of the socket finishes at the level of the contralateral knee. With the addition of the prosthetic knee this makes the prosthesis sit proud, even if a polycentric knee is chosen. The shin tube will then need to be slightly shorter so that on standing the leg length is equal. These issues should be discussed with patients especially at the pre-amputation stage.

Suspension of the prosthesis

Modern sockets are usually of the plunge fit type with the liner suspending over the condyles and therefore contoured on the inside but tubular on the outside allowing ease for donning. Lateral or anterior windows can also be made in the socket with inserts which are held in place by Velcro®. This will allow the broader condyles to locate in the bottom of the socket—the Canadian type. Some patients may also be able to use a liner with seal suspension.

Weight bearing

One of the advantages of this level of amputation is that it can allow 100% weight bearing at the end of the stump, on the rounded femoral condyles. Therefore, the prosthetic socket does not need to rise as high as the ischial tuberosity.

Ankle disarticulation prosthesis

An ankle disarticulation (Symes) is an infrequent amputation but can produce very good end bearing on the distal end of the stump, as the heel
pad forms the actual end of the stump and is sutured anteriorly. Due to
the bulbous distal end of the stump, suspension of the prosthesis can be
achieved by suspending the socket above the malleoli.

Often plunge fit sockets are made using Pelite™ as the liner. The liner is
split throughout the middle section to allow the bulbous end of the stump
to slide through the material to reach the locating end. It is then fitted inside
a laminated socket. An open-back Symes socket can also provide a comfortable fitting with a Velcro® strap round the central portion holding the
liner on to the anterior laminated carbon fibre reinforced shin piece.

Pass out of a prosthesis

Before a prosthesis is delivered to a patient it is important that the following
have been assured as much as is possible: comfort, stability, prosthetic alignment, technical standard, and appearance.

In the passing out of a prosthesis the prescriber must observe the subject
both standing on the prosthesis and walking. The subject should be observed both from the side and the front and back.

The comfort of the device is a prerequisite to use. The socket comfort
score out of 10 should be recorded for every patient.[12]

Upper limb prosthetic rehabilitation

Pre-amputation consultation whenever possible should take place as this prepares patients for living life as an UL amputee. Availability of equipment and the need for carers, even briefly post discharge, can be discussed. Advice from the occupational therapist is invaluable.

Stump shrinkers are not available 'off the shelf' for UL amputees but Tubifast® can give some support without being restrictive. Stump bandaging is not advised. Preoperatively and immediately postoperatively exercise and movements of proximal joints should be encouraged. This will encourage oedema to resolve and remind the patient that they still have a portion of useful arm remaining.

Careful physical examination to elucidate any problems with proximal joints is very important. For traumatic UL amputations, coexistent shoulder injury, for example, tendinitis, tendon tear partial, or full or bursitis, may be present. This could restrict the patient's ability to use a prosthesis and could be a source of ongoing pain. Note should be made of any scarring and unhealed areas which will dictate that time will be needed before casting. Any restriction in range of movement of proximal joints should be identified and thought given to the need for physiotherapy and patient education regarding daily exercises. Good liaison with orthopaedic surgeon, plastic surgeon, and oncologist will result in the best care for the patient.

Many UL amputees choose not to wear a prosthesis in the long term. This can be due to reasons of weight of the prosthesis, lack of sensory feedback, difficulty donning and activating, and cosmesis. There is a higher rate of prosthetic arm rejection with a more proximal arm amputation. One study identified that almost 34% of proximal UL adult amputees reject their prosthesis. Children have a higher rate of rejection of both body-powered and electric prostheses as high as 45% and 35% respectively.

A UL prosthesis will include a socket, an elbow unit (for transhumeral amputees or more proximal amputations), a wrist unit to allow rotation of a terminal device, and finally a terminal device.

A UL prosthesis can be passive or functional:
- Passive refers to a cosmetic hand. It should be noted that even a cosmetic prosthesis can provide some function for pushing and steadying.
- Functional can be body powered (with an upcord and harness system using excursion of the shoulders to make the upcord work) or externally powered. Body-powered terminal devices can be voluntary opening or voluntary closing. A voluntary closing terminal device allows the user to 'feel' the strength of force they are applying.

Myoelectric, using residual muscle activity in the remaining residuum, is the most common type of externally powered prosthesis. It is also possible to have a hybrid UL prosthesis: a body-powered elbow and an externally powered terminal device. Apart from myoelectric control it is also possible to use a linear actuator. The use of a linear actuator allows the terminal device to be opened or closed and also allows proportional control. Proportional control refers to the ability to open or close the terminal device according to how fast you open or close the actuator. A small movement can activate a linear actuator as compared to a body-powered prosthesis where a greater body segment movement is needed to move the terminal device. A cable pull switch or harness pull switch using a linear actuator can also be useful alternatives or in combination with myoelectric control.

Terminal devices

There are a range of terminal devices available for UL prosthetic users. Snooker cue holders and nail scrubbers, mechanical or powered split hooks, prehensors, passive hands, mechanical and electric prosthetic hands, and quick-change wrist units. There are also devices to help participation in sport, for example, holding a bicycle handlebar, throwing, canoeing, and weight lifting.

Electric components are heavier, require a battery to be housed in the socket or nearby, are more costly to purchase, and are more expensive to repair. Nonetheless, there are a range of first-generation prosthetic electric hands, griefers, and now multi-articulated hands available. The latter offer a range of grips with or without a motorized thumb and availability of a wrist flexor/extensor unit also.

Transradial amputation

The most preferred length of the remaining stump is at the junction of the middle and distal third of the radius and ulna. This affords a long enough stump to control the prosthesis but also allows enough room for the distal socket to have rotation units and a terminal device added.

The socket can be suspended over the humeral condyles for a transradial amputee or if the stump is long enough, with a locking liner in a more established patient (Fig. 41.4).

For improved function, many amputees will report that they find a comparatively shorter socket forearm helps with control and function.

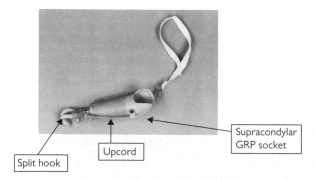

Fig. 41.4 An upper limb prosthesis for a patient with a transradial deficiency—shown is the socket, supracondylar suspension, a split hook 'hand' and an operating 'upcord'. GRP, glass reinforced plastic.

At this level the shoulder and elbow are present and this is a significant advantage. According to the length of the remaining stump, there may be preserved pronation and supination. In general, at this level there will be preserved wrist flexor and extensor muscles and these can be used to activate a myoelectric prosthesis.

Transhumeral amputation

The most preferred length for this level is anywhere within the middle third of the humerus. It is important that there is secure fixation of the triceps and biceps muscles distally to the humerus to allow adequate humeral movements. A long stump which leaves less than 10 cm from the olecranon will result in a more distally placed prosthetic elbow and have a negative impact on cosmesis. A very short humerus less than 4 cm from the axillary fold may mean that the patient is best treated prosthetically more like a shoulder disarticulation level—with the humerus being contained inside the socket but not being of use to aid control or suspension.

The prosthesis at the transhumeral level will require a socket typically suspended over the shoulder or a locking liner with shoulder cap (Fig. 41.5). Activation of a terminal device will require a loop under the contralateral arm with an upcord to open and close the device. An elbow unit allowing internal and external rotation as well as flexion and extension is of great use to position the terminal device for use. In general, a body-powered elbow joint will be chosen as these are much lighter than an electric elbow. As for transradial amputees, there is a large range of terminal devices available, which are task specific.

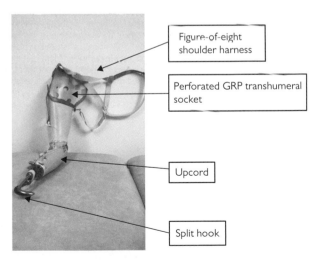

Figure-of-eight shoulder harness

Perforated GRP transhumeral socket

Upcord

Split hook

Fig. 41.5 A transhumeral prosthesis with body-powered elbow and terminal device. GRP, glass reinforced plastic.

Shoulder disarticulation amputation

The benefit of a functional prosthesis at this level is questionable. Not only does the elbow require prosthetic replacement but also the hand and there is absence of a shoulder joint. A cosmetic prosthesis may be requested initially but is quite often discarded. Advice from the occupational therapist about donning any prosthesis is invaluable and most patients will don the prosthesis while lying on the bed. The socket at this level is much more encompassing of the remaining shoulder and will often require additional strapping around the chest to give suspension. As for the aforementioned amputation levels, a body-powered elbow and terminal device can be provided. The lack of a shoulder joint at this level restricts any real use a prosthesis could be and means that a patient would have to rotate the upper body to allow positioning of the prosthetic arm above a table ready for function.

Wrist disarticulation

At this level there is full length of forearm remaining but despite the preserved pronation, supination, and a stump end which is tolerant of pressure, there is a cosmetic and functional sacrifice if a prosthesis is to be made. The prosthesis will be poorly proportioned compared to the other side. The prosthetic wrist will lying distal to the wrist on the sound side and terminal device extending well beyond the tips of fingers on the sound side. The increased length of the forearm when the prosthesis is worn also makes functioning with the terminal device more difficult.

Partial hand amputation

The impact on function depends on the level of loss, number of digits lost, and absence of a thumb. The latter is most disabling and may benefit from fabrication of an opposition plate by the prosthetist or even osseointegration of the thumb. At present, functional prosthetic replacements at this level are cumbersome and very expensive. Many patients 'learn to live' with this level of loss. Future developments in prosthetics at this level may see lighter, more compact, and more cosmetically acceptable options available on the market.

Outcome measures

There is a need for systemic and comprehensive approaches to outcome measurement in amputee care and rehabilitation. The ICF has a useful framework which can be used in clinical practice in the evaluation of patient outcomes. The framework divides outcome measures into four broad domains: activities, body function, participation, and contextual factors. It may be that certain outcome measures actually span more than one domain. Recording a patient's ability to transfer or mobilize with a prosthesis, manipulate items (UL amputees), self-care, and achieve good balance is important to benchmark. A variance of outcome from that expected should be discussed by the MDT. Any outcome chosen should be appropriate and validated for use in the amputee population. Outcome measures should be recorded at key stages during non-prosthetic and prosthetic rehabilitation and used to describe a patient's level of functioning. Where a patient is scoring at the ceiling of a certain outcome measure, then a different more appropriate measure should be chosen, for example, the 2-minute walk test for amputees with peripheral vascular disease and the 6-minute walk test for traumatic LL amputees.

Activities outcomes

Special Interest Group in Amputee Medicine (SIGAM) Mobility Grades

A   Limb wearing abandoned or use of cosmetic limb only.

B   Therapeutic wearer wears prosthesis only for transfers, to assist nursing, walking with the physical aid of another, or during therapy.

C   Walks on level ground only, less than 50 metres, with or without use of walking aids: a = frame, b = crutches/sticks, c = 1 crutch/stick, d = no stick.

D   Walks outdoors on level ground only and in good weather, more than 50 metres, with or without use of walking aids: a = frame, b = crutches/sticks, c = 1 crutch/stick

E   Walks more than 50 metres. Independent of walking aids except occasionally for confidence or to improve confidence in adverse terrain or weather.

F   Normal or near normal gait.

The Locomotor Capability Index, Amputee Mobility Predictor (AMPPro and AMPnoPro) and timed walking tests, 2 minutes, 6 minutes, and the TUG test can benchmark mobility.

The Barthel Index is useful for recording function simply for everyday activities. The Southampton Hand Assessment procedure (SHAP) is a timed measure for use in recording UL amputee function with a prosthesis and also the Assessment for Capacity for Myoelectric Control (ACMC) is useful for benchmarking ability.

Body function outcomes

The numerical rating score for pain and Socket Comfort Score are invaluable for recording level of pain and comfort and comparison with time. The McGill Pain Score is a more in depth way of describing and recording pain. The Hospital Anxiety Depression Scale is useful for recording level of anxiety and depression.

Participation outcomes

The Prosthetic Evaluation Questionnaire is useful for benchmarking QOL. Trinity Amputation and Prosthetic Scales (TAPES) describe adjustment and experience as an amputee, the EuroQol-5D provides a single value for health status. The General Health Questionnaire-12 measures functional health and well-being and can be completed quickly.

Contextual outcomes

The Canadian Occupational Performance Measure (COPM) is patient centred and measures patient satisfaction with their occupational performance and allows the patients and the occupational therapist to set realistic goals.

Psychological issues after amputation

Adjusting to life after amputation of a limb will be challenging for most patients. Where there has been time to prepare the patient with adequate counselling and advice this can ease anxiety and distress. After amputation, the rate of clinical depression can be as high as 35%. Patients may also suffer grief, anxiety, and disruption of body image. The latter requires the patient to be able to reconfigure their new body image, including the crutch or stick and the prosthesis, in order to accept the change and move forward. A patient who has had traumatic loss of a limb may also have symptoms of PTSD. The three cardinal features of this disorder are (1) avoidance of trauma reminders, (2) re-experiencing the trauma, and (3) symptoms of hyperarousal when thinking about the incident. Patient experience can be benchmarked with the Prosthetic Evaluation Questionnaire (PEQ) which has three psychosocial and one well-being scales. In addition, the TAPES has three psychosocial and three satisfaction scales. For treatment of all of the above-mentioned issues, access to a psychologist for CBT and coping strategies is essential.

Surgical advances

Osseointegration and targeted muscle reinnervation (TMR) are surgical advances which may be of benefit for some LL and UL amputees. These processes are not routinely available and the risk of superficial and deep infections and implant failure should be discussed with the patient. The long-term consequences are unknown.

Osseointegration

Osseointegration has been performed on both UL and LL amputees. It is the direct fixation of an implant (usually titanium) into the bone and allows the suspension of a prosthesis from the abutment without use of a socket. There is a failsafe component incorporated to reduce the chance of bone fracture should there be, for example, a fall. It is currently available in Germany, Sweden, the Netherlands, and Australia. Definite risks of superficial and deep infection, loosening and mechanical failure means that patients suitable for this procedure need to be carefully chosen. Potential candidates should undergo full multidisciplinary assessment including psychological assessment.

Targeted muscle reinnervation

TMR is the surgical redirecting of the remaining nerves from the UL to the pectoral and serratus chest muscles. This allows for increased numbers of surfaces sites which could stimulate highly sensitive electrodes within a socket, to allow movement of a prosthesis in a much more intuitive way—a thought-controlled prosthesis. It is now possible to combine osseointegration and TMR.

Paediatric amputee rehabilitation

Congenital limb deficiency

The incidence of congenital limb deficiencies varies worldwide but averages around 1 per 2000 live births. Usually the arm is involved in isolation (70%), the leg alone (18%), or both arm and leg (12%).

Normal limb development happens when mesenchyme condenses leading to chondrification during the 6th week, by 8 weeks the limbs are in their proper position and limb rotation occurs during the 9th week. Primary ossification centres develop during the 12th week and the distal femoral ossification centre at 36 weeks. The physis is where endochondral ossification occurs and results in rapid longitudinal growth.

Limb deficiencies can be grouped into either transverse or longitudinal. The transverse deficiencies look like a stump and should be described according to the segment where the limb has stopped developing and the level within the segment. They usually affect the UL. In general, the more distal an UL transverse deficiency, the less likely a prosthesis will be found to be helpful.

Longitudinal deficiencies are named according to the absent bone or partially absent bone and from proximal to distal. Longitudinal deficiencies are in general more complicated to manage and may also include an arm and a leg on the same side. Therefore care must be taken to examine the baby/child carefully. Experience in managing children with limb deficiencies is essential and due to the relatively infrequent nature of these, it is important that prosthetic and amputee centres build up good knowledge and excellent communication with paediatricians, plastic surgeons, and community and hospital therapy teams. Longitudinal deficiency of the tibia or fibula may be associated with an abnormal knee joint, shortened leg, and unstable ankle with or without deficiency longitudinal deficiency of the foot. Longitudinal deficiency of the femur previously known as proximal femoral focal deficiency (PFFD) can be associated with an unstable knee, and poorly developed hip and foot (Fig. 41.6). There is frequently also a complete or partial fibular deficiency that results in a valgus foot with absent rays. There are various treatment options. Any limb length discrepancy, joint instability, inadequacy of musculature, and malrotation will direct treatment choices. Occasionally an extension prosthesis will suffice; however, osteotomy, rotation, ankle disarticulation, or even a rotationplasty may be needed. A rotationplasty is an alternative to managing certain patients as a transfemoral amputee. By rotation of the tibia by 180° so that the toes point posteriorly and the ankle functions as a knee, a prosthesis can be made which enables the use of a transtibial prosthesis. Various modifications of this rotationplasty have been described. A rotationplasty may be cosmetically unacceptable to patients and it may also derotate in the longer term requiring revision. Careful counselling is required. Some studies for rotationplasty do show a better QOL and level of functioning as compared to an amputation.

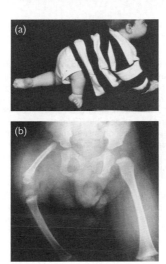

Fig. 41.6 (a) Clinical photograph of an infant with a right longitudinal deficiency of the femur. The length of the whole right leg equals the length of the thigh on the normal side—posing no problem to crawling! (b) Anteroposterior radiograph of the same child showing a right longitudinal deficiency of the femur with a poor-quality hip joint—a predictor of final function.

All children who use prostheses will need regular follow-up so that the length of prosthetic limb matches growth on the contralateral side. In addition, any increasing valgus or varus deformity around a joint can be referred to an orthopaedic surgeon for opinion on the need for intervention (e.g. epiphysiodesis).

It is often helpful for parents to meet with other parents who have a child with a similar condition, this can be very reassuring. There are also support groups such as STEPS and REACH in the UK that provide helpful information and back-up.

Long-term prosthetic issues

Bony overgrowth

This is also known as terminal overgrowth and occurs when the amputation level cuts through bone. It results in a bony spike protruding from the end of stump. The spike can be angulated and even have a number of prongs terminally. It appears to be most frequent in transhumeral amputations and transtibial amputations. It is most likely to occur in children before they reach skeletal maturity. Where possible, amputations in children should be done as disarticulations rather than transections to avoid repeated revisions for bony overgrowth in the future. Prosthetic adjustments can delay surgery for some months but ultimately revision of the stump may be needed.

Autologous bony capping is a surgical option which aims to cover the end of the bone to prevent bony regrowth.[13]

Skin complications

The skin next to the socket accepts load in various pressure-tolerant areas and if there is uneven loading then shearing and blistering of the skin can occur. Weight increase or decrease can lead to pressure areas developing on the skin which can become problematic.

All amputees should be advised of the need to keep the stump skin clean and in as good condition as possible. Chlorhexidine wash can be helpful if recurrent bacterial skin infections are occurring. Regular sock changes and the use of antiperspirant can be useful for sweating. Early follow-up of new amputees and access to a prosthetist promptly is important for all prosthetic users, especially those with diabetes mellitus.

Epidermoid cysts

These occur most frequently in the groin of transfemoral users or behind the knee of transtibial amputees. They classically swell periodically and may burst releasing a purulent or serosanguineous liquid. Many patients will require antibiotics when the cyst is at its largest. Sometimes cysts may join together and communicate. The fit and alignment of the prosthesis should be checked and this can eliminate the problem for many patients. Occasionally, surgery to excise the area is needed and should be a last resort.

Fungal skin infection

This is one of the most common skin problems presenting in established prosthetic users. This is usually seen as a classical red scaly rash with satellite lesions. Treatment with a topical antifungal and attention thereafter to frequent sock changes, cleaning, and drying of silicone or polyurethane liner or antiperspirant is essential.

Contact dermatitis

This may arise on the stump due to contact from an allergen applied to the skin by the patient, such as soap, or an allergy to glue, foam, resins, or varnishes. Patch testing can identify the allergen in some cases. Avoidance of the irritant and/or short-term use of a moderately strong topical steroid cream can result in cure.

Choke syndrome

This is a congestion of the distal end of the stump which results in a verrucous type appearance and skin breakdown. It is caused by a tightly fitting socket which does not allow venous outflow and congestion thus develops. Treatment includes socket revision and use of a distal touch pad in order to encourage venous return.

Painful neuroma

This is a ball-shaped mass at the end of a nerve, it is a disorganized growth of nerve cells and is frequently found in amputation stumps and is usually not painful. On some occasions, pressure over a neuroma can result in neuropathic-type pain which can become very problematic for a patient. The initial treatment is modification to the socket if possible to reduce pressure and off load. An ultrasound scan to locate and subsequent local anaesthetic and/or steroid injection can relieve the pain in the short term. Anticonvulsant and antidepressant medication may also be tried. Surgical excision of the neuroma and transposition of the nerve stump into a vein may be better than relocation into proximal muscle. In addition, nerve capping using a silicone implant attached to the epineural sleeve has also been used with good success. Implantation of the cut nerve into bone or muscle has also been shown to work well.

Musculoskeletal complications

LL amputees spend a greater percentage of time on the contralateral limb as the amputated limb during ambulation. There are also a range of gait deviations which are likely to explain the increased risk of knee and hip OA on the sound side in LL amputees. This risk is higher for transfemoral amputees as compared to transtibial amputees. LL amputation is an additional risk factor for osteoporosis. Up to 80% of all long-term prosthetic users have a bone density reduction of 30% on the amputated side hip joint. Low back pain is also experienced more in LL amputees as compared to the general population. Encouragement to pursue symmetry in gait, leg length, and good posture and avoidance of hopping and obesity should be given to each patient.

Symptoms of overuse including bursitis, tendon tears, partial and full, and OA in the remaining arm have been reported by as many as 50% of UL amputees.

References

1. British Society of Rehabilitation Medicine (2018). *Prosthetic and Amputee Rehabilitation: Standards and Guidelines*, 3rd edn. British Society of Rehabilitation Medicine, London.
2. National Confidential Enquiry into Patient Outcome and Death (2014). *Lower Limb Amputation: Working Together.* ℘ https://www.ncepod.org.uk/2014lla.html.
3. United National Institute for Prosthetics and Orthotics Development (2012). *Annual Report 2011–2012.* Salford University, Salford. ℘ http://www.limbless-statistics.org.
4. Klarich J, Brueckner I (2014). Amputee rehabilitation and preprosthetic care. *Physical Medicine and Rehabilitation Clinics of North America* 25, 75–91.
5. Karanikolas M, Aretha D, Tsolakis I, et al. (2011). Optimized perioperative analgesia reduces chronic phantom limb pain intensity, prevalence, and frequency: a prospective, randomized, clinical trial. *Anaesthesiology* 114, 1144–1154.
6. Vllasoli TO, Zafirova B, Orovcanec N, et al. (2014). Energy expenditure and walking speed in lower limb amputees: a cross sectional study. *Ortopedia Traumatologia Rehabilitacja* 16, 419–426.
7. Smith DG, McFarland LV, Sangeorzan BJ, et al. (2004) . Postoperative dressing and management strategies for transtibial amputations: a critical review. *Journal of Prosthetics and Orthotics* 16, 15–25.
8. National Institute for Health and Care Excellence (NICE) (2015). *Diabetic Foot Problems: Prevention and Management.* NICE Guideline [CNG19]. NICE, London. ℘ http://www.nice.org.uk/guidance/ng19.
9. Vanross ER, Johnson S, Abbott CA (2009). Effects of early mobilization on unhealed dysvascular transtibial amputation stumps: a clinical trial. *Archives of Physical Medicine and Rehabilitation* 90, 610–617.
10. Michael JW (1990). Overview of prosthetic feet. *Instructional Course Lectures* 39, 367–372.
11. Geertzen J, van der Linde H, Rosenbrand K, et al. (2015). Dutch evidence-based guidelines for amputation and prosthetics of the lower extremity: amputation surgery and postoperative management. Part 1. *Prosthetics and Orthotics International* 39, 351–360
12. Hanspal RS, Fisher K, Nieveen R (2003). Prosthetic socket fit comfort score. *Disability and Rehabilitation* 25, 1278–1280.
13. Benrd L, Blasius K, Lukoschek M, et al. (1991). The autologous stump plasy. Treatment for bony overgrowth in juvenile amputees. *Journal of Bone and Joint Surgery British* 73, 203–206.

Index

Note: Tables, figures, and boxes are indicated by an italic *t*, *f*, and *b* following the page number.